Blood and Nation

Contemporary Ethnography

Series Editors
Dan Rose
Paul Stoller

A complete list of books in the series
is available from the publisher.

Blood and Nation

The European Aesthetics of Race

Uli Linke

PENN

University of Pennsylvania Press

Philadelphia

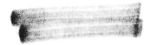

10 9 8 7 6 5 4 3 2 1

Published by
University of Pennsylvania Press
Philadelphia, Pennsylvania 19104-4011

Library of Congress Cataloging-in-Publication Data
Linke, Uli.
Blood and nation : the European aesthetics of race / Uli Linke.
p.   cm. — (Contemporary ethnography)
Includes bibliographical references and index.
ISBN 0-8122-3477-4
1. Blood—Social aspects—Europe.   2. Blood—Symbolic aspects—
Europe.   3. Body, Human—Social aspects—Europe.   4. Body,
Human—Symbolic aspects—Europe.   5. Europe—Politics and
government.   6. Europe—Race relations.   I. Title.   II. Series.
GT498.B55L56   1999
305.8′0094—dc21   98-41467
                                                              CIP

Contents

Preface

While mainstream Germans, like other Europeans, talk about immigration in terms of rivers and floods . . . far-right Germans speak of filth. One neo-Nazi leader in Chemnitz, talking about immigration in 1992, said: "In the Hitler era, Germany was something good, something clean, something big and powerful. Now we're covered with dirt." Another Chemnitz extremist said, "We're going to clean up this country. No foreigners, no filth, no drugs, no pornography, and work for everyone." These metaphors of pollution expose not only contempt for immigrants but also a fixation on a pure nation, which has few close parallels in Britain or in the United States.

Timothy Christenfeld, "Alien Expressions," 1996

My aim in this book is to show, with examples taken from my research on violence in Germany and from the articulations of various discourses of blood in European history, how an aesthetics of race expands from conventional points of reference in language into an organizer of cultural frames in modern state politics. Such frames, as they are articulated in Western cultural fantasy, give rise to discursive forms of violence in a succession of historical epochs, which culminate in the practice of genocide under fascism and in the renewed attempts to annihilate foreigners in post–cold war Germany.

Central to my analysis is the metaphorization of the racial body, which I investigate through the accompanying visions of blood in European history. The complexity of such images, their recurrence across different domains of experience, and their persistence through time are diagnostic of the profound cultural significance of blood, both as bodily discharge and as internal flow. Blood, with its diverse fields of meaning and discursive manifestations, consists of a dominant metaphor or gestalt, mapping fundamental cultural assumptions about gender, sex, and race.

The cultural premises that structure the historic significance of blood are grounded in schematic images of the volatile body: both as embodied subjectivity and as corporeal projection, the body is perceived as perpetually threatened by contagion. In the texts I examine, these visions are rendered tangible through metaphors of blood. Blood appears as an organizing metaphor in allegories of the European male body, the virile (life-giving) body of mythical protagonists, the medieval body of Christ in central Europe, the medicalized (purged) body of men in early modern Germany, the twentieth-century fascist body with its militarization of male flesh, and the citizen's body in postwar Germany with its nationalistic emphasis on interiority, closure, and cleanliness. This type of body, which essentializes masculinist corporeality, stands opposed to the liquid female body with its imputed contaminating influences. This imagined feminine threat appears in early European texts in menstrual metaphors, in mythical renderings of women's bleeding bodies, in the medieval and modern German visions of Jewish bodies, and in the symbolization of the immigrant body in contemporary Germany, defined by abject qualities of wetness, liquidity, and dirt.

I trace the transformation of these conceptual models from antiquity through modern times, thus illuminating the historical emergence of European (and specifically German) ideas about racial purity and contamination. Throughout, I ask how images of gendered violence and violence toward women are reproduced in the German imagination as central icons of a symbolic universe of nationhood that works to suppress difference. German racial ideologies are not just radical interpretations of the Other. They are connected to male repulsion toward and domination of women through metaphors relating to blood imagery. Working historically, I document blood and liquidation imagery in the development of anti-Semitism and anti-Jewish violence, linking images of menstruation to the emasculating potential bound up with female sexuality —which then become the legitimating basis for violence against women and against all things female in modern Germany. My work suggests that metaphors of liquidity also apply to the contemporary public discussion of immigration, thus opening up the potential for "othering" non-Germans. In this book, I link the "rationality" of ordinary political discourse on national immigration policy to the "irrationality" of a racialist and misogynous discourse, suggesting that they are one and the same.

*   *   *

My interest in racial aesthetics began after I had completed several months of fieldwork in Germany during the early 1980s. I was surprised to find that in the course of their everyday life, Germans expressed an intense fear of cultural alienation, a notion contained in the spatial

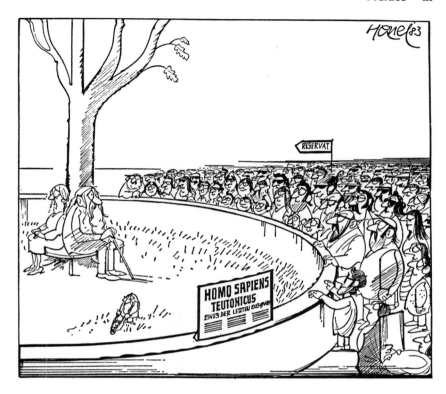

Figure 1. *The German Exhibit or Homo Sapiens Teutonicus: The Last of Its Kind.* From *Frankfurter Allgemeine Zeitung*, no. 2 (3 Jan. 1984), p. 3. Copyright Walter Hanel. Reproduced with permission.

metaphor of *Überfremdung*, literally "over-foreignization," a term used to refer to the estrangement of a people from their cultural heritage through the imposition, the "grafting on," of alien traditions. Such an anticipated loss of culture, according to the German view, could eventually result in biological extinction. As a metaphor, the word *Überfremdung* depicts the terror of submersion in difference—the erasure of identity through racial inundation and saturation with foreignness.

These fears about race and death find visual expression in the media. In one instance, a satirical depiction (Fig. 1), an elderly German couple is placed on a reservation—a preserve for the endangered German species. Sitting beneath an ancient oak tree, the symbol of Germany's national ancestry, the old man and his wife await extinction. In the open-air exhibit, entitled *Homo Sapiens Teutonicus: The Last of Its Kind*, the old

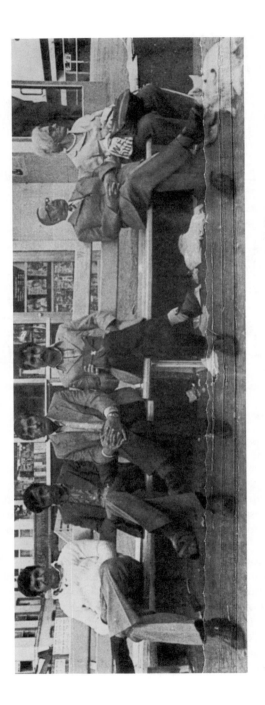

Figure 2. *Foreigners in Germany*. From *Die Zeit*, no. 8 (17 Feb. 1989), p. 4. Photograph copyright Günther Kipphan. Reproduced with permission.

couple is the target of scrutiny by crowds of dark-skinned people. Their Semitic (perhaps Turkish) features, black facial hair, and dark glasses mark these onlookers as oriental "Others," who eye the Germans with a level gaze, a covert act of domination. This motif of racial inundation is persistent. Another example, a photograph (Fig. 2), conveys this German sense of social marginalization—of being pushed to the fringe by immigrants. Entitled *Foreigners in Germany,* the photograph reveals the public iconography of racial difference through opposition and contrast: an elderly German couple, clutching the leash of a small white dog, is positioned uncomfortably at the edge of a bench, a space they reluctantly share with four dark-skinned men who engage the camera directly. This tableau of interracial posturing affirms the public sense of threat: the German fear of a racial apocalypse, of being pushed to the margins of the national body politic by immigrants and foreigners.

During the course of my research, I discovered that the German experience of "over-foreignization" and the anticipated threat of biological extinction were often reiterated by other metaphorical visions. Images of natural catastrophes were most often used to convey the anticipated social crisis. The demise of German culture was consistently described in terms of the destructive potential of fluids, water in particular. Among the most common figures of speech for the migration of foreign nationals to Germany were "flood," "stream," "wave," "flow," "torrent," and "deluge." Such liquid metaphors always carried a programmatic message: "Secure Germany against the flood of job-seeking Turks"; "Build dams against the wave of Turkish migrants"; "Contain the flow of foreigners." Interestingly, the prevention of racial inundation was translated in the realm of metaphor into the immediate containment of "water." On the verbal level, this imagery was conveyed in the form of imperative commands, coupled with key terms like "secure," "block," "protect." As I proceeded with my research, it occurred to me that such metaphors of water might well be circumlocutions for blood. It has been suggested elsewhere that *blood,* once taboo in some contexts, finds expression in terms of other fluids or liquid substances: foam, sweat, whirlpool, river, stream.[1] If this interpretation is correct, the German anticipation of over-foreignization and cultural extinction (circumscribed as the destruction by water) expresses a hidden fear of blood pollution.

After I had uncovered some of the more prominent image clusters, I turned to texts from Nazi Germany to analyze changes in the use of metaphor through time. I immediately began to notice some points of contrast. During the 1930s and 1940s, political practices were focused on the protection of the German social body and the preservation of the "purity" of blood. The primary focus of symbolic activity did not revolve around a fear of cultural alienation but one of biological contamination. It was this notion that appeared in the spatial metaphor of *Unterwanderung*, literally "subversive foray from under ground," a term that sketches in a figurative sense the gradual but invisible movement of an outside force toward the inside of a bounded entity. *Unterwanderung* creates an image that alludes to the subversion of the German population by the penetration of the body. The metaphor locates the permeability of physical boundaries in a sphere or realm that is spatially "below," that is, beneath the body's surface, in its interior regions, where Nazi ideology situated the mythic roots and ancestral blood-origins of the Aryan nation. Until the 1940s, the interior of the body served as a symbolic site of terror and annihilation. In the postwar period, this image was slowly reconfigured. By the early 1980s, German public sentiment had begun to locate the crossing of cultural boundaries in a symbolic realm conceived as "above": the presumed sphere of contamination was transposed outward to the nation's cultural surface or skin.

The inversion of such metaphorical conceptions might attest to the dynamics of historical change. In the 1940s, ethnic minorities living in(side of) Germany had become the focus of hatred and fear. Correspondingly, an organic image was applied to the concept of the nation, and blood, an internal body fluid, came to be infused with symbolic significance. In the 1980s, the target of abuse shifted to those foreign nationals who had entered German territory in search of work or political asylum: they were regarded as outsiders, "outlanders" (*Ausländer*), foreigners. This movement of migrants into Germany was conceived in terms of the destructive potential of water, a natural liquid external to the body.

My research thus revealed several differences in the choice of metaphors. The concept of *subversion by blood* locates the transgression of racial boundaries in a sphere that is spatially below and at once inside. In contrast, the image of *submersion by water* points to the realm above and outside as the source of danger. The focus on blood served to interiorize the source of racial contagion: the flow of blood, regarded as dangerous and threatening, issued from inside the nation's body. Contact with the contaminating substance was rendered inevitable by its proximity: since one could not escape or flee from the contagion, it had to be eradicated. In contrast, the focus on water acts to exteriorize the locus of contamination. It is displaced from the body to the natural environment. But inundation by water likewise poses a threat to the center—not from within (as in the case of blood) but from its outermost margins. The social goal is to establish as great a separation as possible from it, without being engulfed or overwhelmed.

Despite this opposition of symbolic codes, the same logic is operative in both cases. Germans tend to express ethnic and racial differences in terms of fluids: liquid metaphors always prevail. In the German imaginary, the fundamental tension is between corporeality and liquidation. The potential site of confrontation is the body. Its solidity, its physical boundaries, and its internal integrity are always deemed threatened by dangerous internal or external flows. The aim of German political practice appears to be focused on eliminating such contaminating matter. These observations led me to investigate the concept of blood in popular articulations of race in European history and to seek out the various locations of blood and contagion in German racial ideologies.

* * *

In this book I aim to establish a genealogy of European racial aesthetics as revealed through metaphors of blood. My work traces the concept of blood and its metaphorical significance through several epochs of European cultural history. Chapter 1 begins with an analysis of the protohistoric emergence of the metaphorical field in central Europe, followed by an examination of the mythic implications of blood for European social organization, with particular reference to premodern concepts of kinship, womanhood, and masculinist physicality. Chapter 2 looks at the semantics of blood in early northern Europe, where the evidence from early German language and ritual practice attests to a radical shift in cultural attitudes toward blood: linked to vegetative images (soil, roots, flowers), gendered sexualities, and protoethnic boundaries, blood is no longer a mere marker of kinship categories. Chapter 3 shows how blood became a focal point and, sometimes, an agent of male domination in the early medieval period, as revealed by mythological narratives about world origin and human genesis. In Chapter 4, I continue with an examination of blood symbolism in late medieval Europe, where the connotations of blood shifted from reproductivity and gender to locality, community, and ethnic origin. The medicalization of blood ideologies in modern Europe is my next topic. In Chapter 5, I trace the route by which blood would become a signifier of a physical or biomedical concept of race. In Chapter 6, I analyze the political implementation of such popular conceptions of blood in fascist Germany, where blood purity became the dominant ideology of the state. In the final chapter, I turn to postwar Germany and examine the resurgence of blood images in contemporary German politics. I conclude by documenting the persistence of the racial aesthetic in cultural articulations of violence and anti-immigrant sentiments in post-unification Germany. My research suggests that it is precisely the historical density of corporal metaphors—propelled by fears of female bodies—that sets into motion the perpetual articulation of a cultural aesthetic focused on blood, contamination, and race.

Acknowledgments

Ideas do not emerge from a vacuum. Many of my instructors, colleagues, and friends generously offered me assistance, both in locating relevant source materials and in providing useful suggestions. I am deeply indebted to Alan Dundes, my mentor and dissertation chair, whose intellectual fervor and scholarship were a constant source of inspiration. I am grateful to John Lindow for his careful reading of several early versions of this manuscript, and for his help with the translation and interpretation of the medieval texts. My thanks also go to Stanley Brandes, who kindly shared with me his expertise in the field of symbol and metaphor. For their constructive criticism and editorial comments I am grateful to Paul Friedrich and Gary Holland. Although this work was begun at the University of California at Berkeley, I owe much to the intellectual influence of David Parkin, who took me under his wing while I was at the School of Oriental and African Studies in London. During a two-year appointment at the University of Toronto, I received insight and encouragement from Ivan Kalmar whose unwavering belief in the importance of this project strengthened my determination to begin the long process of revision. Finally, I must express my deep sense of gratitude to Thomas Hauschild, at the Institute of Ethnology at Tübingen University, where the final draft of the manuscript was completed. I am grateful for his courage in accepting my work as a contribution to historical anthropology.

I owe a great deal to conversations with Omer Bartov, John Borneman, Erika Dettmar, Heide Fehrenbach, Michael Herzfeld, Utz Jeggle, Gudrun König, Ruth Mandel, Carolyn Nordstrom, Jeffrey Peck, Donald Pitkin, Robert Rotenberg, Neil Smith, Paul Stoller, Bernd Jürgen Warneken, and Eric Wolf. I must also single out two colleagues, because many of their ideas became my own, and without their encouragement this work would not have been finished: David Merritt and Allen Feldman.

This book has been a long time in the making, and diverse sources of funding have been essential to its completion. The initial research for this project was funded by several grants from the Robert H. Lowie Fellowship Foundation (University of California at Berkeley) and a generous stipend from Phi Beta Kappa. Fieldwork in 1988–1989 was supported by a fellowship from the Social Science Research Council (Berlin Program). Additional research, analysis, and write-up of the findings have been enabled by several grants from the Rutgers University Research Council and a series of competitive fellowships from the Rutgers Center for Historical Analysis (RCHA), the Center for the Critical Analysis of Contemporary Culture (CCACC), and the Institute of Ethnology at

Tübingen University, where I spent six months as a visiting faculty member in 1997 and 1998.

Since this work was written over the course of several years, some parts have previously appeared in print. A first draft of Chapter 1 was published in the *Journal of Indo-European Studies* 13, nos. 3–4 (1985): 333–76. A later version of this text appeared in *Comparative Studies in Society and History* 34, no. 4 (1992): 579–620 with substantial revisions. Different segments of Chapter 3 were published in the *Journal of Psychohistory* 16, no. 3 (1989): 231–62; in *From Sagas to Society* (G. Pálsson, ed.), pp. 265–88 (Enfield Lock: Hisarlik Press, 1992); and in *Denying Biology* (W. Shapiro and U. Linke, eds.), 129–65 (Lanham: UPA, 1996). A short version of Chapter 7 appeared in the *American Anthropologist* 99, no. 2 (1997): 559–73 (copyright American Anthropological Association). The quoted excerpt in the Epilogue was reproduced from *Konkret: Politik & Kultur* 1 (1994): 42 (Hamburg: Konkret Verlag). I am grateful to the above presses and editors for their permission to reprint revised portions of these texts.

Part I
Blood Images
in Early Europe

Chapter 1
Artifacts of Gender
Prehistoric Images of Blood
and Reproduction

> What are we to make of the red symbolism which, in its archetypal
> form in the initiation rites, is represented by the intersection of two
> "rivers of blood"? This duality, this ambivalence, this simultaneous
> possession of two contrary values or qualities, is quite characteristic
> of redness in the Ndembu view. As they say, "redness acts both for
> good and ill."
>
> Victor Turner, *The Forest of Symbols*, 1967

Ideologies of reproduction are social facts, collective representations of
the dramatic ways in which human beings construct and appropriate
gender for the imaging of social reality. Such symbolic universes are
often centered on the body.[1] As a template of cultural signification, the
body becomes a model through which the social order can be apprehended. For instance, gender hierarchies are sometimes envisioned by
means of anatomical or physiological paradigms.[2] However, the operation of societal power is generally focused on women's bodies and bodily
processes. Women, according to a widespread (and controversial) paradigm, are grounded in nature, by virtue of the dictates of their bodies:
menstruation, pregnancy, and birth.[3]

The conception of female sexuality and procreation as "natural" (that
is, wild, untamed, raw, dangerous) seems at times to justify existing
orders of power and domination. Textured in images of mastery over
nature, cultural representations of gender stress the legitimacy of male
authority.[4] Men, as divine or sacred actors, establish symbolic monopoly
over human reproductive processes by the simultaneous denigration
and emulation of female sexuality. Blood is a focal metaphor in these
imageries of power.[5]

Studies of men's rituals, in which women's reproductive processes are simulated by inducing heavy flows of blood, suggest that cultural attitudes toward menstruation are fundamental to gender stratification.[6] Gender relations are deeply rooted in male competitions in which the procreative power of women and their labor are reduced to currencies of masculine achievement.[7] This expropriation of female labor sets into motion the transformation of reproductive bodies and blood as male symbolic capital.[8] The harnessing of women's procreative power in rituals of bloodletting or blood sacrifice confers value, status, and privilege as idioms of manhood and validates the existence of such (male-propagating) orders as brotherhoods, lodges, secret cults, and patrilineal descent groups.[9] Men's quest for immortality and power thus finds expression in the exclusion of women from processes of social reproduction.

This chapter examines cultural conceptions of gender in Indo-European prehistory. I explore prehistoric notions of what constitutes manhood or maleness in relation to femaleness, with particular emphasis on the underlying ideologies of reproduction as articulated in the (symbolic) imaging or presentation of kinship, marriage, and descent. The prevalent gender images are shown to be embedded in blood metaphors. The crucial question is whether culturally constructed differences between men and women can be documented for prehistoric social systems. Categories of cognition typically have some linguistic, material, or spatial dimensions that can be made visible. A number of studies have provided support for this assertion by demonstrating the accessibility of seemingly elusive subjects like social organization, prestige, and ideology.[10] Several decades ago, historical linguists, deploying language and texts as their tools, began to explore the semantics of gender in their more general efforts at deciphering prehistoric social life.[11] Archaeologists, likewise, recognized the possibilities for gender research in their analysis of material remains, ranging from burial patterns, grave goods, architecture, art, and pottery to food disposal scatterings.[12]

Speculations about past systems of meaning are, however, never unproblematic. As in all attempts at prehistoric reconstruction, one cannot establish absolute verities but only degrees of probability. The plausibility of a postulated or inferred system of meaning depends on such criteria as internal consistency, correspondence with textual evidence, and the degree to which the analysis adds to our understanding of similar conceptual frames. Furthermore, in the absence of ethnographic or ethnohistoric commentary, the recovery of semantic artifacts and ancient meanings is sometimes guided less by a systematic methodology than by a sense of intuition: "In research into prehistory, as in structural analysis, there is no simple, programmable procedure for discovery, for hitting on the variables that are going to have discriminating power. On the contrary, one develops a feeling for the subject, learns languages, analyzes texts, reads secondary sources, tries out approaches and new models, and, in the course of it all, gradually sorts and sifts out variables and hypotheses that are increasingly realistic and sensitive to one's materials" (Friedrich 1978: 9).

My investigation of blood symbolism in the remote Indo-European past led to a gradual isolation of several themes that are themselves redolent and charged with meaning: violence, aggression, death and winter (the female affine); and fertility, birth, life and spring (sister and wife). These themes constitute a conceptual or ideational landscape in which the integrity of the reproductive body, marked by the presence or absence of blood, stands out most clearly. Women in proto-Indo-European society constituted a class of beings who were symbolically marked: their bleeding bodies (during menstruation, defloration, and birth) were associated with death, the pollution of the corpse, the danger of annihilation. Female procreative power, that is, the ability of women to reproduce life naturally, through the body, was thus denigrated and negated. My research suggests that we find these representations of womanhood (that is, carnality, death, blood) encoded in the kinship terms for women: sister, female affine, and wife. Proto-Indo-European men comprised a separate class of beings who administered the realm of social reproduction, a domain from which women were excluded. Ancestral origins and intergenerational continuities were traced through men, from father to son. Building on my earlier work,[13] I document that proto-Indo-Europeans conceptualized the essence of such male-propagating linkages, the very substance of patrilineal descent, in terms of blood. Blood, as the dominant symbol of women's reproductive labor, was appropriated to represent the propagation of society by men. In this context, blood was transformed and disguised as male symbolic capital: a substance of power and immortality.

The Indo-Europeans: Archaeological Theories and Constructs

The source material for my analysis derives from the verbal artifacts and semantic remains of what has been termed proto-Indo-European, an archaic (reconstructed) language associated with a congeries of prehistoric tribal cultures whose original territory converged on the Black Sea area somewhere between 6500 and 2500 B.C. During this period of presumed (partial) linguistic unity, members of the Indo-European community extended their domain beyond Anatolia to the Balkans and central Europe—meeting there the resistance of native peoples in western and northern Europe.

Identification of the original homeland of the Indo-European peoples and the mechanisms of their migratory dispersal are still uncertain. The movements of a prehistoric people are generally difficult to trace in the archaeological record. Attempts to interpret this evidence have produced multiple theories about the origins of the ancestral proto-community: potential sites have been postulated in regions as diverse as southern Russia, Anatolia, and the Balkans.

Romantic conceptions of prehistory favored the idea that common Indo-European rose from the steppes. This assertion found resonance among some archaeologists,[14] who discovered traces of early settlements, dating from 4500 to 2500 B.C., in the steppe-forests of the southern Ukraine and south Russia. Such settlements, however, are few; evidence for habitation is scarce. The existence of people in this region is documented primarily through mortuary practices: the burial of the dead in an earthen or stone chamber; the frequent use of ocher and other red minerals, probably as symbolic blood offerings; the entombment of grave goods, which included weapons (stone battle-axes) and animal remains (sheep, goat, cattle, and horse); the marking of burial sites by erection of a grave mound or low tumulus (Russian *kurgan*). Based on the archaeological findings, the corresponding culture has been typified as warlike and pastoral, highly mobile, with technologies that included wagons drawn by oxen and the harnessing of horses. These people probably originated in the eastern steppe, perhaps in the Volga-Ural region, and from there pushed westward to the steppe-forests and foothills between the Caspian Sea and the Carpathian Mountains. According to the steppe hypothesis of Indo-European origin, the proto-speakers are conceived in terms of this patriarchal warrior culture of horse-riding nomads, who swept into east-central Europe from the steppes of southern Russia in a wave of conquest, superimposing themselves in a series of stages on indigenous farming communities. They brought with them knowledge of bronze metallurgy used for weapons, an ideology of hierarchy, and a male-dominated pantheon of horse-riding sky gods.

The archaeological evidence for colonizing expansion by nomadic warriors derives from the documented social transformation of southeastern Europe. Under the incursion of the steppeland nomads between 4000 and 2500 B.C., a society identified as peaceful, egalitarian, and essentially matrifocal (female centered) abruptly disappeared.[15] Indigenous burial practices changed in a manner suggesting recurrent episodes of invasion: mounds and tombs became morphologically identical to those of southern Russia. The graves were typically confined to the burial of privileged males, whose bodies were accompanied by arrows, spears, knives, and other symbolic representations of power, such as horse-headed scepters. The sacrificial execution of a woman after her husband's death (the rite of suttee) is indicated by some burials, revealing the patriarchal character of the invading warrior-pastoralists. The steppeland nomads subverted the local farming populations of southeastern Europe, bringing with them a new religious ideology centered on warlike sky gods and sun worship. This cultural focus is reflected in the inscriptions of Alpine stone stelae that depict horses, wagons, sunbursts, and especially weapons (axes, spears, arrows, and daggers) characteristic of the warlike proto-Indo-Europeans.

The notion of an aggressive Indo-European ancestry, propagated by the invasion of nomadic warriors, has been challenged. Some archaeologists propose that the prehistoric mechanism for cultural domination was not conquest but rather the gradual and peaceful spread of farming, beginning as early as 6500 B.C.[16] The dispersal of Indo-European languages has been correlated with the adoption, over generations, of an early agricultural economy, propagated by a "wave of advance" through successive geographical displacements. The very transition from foraging to farming engendered an increase in food production and, subsequently, population growth, a process that exploded the need to colonize unfarmed habitats. According to this theory, Indo-European became the dominant language because its speakers enjoyed greater economic and demographic success than the indigenous hunter-gatherers, who were forced to either assimilate or seek refuge in isolated settlements. Based on the evidence from radiocarbon dating of grain found at archaeological sites, which has been used to trace the spread of farming technologies into Greece and the Balkans after 7000 B.C., the origins of the proto-Indo-European speakers have been shifted from southern Russia to eastern Anatolia (in the Near East). As suggested by the language-farming hypothesis, prehistoric steppe settlements represent a secondary migration from a territory southwest of the Black Sea.

Independent evidence for the Anatolian origins of the proto-Indo-Europeans at 7000 B.C. has been uncovered by historical linguists (see Gamkrelidze and Ivanov 1985a, 1985b), whose studies point to a greater contact between early Indo-Europeans and Semitic peoples than was previously assumed. Their work has adduced technical arguments, such as linguistic correspondences in consonant patterns, especially traces of a shared vocabulary with neighboring Semitic and Kartvelian (Caucasian) languages, to argue for a longstanding geographical proximity. The research would suggest that even before the proto-Indo-Europeans reached the Russian steppes, they had a homeland in eastern Anatolia, where contact took place with Semitic speakers to the south and east.

In contesting the traditional assumption that a single major process, either conquest or farming, caused Indo-European domination, some archaeologists have argued convincingly that prehistoric dispersal mechanisms were probably varied. The propagation of a proto-Indo-European language might have been promoted by a number of practices: population movements through migration; the trading of economic or prestige objects, such as the directional exchange of metals and domesticated animals; secondary farming (livestock, horses, woolly sheep); pastoralism; and conquest.[17] The Indo-European settlement of prehistoric Europe may have taken place gradually and in successive stages:[18] the introduction of agro-pastoral farming from the Near East (Anatolia) into central Europe, the Ukraine, the Balkans, and southern Italy, after 6500 B.C.; agricultural intensification through the development of the plow, dairy production, and weaving (secondary products revolution), as well as the adoption of proto-Indo-European as a language of exchange, technology, and communication in western and northern European communities as early as 4800 B.C.; finally, elite dominance by nomadic pastoralists from the eastern steppes, between 3800 and 2500 B.C.

By the beginning of the classical period, perhaps even earlier, Indo-European languages were distributed over the entire continent, except for a few marginal areas. Residual pockets of non-Indo-European languages (e.g., Aquitani, Basque, Etruscan, Iberian, Lingurian, Tartesian, and Pictish; Sicel, Rhaetic, Messapic, and East Italic) attest to the presence of noncolonized peoples in prehistoric Europe.[19] Much of the Iberian Peninsula, parts of Italy, southern France, the Mediterranean islands, the Atlantic coast, and some parts of Britain were apparently inhabited by non-Indo-European speakers during most of the colonizing period. Likewise, in northern and eastern Europe, Finno-Ugric-speaking peoples were still assimilating indigenous (non-Indo-European) populations up to the very end of the first millennium B.C. Such observations imply that in remote antiquity, the dispersal of proto-Indo-European languages was far more restricted (and perhaps more localized) than archaeological sources would suggest. Furthermore, we need to remember that the construction of a proto-language is a hypothetical reality, perhaps consisting not of a single, unified mode of communication, but rather of a cluster of closely related dialects: "If there was ever a single proto-language, most linguists are convinced that even at that stage, it must have been differentiated into several dialects, since it was a language spoken without any central authority, and since the unifying and standardizing effect of literacy and all that goes with it was totally absent" (Zvelebil and Zvelebil 1988: 575–76).

Reconstructing Culture: Language Patterns and Semantic Artifacts

Some insights into early Indo-European origins and culture may be gained from a reconstruction of the proto-language (dialects). A survey or inventory of prehistoric linguistic categories can promote identification of a particular geographical territory by classifying landscape markers; the naming of vegetation, animals, birds, and modes of subsistence; and the descriptions of technology, types of settlement, architecture, social systems, and mythology.[20] An analysis of the proto-Indo-European verbal repertoire thus provides us with a partial cognitive map of several related conceptual domains: natural environment, economy, social structure, and possible patterns of collective representation.

Such a semantic inventory relies on the careful analysis of the histories of several linguistic forms, that is, on the construction of pertinent etymologies. An etymology traces the evolution of a word and its transmission from one language to another, leading ultimately to the reconstruction of a hypothetical proto-term. Through the formulation of etymologies we derive diagrams of those systematic correspondences of phonemes and morphophonemes that appear in a set of related languages.[21] When the history of cognate words is thus traced, we achieve an approximation to the overt linguistic forms that formerly existed as semantic categories in a prehistoric system of verbal discourse.

Linguistic markers of the contemporary landscape unfortunately contain few clues as to where the early Indo-Europeans were situated. A reconstruction of the proto-language suggests that Indo-European speakers knew plains and mountains, rivers and lakes. The weather vacillated enough to give them words for snow and ice. Only three seasons—winter, spring, and summer—are reconstructible. The botanical evidence hints at a conception of forest: several trees (birch, willow, elm, ash, oak, yew, pine) were set in the contemporary landscape. An assortment of wild animals (wolf, bear, lynx, elk, deer, beaver, otter) were known to proto-Indo-European speakers. The most commonly reconstructed bird names include the eagle and possibly some other larger bird of prey, as well as the goose, crane, and duck. In the categories of insects, reptiles, and fish, we find the honeybee, wasp, snake, turtle, salmon, trout, eel, and carp. We thus arrive at a landscape that included enough trees to provide forest environments for a variety of wild animals. A riverbank or lakeside orientation is discerned from the identifiable list of animals and birds, although this is hardly surprising in terms of a prehistoric settlement.

The subsistence economy for the proto-Indo-European population was based on stockbreeding with some agriculture. Domesticated animals (cow, ox, steer) and their use as food (meat, marrow) are well documented in the proto-vocabulary. Terms for wool, hide, and dairy products (cheese, butter) have been linked both to cattle and to the breeding of sheep and goats. The use of oxen for traction is indicated by the reconstructed terms for yoke and plow. Wheeled vehicles would most likely have been drawn by oxen at the time of the earliest Indo-Europeans. The importance of cattle is also reflected in words for cattle raiding in some Indo-European languages and in the use of the cow in Sanskrit and Greek as a special beast of sacrifice. Included in the concept of movable possessions were the pig, horse, and dog. In contrast to this evidence for animal domestication, the vocabulary related to agriculture is somewhat more limited. On the basis of the available lexical residue, at least some agriculture, as suggested by words like plow, sickle, and field, was known to the proto-Indo-Europeans.

The vocabulary concerning settlement and architecture is so generic that it offers only the vaguest image of a proto-Indo-European community. In addition to the words for house (post, doorpost, wall, clay, dough) or hearth, other terms designated a small settlement whose members were related: a village may have been composed of a body of houses belonging to an extended family or a collection of houses inhabited by the members of a clan. Some form of fortified settlement or refuge probably existed in the proto-Indo-European landscape.

Basic technologies were an integral part of the proto-Indo-European subsistence economy. A variety of words for different types of containers and bowls are reconstructible, revealing knowledge of pottery. The vocabulary of metallurgy is poorly and controversially represented: the primary utilitarian metals appear to have been copper and bronze, although a strong case can be made for an acquaintance with silver. Secondary technologies linked to agriculture and stockbreeding are also attested. There is linguistic evidence for weapons used in hunting, raiding, and war; the most unequivocal reconstructions concern the bow, bowstring, and arrow, all of which support the existence of archery within the proto-community. A thrusting or hurling instrument such as a dagger is usually postulated in connection with other weapons (sword, spike, stone ax). The word for stone ax is cognate to words denoting sky, hammer, and missile, which are frequently associated with the Indo-European gods of thunder and bolts of lightning.

The linguistic evidence suggests that the social system of the proto-Indo-Europeans was androcentric and patrilineal: social membership was conferred by birth and traced through a genealogy of men. Although we cannot reconstruct a common word for marriage, we find that Indo-European languages employ the term to lead when expressing (from the groom's perspective) the act of becoming married. The residence rules of the early Indo-European community were patrilocal: upon marriage, a woman was required to live in the house of her husband or with his relatives. Within the family, the father assumed the role of stern disciplinarian, as did his brothers, who—in a patrilineal system —all competed for positions of authority over their younger kinsmen.

Beyond the immediate household and extended family, several institutions become apparent from an inventory of the proto-language. Individuals tended to belong to larger social units: upon birth, they assumed their hereditary membership in a clan and there submitted to the leadership of a chief or lord, the master of the clan. Other terms reveal the existence of military organizations or some form of warrior sodality among the earliest Indo-Europeans (campaign, people under arms, and so forth). The underlying vocabulary of strife or violent (political) conflict can also be seen in the proto-Indo-European terminology for blood revenge and blood payment.

The reconstructive research suggests that Indo-European peoples tended to organize the social divisions of their communities through a tripartite conceptual system.[22] Society was divided into three classes: priests, warriors, and herder-cultivators. This model is recoverable from mythology with its distinctive realms, groups of deities, and characteristic powers of divine figures; it also permeates other societal domains:[23] medical practices, canonical recitations, and ritual animal sacrifices.

Blood and Body

An inventory of the proto-language reveals that Indo-European concepts of manhood in the domain of warfare, kinship, and ritual were conveyed through idioms of blood. In particular the representation of men's social power, the determination of origin and ancestry by patrilineal descent (that is, the very principle on which the continuity of Indo-European society depended), relied on blood as its dominant symbol: a man's lineage or clan membership was signified by blood. This expropriation of blood as a symbolic medium for the imaging of (male) social reproduction marked the exclusion of women from power. The underlying conceptual scheme was accommodated linguistically. We find that the proto-Indo-European vocabulary contained distinct categories of women in opposition to men, which rendered separate stages of the female procreative cycle socially meaningful: sister (premenstrual), female affine (menstrual), wife (birth giving). However, such a successive reformulation of identity and kinship status further promoted women's dissociation or fragmentation from a unitary and enduring body of men.

The articulation of such gender differences through blood metaphor can be made evident in prehistoric language patterns. My work suggests that proto-Indo-Europeans promoted a dual image of blood (loss and containment) that was framed by cultural assumptions about reproductivity and power. Women in proto-Indo-European society, through the collective apprehension of their corporality as fragmented, open, and bleeding, were disembodied, stripped of their procreative power. Men, in contrast, through the cultural perception of their physicality as whole, closed, bounded, and blood retaining, were embodied and imbued with generative potential. Within the confines of the body (there concealed from view), blood, the seat of masculine power, was called *ēs-r̥- (inside blood). The flow of blood that penetrated the boundaries of flesh and skin to emerge as a visible substance, the sign of dissipating power and female sexuality, was termed *kreu̯- (outside blood). This fundamental dichotomy in the Indo-European conception of blood is probably unique.[24] There exists little evidence for such a terminological opposition elsewhere.[25] Few languages contain in their verbal repertoire two separate terms for blood. And in such cases, meaning is focused on other concerns, for instance, the amount of blood spilled (marked by singular/plural) or the causes of bloodshed, as by ritual and secular means (sacrifice vs. homicide).[26] Early Indo-European notions of blood, as well as of society, were permeated by corporeal images. Social meanings were centered on the body. The corresponding demarcation of the inside and the outside blood was subsequently associated with life and death, nurturance and danger, procreation and annihilation. I argue that these concepts of blood formed the basis of a number of metaphorical extensions in the domain of gender, kinship, and descent, where they surfaced in images of linkages and end linkages, manhood (procreator) and femaleness (sisterhood, erotic femininity, motherhood), inclusion and exclusion from membership in social groups. I document these symbolic meanings of blood by a brief exploration into historical semantics.

The Signification of Blood

The linguistic evidence suggests that the proto-Indo-European conception of bleeding and loss of blood was closely interwoven with images of bodily harm. We find that outside blood (*kreu̯-) is correspondingly a term loaded with negative connotations. In Indo-European thought, bleeding implied wounding. The visible appearance of blood was therefore presented in a symbolic sense as linked to physical injury and to acts of violence against the body. Such connotations of aggression permeate the semantic field of *kreu̯-, which is made explicit by the meanings of its presumed derivatives in a number of Indo-European languages (Table 1). These include heartless, bloody, cruel, gruesome, gory, fierce, horrid, bloodthirsty, source of horror, the one who wields a bloody weapon, making men bloody, shedder of blood, performer of a gory act, slaughterer. The common meaning of these derivative terms suggests that the presence of blood outside the body was associated with aggression, in particular with the infliction of pain and deadly wounds, actions which by implication inspire feelings of fear, horror, and loathing.

Additional etymological evidence supports the semantic equivalence of bleeding and wounding in the Indo-European world view. One finds explicit data linking blood effusion to the external penetration of the body. A number of derivatives of the nominal root *kreṵ-, outside blood, confirm the accuracy of such a notion. Among those are terms denoting beat, whip, crush, damaged, wounded, chip, fragment, splinter, bloody. Although these terms make explicit the conceptual link between the flow of blood and violence by alluding to the physical destruction of the body, other derivatives convey the same idea by focusing meaning on the downward movement of the already injured body (Table 1). Examples include crash, fall, brake, burst forth, tumble, steep, twisted, collapse. Other cognates are corpse, decay, and death.[27] According to this imagery, the wounded body, by bleeding, becomes devoid of life and is thereby eventually destroyed.

The semantic or symbolic equivalence of bleeding and wounding may well be universal. This type of equation has been documented outside the Indo-European context by ethnographers,[28] and it has received considerable theoretical attention. Psychoanalytic interpretations have linked conceptions of bleeding to sexually aggressive acts like defloration and to men's projective fantasies concerning such actions.[29] Scholars who follow this approach have argued that the implicit meanings of female genital bleeding closely resemble socially standardized attitudes toward bloodshed in warfare or hunting, as well as other forms of violence against the body.[30] Whereas such images of aggressive violence are readily apparent in contexts of defloration, cross-cultural surveys have uncovered relatively little evidence for the explicit association of female menstruation with an inflicted wound. The linguistic documentation is scarce. For example, in Zulu, an African language, the term for blood (*i-gazi*) denotes bloodshed in some contexts; the word is a cognate of to menstruate and to wound.[31] The conceptual link is explicit in the language of West Greenland Eskimos: the standard reference for blood (*auk*) appears in such expressions as wounds him mortally, bleeds (from a wound), has a flux of blood, menstruates, strikes him so that it bleeds.[32] Likewise, the Chinese term for outside blood (*xuebeng*) denotes blood from the uterus as well as blood from a wound, thereby equating destructive bloodletting with menstruation.[33] The only ethnographic connections, however, were reported for the Maria Gond of India, who

TABLE 1. Blood and Violence: The Semantics of *kreu̯-

Sanskrit	*krūrá*	wounded, bloody
	krūrá-	cruel, bloody
Vedic	*kravaná-*	shedder of blood, performer of a gory act
Avestan	*krūma-*	cruel, bloody, gruesome
	xrūra-/xrūta-	bloody, fierce, gory, horrid
	xrvīšyant-	bloodthirsty, source of horror
	xruvi-dru-	the one who wields a bloody weapon
	xrūnar-	making men bloody
	xrūnya-	bloody mistreatment
Russian	*krov'*	blood
	krovávyi	bloody
	krochá/kruch	chip, fragment, splinter
	krutój	twisted, steep
Lithuanian	*kraũjas*	blood
	krùvinu	make bloody
	krušu/krùšti	crush
Latvian	*kruts*	falling down steeply
	kràulis	crash, downfall
	krusu	crush
Old Prussian	*krawian/crauyo*	blood
	krut	to fall
	kruwis	fall
Old Norse	*hrun*	collapse
	hrjóta	brake, burst forth, crash
	hrynja	to fall, crash, stream forth
	hrør	corpse
Old English	*hrēosan*	tumble, crash, downfall
	hryre	decay, death
Cymric	*crau*	blood
Latin	*crūdēlis*	cruel, heartless
Greek	*kroúō*	beat, whip, crush
	kroiós	damaged, broken
Breton	*kriz*	cruel
Middle Irish	*crú*	blood
Cornish	*crow*	blood

References: Buck 1949: 206; Frisk 1970: 27–28; Grimm 1868: 701; Mayrhofer 1956: 280; Pokorny 1959: 621–22; Schwartz 1982: 190–92; Vasmer 1953: 665, 669, 671; de Vries 1961: 251, 258, 263, 264.

believe that the vagina once contained teeth and that when these teeth were removed, the wound never healed completely; and for the Arunta of Australia, who attribute the menstrual flow to demons who scratch the walls of a woman's vagina with their fingernails and make them bleed.[34] Given the evidence, some scholars therefore attempted to explain the origins of such connotations of aggression symbolically by reference to male menstruation or procreative envy, thus suggesting a possible connection between women's uterine blood and men's infliction of wounds to simulate such bleeding.[35] The denigration of female sexuality (through its association with death and violence) is thereby linked to the expropriation of female reproductive power by men.

Sociological studies likewise document that the symbolism of uncontained (menstrual) blood nearly always has an explicit reference to violence, to killing, and, at its most general level of meaning, to breach, in both the social and the natural orders.[36] Rooted within this conceptual web, shedders of blood, such as hunters, man slayers, and circumcisers, are typically perceived as liminal beings whose actions are functionally equivalent to the loss of blood by menstruating women. In other words, female blood givers are identified with male blood spillers. This symbolic equation is well documented for the Ndembu of Zambia in Central Africa.[37] There, blood and its color are dominant symbols of the hunter's cult, representing the wounds or the death of animals, the red meat of game, and the unity of all initiated hunters. Blood stands for the hunter's power to kill; it also symbolizes the act of homicide. Moreover, in the boys' initiation ritual, the emblems of hunting and murder become symbols that stand for the blood of circumcised boys. Such acts of bloodletting by men, expressive of violence, death, and social transformation, are transferred to menstruating women: "The field context of these symbolic objects and items of behavior suggests that the Ndembu feel that the woman, in wasting her menstrual blood and in failing to bear children, is actively renouncing her expected role as a mature married female. She is behaving like a male killer, not like a female nourisher" (Turner 1967: 41–43). In sociological terms, the Ndembu interpret the appearance of menstrual blood as an abrogation of the responsibilities of womanhood (pregnancy and child production), which is sanctioned negatively by recourse to cultural sentiments regarding bloodshed. Although sociological theories emphasize the coercive function of blood symbolism, which is to achieve women's compliance with collective sentiments, psychological theories seek to uncover the locus for such repressive ideologies in male fantasies of procreation. But the issue here is not one of gathering worldwide documentation for the symbolic equivalence of blood and violence so much as demonstrating its relevance to the meaning of proto-Indo-European *kreu-, outside blood. The coercive denigration of female sexuality in proto-Indo-European society is attested by additional sets of terms that associate menstrual or outside blood with a state of rawness (naturalization of the body), the loss of fluid (death), and coldness and solidity (corpse).

In proto-Indo-European cosmology, the imagery of bleeding provided a central metaphor of a physiological and social transition of the body. The visible appearance of blood had connotations of abuse, disfiguration, and wounding. It signaled the destruction of the body. Bleeding meant dying in symbolic terms. The initial stage of this transitional process was marked by rawness, an Indo-European circumlocution for the body once it had been injured and stripped of its skin, with its flesh exposed and bleeding. In his work *Le cru et le cuit* (1964), Lévi-Strauss repeatedly associates rawness with what he calls the natural world as opposed to the cultural realm of the cooked. Such an interpretation would lead us to believe that the body, as it bleeds, is naturalized, that is, brought into closer proximity to nature, death, and the carnal—a view essentially supported by the Indo-European linguistic evidence. The intrinsic connection between the flow of blood and rawness is expressed by a set of terms denoting raw flesh, bleeding, crude, raw blood, bloody, piece of bloody flesh (Table 2). These symbolic associations reveal a conception of the world according to which danger and destruction entered the body from without. Death lurked in the external realm, outside one's physical manifestation. The visible presence of blood was thus perceived as a prelude to death, for it impressed upon the body the visible signs of dissolution, of the breaking or rupture of physical form.

Additional evidence reveals that the process of dying connoted discontinuity in Indo-European. The body died when the flow of blood came to a halt. Metaphorically speaking, death was marked by the absence of internal fluids. The appearance of blood, signifying a loss of vital liquid, was therefore linked to death. Perhaps for this reason the image of the bleeding body once played an important role in rituals pertaining to the dead. The body of the dead, conceived as dry, was in need of liquid, preferably actual life liquid such as the blood of animals or humans, which would help it regain the state of the living otherwise known as wet.[38] Archaeological findings reveal the antiquity of such conceptions. Excavations have shown the presence of red liquids or pastes in human graves dating as far back as prehistoric times; pits as receptacles for sacrificial blood appear in proto-Indo-European burial sites as early as 3500 B.C.[39] The symbolic importance of blood in funeral rites persisted at least until the end of classical antiquity. The evidence from Greece and Rome reveals that the dead were commonly offered blood libations at the graveside, which were poured through an opening into the earth below.[40] Actual blood or blood substitutes, made of red ocher, clay, or other reddish minerals, were sometimes applied to the body and in particular the head of the deceased.[41] Textual sources furthermore do not limit the special use of blood to rituals pertaining to the dead. Blood belonged to the lower regions, the nether world, to the demons and the gods of death.[42] Additional evidence associating blood with sinister elements exists in both Greek and Vedic texts.[43] Hittite mythology contains similar notions. There, blood, the preferred drink of the underworld's

TABLE 2. Blood and Death: The Semantics of *kreu̯-

Sanskrit	krūdáyati	makes thick, harden
	kravís/kravyám	raw flesh, blood
	krūrá-	bloody, raw
Skythian	xrohukasi	shining ice
Tocharian	krost	cold
Avestan	xrŭždra-	hard
	xrū-	raw flesh
	xrūmant	bloody flesh
	xrūm	piece of bloody flesh
Sogdian	wi-xrūn	blood from a wound, gore
Middle Persian	gu-xrūn	gore, thick coagulated blood
Greek	krúos	frost, icy cold
	kruerós	ice cold, gruesome
	kréas	raw flesh, meat
Latin	crusta	crust, solidified blood on a wound
	cruor	raw, thick blood
	crūdus	bleeding, raw, crude
Old Irish	crúaid	hard, solid
Old High German	hroso	ice, crust
	hrō	raw, crude
Old Norse	hriósa	shiver
	hryðja	rain and snow
	hrár	raw, crude
Norwegian	ryggja	shiver
Old English	hrīðig	covered with snow
	hréaw	raw, crude
Lithuanian	krušá	hail
Latvian	kreve	coagulated blood
	kru-es-is	frozen mud
	krusa	hail

References: Buck 1949: 206; de Vries 1961: 251, 258; Frisk 1970: 11–12, 28–29; Klein 1967: 373; Mayrhofer 1956: 277, 280; Pokorny 1959: 621–22; Schwartz 1982: 191, 192; Vasmer 1953: 665.

inhabitants, assumed an important role in rituals for communicating with them.[44] Thus blood was attractive to certain powers, but only those associated with unpleasantness, war, and death.[45]

Within the semantic field of outside blood (proto-Indo-European *kreu̯-), death was made comprehensible not only by reference to the transformation of the bleeding body but also in terms of the changing quality of blood itself. We find this expressed by the following cluster of derivatives: makes thick, harden, solid, gore, coagulated blood, crust, solidified blood on a wound (see Table 2). The common meaning of these terms suggests that dying was semantically equated in early Indo-

European thought with a process of solidification: the body upon death was transformed into a corpse. Proto-Indo-European *kreu- makes explicit this transformation of blood from a liquid to a solid substance. In this sense, it should be understood as a metaphor for the passage of life.

The solidification of blood was further associated with ice and cold, which are the very attributes of the dying body and of death. Traces of this metaphorical extension from outside blood to freezing persist in a set of derivatives denoting ice, crust, frozen mud, shiver, cold, frost, gruesome (see Table 2). These terms link the cessation of the flow of blood to the absence of warmth. The process of dying was thereby expressed in terms of both the solidification and the cooling of blood.

Ice, cold, and frost as metaphors of bleeding (and female menstruation) associate the destruction of the body with the changing seasons of the year, and with winter in particular. The semantic link of outside blood with winter is clearly indicated by terms denoting rain and snow, covered with snow, hail (see Table 2). The conceptual link between the dying body and winter probably made sense in light of what could be empirically observed in the case of vegetative growth. In winter, most plants inevitably pass through a season of saplessness, of rest and apparent death. In many parts of the Indo-European world, this period coincides with the onset of frost and cold. Thus, the cooling and solidification of blood in death could be logically construed as signs of the same sort of freezing process that produced the apparent death of plants.

Such notions of the seasonal transformation of creative fluids (from liquids to solids) probably also reflected cultural interpretations of menstruating women. The cyclical renewal of female fertility (typically equated with the rhythmic appearance of blood) was modeled after images of vegetative growth and reproduction. According to the evidence from attempts at cultural reconstruction, proto-Indo-Europeans believed that a woman's menstrual blood periodically retreated to the womb, where it coagulated to become the substance from which the fetus was formed.[46] Human procreation was thereby linked to the stagnation of female sexual or menstrual blood and linguistically conveyed through images of frozen fluids: the solidification and cooling of blood. The symbolic representation of female procreation in language thus relied on graphic descriptions of winter, the cold time of the year, when the seeds of organic life lay buried in a seemingly dead world of snow and frost. Here, as conveyed through metaphors of blood, the oppositional domains of death and female reproductivity, conception and barrenness, pregnancy and loss of life (mortality), were paired and conceptually assimilated: birth givers were perceived as death givers in proto-Indo-European. This deconstructive symbolism of the outside

TABLE 3. Blood and Life: The Semantics of *ēs-r̥-

Old Iranian	(*ahr(a)-)/*wahunī-	good stuff
Sanskrit	ásr̥k/asra-	blood
Armenian	ariun	blood
Old Latin	aser	blood
Hittite	ešhar	blood
Tocharian A	ysār	blood
Latvian	asins	blood
Greek	ĕar/eīar	blood, life sap, seed, spring

References: Buck 1949: 206; Friedrich 1952: 39; Frisk 1960: 432, 433; Mayrhofer 1956: 66; Onians 1973: 177 n.9, 438 n.1, 512; Pokorny 1959: 343, 1174; Puhvel 1984: 305; Schwartz 1982.

blood served to annihilate or negate the creative power of womanhood and to devalue female sexuality.

Loss of blood, the signifier of death in the proto-Indo-European culture, was the mark of femaleness or womanhood, the sign of dissipating power. Containment of blood, in contrast, signified life. As we will see later, when retained within the confines of the body, blood was equated with the seat of masculine power, the procreative stuff of manhood and patrilineal descent. One aspect of this equation attested by the linguistic evidence is the ascription of positive connotations to inside blood (*ēs-r̥-): warmth, spring, fluidity, propagation, health, vitality, and goodness. Such connotations are conveyed implicitly by terms with the extended meaning life sap or seed of life (Table 3). There exists ample documentation of the Indo-European folk idea that the living body is liquid and in death becomes dry.[47] Dying might have been understood as a drying process and as a final removal of finite body fluids.[48] Therefore it is not unlikely that the movement of blood inside the body was perceived as the very essence of existence. Additional evidence suggests that early Indo-Europeans conceived of inside blood as good. When this blood penetrated the confines of the body, flowing toward the outside, it became a maleficent, evil fluid. The documentation can be drawn from blood symbolism in ancient Iran,[49] where the term for inside blood reflected the ordinary word for good stuff (see Table 3); connotations of evil were relegated to gore and blood from a wound. Accordingly, in Indo-European cosmology, the solidification and cooling of blood signified violence, decay, and death. In contrast, the warmth or fluidity of blood inside the body emerged as a central metaphor for life, procreation, and rebirth.

Proto-Indo-European "outside blood" was embedded in a field of metaphors having as its central theme the destruction of the body, the end of life in death and in winter. Its apparent antonym, "inside blood," alluded to the growth of life and the warmth of spring. This connotation is made explicit in the association of inside blood (that is, sap, seed) with spring (see Table 3).[50] The concept of blood inside the body thus differs sharply from that of blood outside the body. Among early Indo-Europeans, the diminution of finite body fluids and the visible appearance of blood marked in a symbolic sense the time of death in winter, when the movement of liquids came to a halt. Blood was expected to resume its flow at the onset of spring, the beginning of the warm season, the time of regeneration and growth.

Such an interpretation of the cosmology of blood emerged as a dominant discourse in the classical Greek doctrine of the humors, which was formulated as a coherent body of knowledge between the fourth and fifth centuries B.C. by Pythagoreans, Alcmaeon, and Hippocrates.[51] According to the main theoretical assumptions, the human organism contained four fluids, or humors—blood, phlegm, black bile, and yellow bile—in which the qualities of heat, cold, moisture, and dryness were inherent in various paired combinations. The properties of the humors appeared to be related to the seasons of the year. Blood, being hot and moist, was defined as the primary liquid of summer and spring. The cold and thick fluids like phlegm prevailed in winter. Changes in the composition of body liquids and the transformation of their essential qualities in different seasons served to explain the cause of metabolic variations and the disposition to illness. Such notions about blood and the periodicity of body fluids generally informed the major medical concepts up to the late Middle Ages.

Male Sexual Fluids: Blood and Semen

The social relevance of the semantic opposition between the inside and the outside blood can be documented in the realm of Indo-European conceptions of kinship. Proto-Indo-European speakers lived in communities composed of a number of extended patrilineal families; the villages were small, distant and presumably exogamous.[52] According to the rules of residence, women married *out* of their natal homes and moved with their husbands to geographically remote settlements. As women were drawn into the households of their relatives by marriage, they were separated from their own kin. In addition to the residence pattern and the spatial distance between allied families, symbolic boundaries made explicit the social contrast between affines and consanguine kin. Indo-European communities were predominantly patrilineal, and descent was traced through men.[53] The line dividing relatives by marriage from consanguine kin was thus sharply drawn, for membership in social groups, derived from the equation of a man's seed with his offspring, passed from father to son.

At the level of metaphorical discourse, male procreative power was conceived in liquid terms. In several Indo-European languages, the poetic word for male refers to fluids emitted (i.e., the seed). Examples include Sanskrit *vár* (water) and its cognate terms, with the meanings rain, dew, powerful and virile man, stallion, bull, aurochs, boar, shedder of seed.[54] Another example, although from a different root (Old Norse *verr* or *ver*), reveals the semantic equation of water, sea, husband. This suggests that at least in a figurative sense male or husband originally referred to this masculine fluid, which was understood as the most important reproductive characteristic of a man.

The principle of patrilineality in Indo-European, deeply embedded in the premise that men alone were responsible for procreation, is best expressed in the proto-Indo-European term for son, which can be derived from a verbal root to give birth.[55] The word for son was thus associated with ideas of female reproduction.[56] Some scholars suggested that this linguistic proximity of giving birth and son not only reflected the close relation between mother and child but also designated the son (in contrast to the daughter) as the true offspring.[57] I propose that the primacy of patrilineal descent in Indo-European world view permits still another interpretation. The cultural assertion of male unilateral creation provided a conceptual framework within which the son assumed the status of procreator. In a symbolic sense, he was to give birth to future generations of his lineage. We have here a linguistic attestation of a case of male procreative symbolism: the societal appropriation of female reproductive power and its emulation by men.

In the Indo-European world, the power men represented or embodied was thought to be concentrated in their semen. It was this masculine fluid that was held responsible for acts of male unilateral creation. Since the generative potential of men was unable to display itself directly, it had to revert to the state of the seed. Men reproduced themselves in seed form. Such a concept often appears as a mythological theme. According to an Iranian creation myth, the first human male, Gayomard, succumbed to the blows of an evil spirit, and his seed entered the earth. Forty years later, it gave birth to the plant *rivas*, which in turn changed into a man and a woman.[58] We find the same motif in a popular European medieval legend, which among French, English, and German poets turned into a narrative about the tree of life.[59] One such version states that when Adam was dying, his son Seth went to the Garden of Eden to obtain from the cherub three seeds of the Tree of Life for his father. But Seth returned too late; Adam had already died. Seth placed the seeds in his father's mouth, and he was buried with them. Some time later, the seeds sprouted, growing into a wonderful tree.[60] In this tale, the dead and barren body, infused with seed, begins to procreate, generating life in the form of a tree, which rises as a symbol of everything creative and thereby manifests the power latent in the masculine seed.[61] In short, the tree represents the reconstituted virile body of men.

The elementary relation between the male body and the tree is characteristically one of procreation through the liquid seed. Both Scandinavian and Iranian mythology focus attention on the sappy tree, the growth of the all-semen-producing-tree from which seed in the form of water, dew, honey, yellow sap, or white and milklike fluid pours into a well beneath the tree; the tree hides its roots in this well and draws its nourishment from it.[62] Similarly, in Indian poetry of the late period, the eternal fig tree bears the name *Ashvattha*, or the seed of all things.[63] Both the Vedas and Upanishads reiterate that "the seed contains the tree, and the tree the seed."[64] Like the body of men, the tree is seen as self-generative and self-perpetuating. It becomes in this sense an unambiguous metaphor for masculinity. Growing from the male seed, the tree also produces semen, thereby giving plastic expression to men's procreative power.

The tree, it would seem on occasion, might have had something to do with the genesis of the world. In many early Indo-European narratives, the ancestral father appears as the guardian of the tree that generates seed in the form of offspring or from its seeds gives birth to men.[65] Human beings are said to descend from trees in Greek folk tales. Such a tree origin of mankind is attested explicitly in Hesychios, where human beings are called the fruits of the ash tree; according to Hesiod, the third or iron generation of humans was born from such a tree.[66] Scandinavian creation myths reveal a similar notion. In the texts of the Edda, a giant ash tree is said to contain the future ancestors of humankind in seed form.[67]

This imagery of the fertile tree seems to have incorporated signs of female physiological processes: the tree gives birth and generates human life as does a woman. Some scholars have therefore argued that the procreative tree may sometimes be interpreted as a symbol of female reproductive power.[68] The significance of this generative symbolism of trees becomes apparent when analyzed with reference to the larger Indo-European social system in which it was embedded. According to the ideology of patrilineality in proto-Indo-European society, membership in social groups passed from father to son; men alone were held responsible for acts of procreation. The tree, rising from the masculine seed as an extension of the male body, provided a symbolic medium for the realization of men's generative potential. Numerous instances of this concept exist in northern European myths, where gods and sacred beasts are said to impregnate a tree: in the *Vǫlsunga Saga*, Odin pushes his sword into the tree, or Odin's boar slits the tree with its horn. In both narratives, the tree gives birth to men.[69] Here infused with masculine fluids, the tree transforms in a metaphorical sense into a substitute womb for men. As symbolic representations of men's creative potential, trees are thus androgynous, possessing both male and female attributes.[70] Additional evidence from images of bleeding trees serves to illustrate this point.

Although the tree in Indo-European narratives grows from the procreative fluid of men and reproduces it in seed form, the liquid contained inside the tree is blood. Blood as sap flows through the tree.[71] Understood as the counterpart of the fluids of plants, blood appears to have been the vehicle of vegetative growth.[72] Thus, when attacked and wounded, plants began to bleed as did the human body.[73] This imagery of bleeding plants or trees surfaces as a recurrent theme in the works of Roman poets. Ovid provides the best example when he describes how Erysichthon violated the sacred grove of Ceres, the goddess of fertility, and attempted to uproot one of her trees. He writes: "There stood among these [trees] a mighty oak with strength matured by centuries of growth, itself a grove. Round about it hung . . . votive tablets and wreaths of flowers, witnesses of granted prayers, often beneath the tree dryads held their festival dances . . . [Erysichthon] bade his slaves to cut down the sacred oak . . . The oak of Deo (Ceres) trembled and gave forth a groan, at the same time its leaves and acorns grew pale . . . when that impious stroke cut into its trunk, blood came streaming forth."[74] Acts of violence against plants thereby produced the same effects as the mutilation of human flesh. The penetration both of the body and of the tree induced the flow of blood.

Indo-Europeans, in their myths and legends, tended to attribute the origin of plants to the violent death of a primeval giant or god. In such narratives, trees typically grow from the body of dead heroes.[75] An early Roman myth accompanying a seasonal fertility rite tells about the goddess Cybele, who loved a shepherd by the name of Attis so passionately that she made him emasculate himself, for then he could belong to none but her. Attis cut himself beneath a pine tree; there, he bled to death, and his spirit retreated into the tree:

From then on in Rome, toward the end of March, a pine tree was cut and brought into the sanctuary of Cybele, where it was swathed like a corpse with wooden bands and decked with wreaths of violets; for the violets were said to have grown from the blood of Attis. To the stem of the tree his effigy was tied, and then it was taken in solemn procession to the temple. The next day a strict fast was observed in preparation for the celebration of the *Day of Blood* (Dies

Sanguis) on the 24th of March. This day became the ritual re-enactment of the death of Attis. With much wailing and lamentation, the effigy was removed from the tree and buried in a tomb, while the priests of Cybele gashed their arms in remembrance of the blood sacrifice of Attis. (Cook 1974: 14–15)

Here, myth and ritual became alternative means for expressing the same cultural idea. Male blood-sacrifice, while promoting the death of the physical body, granted immortality of the spirit by the immediate containment of blood within the tree. Inside blood, presented as male genital blood, exuded life energy and reproductive power, which enhanced the birth of vegetation, inducing the growth of flowers and the tree. Ritual action made tangible the mythological metaphor by celebrating the end of winter in the renewed flow of blood.

Blood and sap, male bodies and trees, were metonymically equated in early Indo-European narratives. When the life of a man had come to a sudden, perhaps unexpected end, it was carried on within a tree.[76] The birth of trees was thereby linked to the death of men.[77] Growing from the barren body, the tree rose from the procreative seed inside it and transformed it into blood. The work of Virgil offers a poetic rendition of this idea, describing in detail how Aeneas, when offering sacrifice to the gods, came upon the grave of the murdered Thracian king Polydorus:

By chance, hard by there was a mound, on whose top were cornel bushes and myrtles bristling with crowded spear-shafts. I drew near; and essaying to tear up the green growth from the soil, that I might deck the altar with leafy boughs, I see an awful portent, wondrous to tell. From the first tree, which is torn from the ground with broken roots, drops of black blood trickle and stain the earth with gore [*nam quam prima solo ruptis radicibus arbor vellitur, huic atro liquuntur sanguine guttae et terram tabo maculant*]. A cold shudder shakes my limbs, and my chilled blood freezes with terror [*gelidusque coit formidine sanguis*]. Once more, from a second [tree] also I pluck a tough shoot and probe deep into the hidden cause; from the bark of the second also follows black blood [*alter et alterius sequitur de cortice sanguis*] . . . But when with greater effort I assail the third shaft, and with my knees wrestle against the residing sand—should I speak or be silent?—a piteous groan is heard from the depth of the mound, and an answering voice comes to my ears. "Woe is me! why Aeneas dost thou tear me? Spare me in the tomb at last; not from a lifeless stock oozes this blood [*aut cruor hic de stipite manat*]. Ah! flee the cruel land, flee the greedy shore! For I am Polydorus. Here an iron harvest of spears covered my pierced body, and grew up into sharp javelins."[78]

These narratives not only demonstrate the importance of the tree in the life cycle of men. They also suggest a basic homology of blood and semen. Both fluids engender the growth of plants. Blood is transformed into generative seed by the death of the male body, and the seed turns to blood within the tree. Even when the life of the solid body came to an end, men's procreative power resumed in liquid form inside the tree, where it was preserved by the perpetual motion of fluids and by the transmutation of semen into blood. Such a transformation of sexual fluids within the tree assimilated the body of men to the reproductive cycle of women, metaphorically conceived in terms of the (seasonal) rebirth of plant life in spring. This metaphorical assimilation of blood, male bodies, and the tree "naturalized" assumptions of the procreative power of manhood.[79] It transformed the symbolism of male unilateral creation into a fact of nature, representing it "ultimately as a natural part of the celestial order" (Cohen 1969: 221). The cultural or symbolic appropriation of women's reproductive potential by men was thereby made to seem immutable.

Imagining the Social Body

Proto-Indo-European peoples, like many central Asian nomads, probably conceptualized their families and clans as metaphorical parallels to the human body. Patrilineal subgroups and kinship statuses were referred to as knees, elbows, thighs, and backbones.[80] The set of terms sharing the component meaning patrilineal kin group [81] seems to be related not only to words for knee, stem, and offspring.[82] It also contains the same root as found in *generation,* which is the semantic equivalent of beget, give birth, procreate, germinate.[83] Thus the backbone, perhaps understood as the stem of the body, and the main joints as well, were thought in some way to be the seat of paternity.

Given the evidence from ancient Greece, it becomes clear that not merely the skeletal structure or image of the *solid* body, composed of flesh and bones, informed early Indo-European conceptions of kinship. The root metaphor for membership in social groups was also drawn from notions of the *liquid* body and the flow of the internal fluids.

Until the discovery of the circulatory system by classical philosophers, all liquids were commonly assumed to move by ebbing and flowing up and down inside the body.[84] This concept of the unidirectional motion of organic fluids was paralleled by the assumption of unilineal (male) descent. The procreative masculine fluid, the seed, thought to be enclosed in the skull and the backbone and specifically identified with the generative marrow, flowed thence down through the genital organs to propagate new life. The liquefiable content of the joints was classed with cerebro-spinal fluid and was thought to contribute to the seed. Like other major body cavities, the joints secrete fluids and also contain marrow; these substances were assumed to melt, perhaps with the spinal marrow, into semen.[85] Whereas the head, the backbone, and the knees were understood as the generative members of the body in Greek mythology, it was the thigh that appeared in Vedic texts as a euphemism for the phallus, and from which the seed was discharged in many of the acts of male unilateral creation.[86] Scandinavian creation myths reveal some parallels. In a passage of the poetic Edda, a giant is said to have given birth from the *sweat* emitted under his left armpit.[87] This example is consistent with the Indo-European paradigm insofar as it asserts that men have the power to generate life from the fluid of the joints.

According to the Indo-European iconography of the male body, the *linear* motion of fluids became the ultimate source of creation. On the microcosmic plane, the flow of semen from the head down through the spine toward the genital organs transformed the backbone into a channel for the vertical movement of seed liquid. Along this linear axis, the body was assimilated to the spinal tree, whose trunk was the medium for the rising sap from the soil to the branches.[88] Thus, on the macrocosmic plane, the structure of universal space was modeled by the image of an axial channel through the tree.[89] This symbolism of the line allowed the tree to rise above time, so that it no longer participated in duration; by the lineal flow of generative fluids within it, the tree conveyed a sense of absolute perfection.[90] The vertical channel through the tree was integrated into the reality of the masculine body, conceptualized as passing along or through the spinal column into the genitals and joints.[91] Such an emphasis on the vertical prolongation of both the body and the tree gave metaphorical expression to the male conquest of temporal limitations (i.e., immortality) ultimately accomplished by the linear motion of the masculine seed.

Proto-Indo-European assumptions of creation and descent were dominated by this concept of the axial channel, the symbolism of the line: male procreative bodies propagated society patrilineally, from father to son. Such linear images of reproduction correspond to an androcentric view of the world, an ideology centered on the generative power of men. In more female-centered societies, concepts of birth and procreation appear to be radically different. For example, in Scandinavian (i.e., Old Norse) mythology, *linear* images of creation are displaced by *cyclical* images of reproduction.[92] This difference in symbolic emphasis, from a focus on the line to a focus on the cycle, corresponds to a shift in the cultural conception of the reproductive role of women: the proto-Indo-European assertion of exclusive male creation was antithetically opposed to a concept of bilateral descent in ancient Scandinavia, that is, a belief in the creative potential of both mother and father, man and woman.[93] Accordingly, in north Germanic mythology, women were envisioned as equal participants in the creation of life. Their generative potential, circumscribed symbolically through liquid metaphors (i.e., blood), was explicitly acknowledged: allusions to female sexual creation were dominated by assertions of a liquid cycle, which probably reflected cultural interpretations of female menstruation. Given the contrastive emphasis on the primacy of paternity in early Indo-European society, it is not surprising that the creation of life was perceived as a male prerogative. Correspondingly, the generative symbolism of female sexual blood was appropriated and transformed into a social metaphor of masculinity: blood came to mark relations of descent through men.

Women Inside the Social Body: Non-Erotic Femininity

Although Indo-Europeanists have commented on the use of body liquids as metaphors of patrilineal descent, they have tended to ignore the centrality of blood in conceptions of kinship. Understood as the liquid of the flesh, blood was one with the cerebrospinal fluid and the seed, the stuff of life and masculine power.[94] According to patrilineal ideology, descent through men thus meant being of the body and of the inside blood. By implication, members of a different patri-clan belonged to another body and to the outside blood. Correspondingly, proto-Indo-European *ēs-r̥- and *kreu̯- are attested in the kinship terminology as markers for women's relationship to men by birth or marriage, blood or custom.

The concept of inside blood served as a semantic construct that marked relations of descent through men. According to the linguistic evidence, it is attested in the term for sister: proto-Indo-European *swesōr-.[95] This kinship category probably referred not only to true siblings but also to members of the classificatory units: own woman or clan sister, or, as some etymologists have suggested, to the more inclusive patrilateral female cousin. Included in the reference, however, were only those women whose social identity was established by birth,[96] which was conceived in terms of blood. How is this sense reflected in the word sister (*swesōr-), a form of exceptional linguistic interest because it seems open to analysis as a compound formed from two elements? The first segment consists of a root for own, the demarcation of a social relationship, which occurs elsewhere in the kinship terminology with the meaning of member of the own group by birth, of the seed, or his.[97] The structural position of sister was thereby defined by reference to a social unit, the patrilineage, in which membership was traced through men.[98] The interpretation of the second element *esōr- is controversial due to discrepancies in the semantic evidence. Some Indo-Europeanists have seen in it simply a term for woman or female.[99] Others have opposed this suggestion on morphological and semantic grounds, instead proposing that the term should be derived from the proto-Indo-European root for blood.[100] The reference to sister would thereby denote "of one's own blood" or "connected by blood." There exists some evidence that these interpretations are not mutually exclusive. In fact, I have argued elsewhere that the Indo-European terms for blood and woman can be derived from the same root.[101] Moreover, proto-Indo-European *$\breve{e}s$-r- specifically referred to blood *inside* the body; it was not a generic term for blood. The category "sister" therefore reflected the compound meaning of own-inside-blood-woman. Because the boundaries of the social body and the membership in social groups in proto-Indo-European society were defined by male descent, the meaning of sister expressed the fact that until marriage a woman belonged to an aggregate of people related by the blood of men.

Given this interpretation, it is perhaps surprising to find that the reference to inside blood was not used in kinship terms for men and did not, for instance, appear in the word for brother. The proto-Indo-European word for brother denoted a fraternity, a group of men, whose members were not necessarily related by blood or birth. The semantic opposition between sister and brother rested on the assumption that all men within the same age grade belonged to a *phratry*, mythically descended from the same father.[102] The sister, in contrast, was acknowledged as a member of the social body only through her link to men. In light of such assumptions, coupled with the ideology of patrilineal descent, the reference to sister as own-inside-blood-woman may perhaps be understood as a symbolic gesture intended to affirm a woman's membership in an exclusive group of men.

Some Indo-Europeanists have argued that the root for own, when used in terms for women, typically alluded to kinship by alliance and did not denote consanguineal kin relations.[103] This would mean that the compound element connected those so designated with another exogamic body or another patri-clan. The clan sister belonged there potentially and did so in fact after marriage.

The linguistic evidence suggests that young women in proto-Indo-European society were removed from the category sister to become prospective wives at the first onset of the menarche, the visible appearance of menstrual blood. The flow of blood changed the identity of a pubescent female from a non-erotic being, the own-inside-blood-woman, with whom sexual relations were prohibited by the incest taboo, to a woman of the outside blood destined to leave her natal village and take a husband from a distant settlement. The geosocial displacement of menstruating (and unmarried) women was probably promoted by the cultural concept of blood in proto-Indo-European: when contained inside the body, blood was identified as the substance of male procreative power, signifying descent through men. The loss of blood in menstruation, which was involuntary and recurring, correspondingly implied a dissipation of social power, a weakening of the collective body, which had to be contained. It only made sense to rid one's own community of the impending threat of death (disempowerment or loss of immortality) by invoking the rule of exogamy. Young menstruating women were married out and bound to men from other clans, whose procreative efforts were to result in the containment of blood. These representations of femaleness, the imaging of women as separable pieces of the social body, constitute symbolic modes of female dismemberment that are expressive of the cultural marginality and fragmentation of women in proto-Indo-European society, a society that (by contrast) promoted the organic unity of men.

Women Outside the Social Body: Erotic Femininity

As a referential system, kinship terminology is relativistic. From the point of view of the male speaker, his prospective bride was a member of another body, thereby belonging to the blood outside his clan. This shift in perspective, which probably coincided with the onset of a woman's menstrual flow, was encoded in language. Seen as a potential spouse and as a legitimate object of erotic desire, a woman was stripped of her identity as sister to become the female outside the social body. Her new status was correspondingly inscribed linguistically by use of the proto-Indo-European morpheme *kreu̯- "outside blood."

The concept of outside blood appears in kinship terms for female affines, the nonmembers of the husband's patriline. It is attested in proto-Indo-European *swekrū-, which is reflected in all principal languages with the meaning "woman of the outside group." [104] *Swekrū- seems to be the antonym of "sister," woman of the inside blood. It consists of a compound formed by the element "own by birth," the acknowledgment of social membership, and a morpheme for head, chief, power.[105] But according to the standard etymology, we recognize in *krū- an alternative form of proto-Indo-European "outside blood." The term *swekrū- therefore reflects the compound meaning own-outside-blood-woman.

Etymologists have traditionally reconstructed *swekrū- with the meaning mother-in-law, a term from which a number of secondary extensions were formed later to include other relatives in the class of affines.[106] Such traditional semantic reconstructions have ascribed to proto-Indo-European *swekrū- the exclusive meaning of husband's mother. Yet in Italic, Celtic, and Germanic kinship terminology, this term also denoted wife's mother.[107] The discovery of additional textual evidence in Avestan manuscripts and the Rig-Veda lend support to the assertion that *swekrū- already designated a man's mother-in-law in proto-Indo-European times.[108] The traditionalist interpretation of *swekrū- implies that this term was originally coined by the bride, who joined her husband's lineage as a newcomer. This assumption seems unlikely, given the subordinate position of women in the proto-Indo-European social system in general, and the outsider, the daughter-in-law, in particular. Nevertheless, while women may perhaps not be credited with creating a special terminology, it is not unlikely that **swekrū-* was a term of reference that they used predominantly.[109] I would argue that Indo-European kinship terminologies evolved from an androcentric view of the world as a reflection of the ideology of patrilineality, which relegated female affines, mother and daughter, to the blood outside the social body.

Marriage eligibility, determined by the onset of menstruation, radically changed the social status of the sister. Once a woman became a bride, she was separated from her own kin to join the familial group of her husband's father in a remote settlement. This transition from own-woman of the inside blood to woman of the outside blood may have been accompanied by ritual practices: "There is some evidence of bride capture. For example the warrior caste in India had a special term for this practice; symbolic bride capture was an integral part of many earlier peasant wedding rites, notably among the Slavs; and it used to be a hallmark of life in the Caucasus. One may realistically postulate that bride-capture figured in [Proto-Indo-European] marriage ritualism and that it may have been an occasionally practiced alternative among the small and probably exogamous communities of the putative [Proto-Indo-European] homeland" (Friedrich 1979: 227–28).

Similarly, it becomes clear, when examining Indo-European expressions for marriage, that a woman did not actively marry; she was led away by a man. She did not accomplish an act; she changed her physical and social condition.[110] Now this is precisely what the semantic field of proto-Indo-European outside blood makes evident. A woman's ritual change in status was marked by the flow of blood. The connotations of aggression, violence, and sexuality intrinsic to the meaning of outside blood referred not only to a woman's menstrual discharge but also to the blood that appeared during the consummation of marriage, in the act of defloration. There is some textual evidence for this interpretation. We find in the Rig-Veda one veiled but highly charged reference to female sexual blood, not menstrual blood, but the blood of defloration: "The 'purple red stain' becomes a dangerous female spirit walking on feet, a witch who binds the husband and makes his body ugly and sinister pale; it burns, it bites, and it has claws as dangerous as a poison is to eat."[111] The blood described in the Vedic passage is not explicitly said to play a role in procreation but appears in a wedding hymn, resonant with expressions of fertility. Interestingly, the text suggests that sentiments of aggression are not merely evoked by the sexual act of defloration and the subsequent appearance of blood. The reference to the paleness of the husband's body alludes to the idea that power, carried by semen, is lost through sexual contact.[112] Even more explicit, however, is the indication that the woman's blood itself presents a danger to the groom. Why should this be so?

Indo-Europeans tended to view the process of sexual intercourse in terms of the interaction of various body fluids, notably blood and semen.[113] Although concepts of the precise nature of these fluids and the manner of their interaction have varied from time to time and from text to text, the underlying paradigm emerges clearly. In proto-Indo-European communities, membership in social groups was determined exclusively by male descent. Because the masculine seed was conceived as a unilaterally effective fluid, men were presumed to derive their procreative power from the ability to produce semen. The generation of male sperm was believed to take place inside the blood. Blood was the source of the seed, according to classical Greek conceptions: Diogenes of Apollonia considered it as *sperma sanguis*, the blood-sperm. Following Aristotle, semen was a product of blood. So also the Stoics derived sperma from the blood.[114] Vedic texts state clearly that blood in men created semen during sexual intercourse.[115] At least in the context of procreation and kinship, Indo-Europeans defined blood as a male sexual fluid. Since it contained the seed, it probably made sense to render a woman's allegiance with her natal clan metaphorically in terms of blood. Flowing inside her body, it was this fluid, signifying patrilineal descent, that appeared visibly not only at the time of menstruation but also during defloration. The consummation of the marriage ritual thus placed men in a competitive position with rival blood or seed givers belonging to the category of affines. When expressed in liquid terms, this meant that blood (the sign of descent) and semen (the sign of sexual intercourse) were alternative means for expropriating women's bodies and for asserting competing claims of paternity and male reproduction. When expressed in symbolic terms, this meant that the female of the outside blood (patri-clan) had to be transformed into a member of the inside blood (husband's clan) to establish the legitimacy of her offspring. A man could therefore not incorporate his bride by mere penetration of her body. He had to shed her blood, for the symbolic change in a woman's clan affiliation was accomplished only by a transfusion or substitution of sexual fluids. As a man gave his seed to the bride, he needed to extract some of her blood. The bloodletting assumed significance insofar as it was intended, in a symbolic way, to expropriate from the bride's body the remaining blood-sperm of her father's line of descent. It is thus possible that the marriage ritual centered on an exchange of blood between bride and groom, perhaps a synecdochal expression of the linkage between their respective clans.

Perhaps this interpretation can shed some light on why the early Indo-Europeans prohibited remarriage for widows. A woman whose husband had died was as a rule subject to severe restrictions. Among some early Teutonic and Greek tribes, she was forbidden to remarry; under Roman law, a widow could not remarry out of the clan of her deceased husband and, as elsewhere, was sometimes subject to the law of levirate, which forced her to marry her dead husband's brother.[116] Such customary rules hint at the importance attributed to a woman's virginity. Only by the loss of blood of defloration could a woman change her clan affiliation in a symbolic sense.

By bleeding, a woman died in an almost realistic sense. The first onset of menstruation and, later, the consummation of marriage marked her death in the category of sister and thereby ended her membership in the paternal lineage: *swesōr- the woman of the "inside blood" assumed the social identity of *swekrū- the female of the "outside blood."

While a woman's change in social status was expressed in terms of blood, the condition of the bride may have been conceived as raw. Among early Indo-European peoples, the newly married woman assumed a marginal position, marked by discontinuity. Although she had been removed from her own kindred, she was not yet a member of her husband's patri-clan. Although she was the end-linkage in her natal group, unable as sister to continue her father's line of descent, the bride had not yet given birth to a new member of the husband's clan.

After marriage, blood appeared in a woman most significantly in the form of menstrual or uterine blood. It was, however, men's sperm which in the early Indo-European world view was credited with the power to obstruct and reverse the rhythmic flow of female blood. Classical theories proposed that menstrual blood retreated to the womb under the influence of the seed, where it coagulated to become the substance from which the fetus was formed.[117] Post-Vedic medical textbooks summarize this process in stating, "from the [sexual] desire semen is born and from semen uterine blood."[118] The cessation of the woman's outward flow of blood signaled a change in state, an interruption of the course of life, that is, a transformation of the female body.

Re-Entering the Social Body: Woman as Birth Giver

In early Indo-European communities, the containment of blood inside the womb engendered the bride's incorporation into her husband's family as wife: proto-Indo-European *uksōr. Derived from a root *ewk- (to become used to by repeated use, learn), this word referred to a category of originally alien women to whom men became accustomed through marriage (as opposed to descent, that is, women as sisters). A

TABLE 4. Blood and Womanhood: The Semantic Categories

Sister	(sw-esōr)	Own-inside-blood-woman	Birth
Female affine	(swe-krū)	Own-outside-blood-woman	Menstruation
Wife	(uk-esōr)	Accustomed-inside-blood-woman	Impregnation

wife entered a new social unit not by birth but through the assimilation of new customs.[119] In the second element of this term we recognize a form already discussed with reference to sister (*swesor-), which we have taken to be blood. The kinship category wife can therefore be rendered as the accustomed-inside-blood-woman.

Unlike the sister, the wife became a member of the inside blood and of the body not by being born, that is, by descent but by sexual intercourse and by giving birth to child. By bearing a child, in particular a son, a woman established her full status as a member of the patrilineal grouping into which she had married. The proto-Indo-European term *uksōr formally declared that the bride, the outside-blood-woman, came under the power of the husband's blood. More specifically, it acknowledged that she once again contained the blood of men. Greek philosophers like Galen felt that after fertilization, uterine blood appeared as the first step in the formation of the fetus and that this blood was created from the male sperm.[120] Similarly, in Vedic texts the male seed is said to be the source of blood; a final solution is achieved in the Tantras by the statement that "the blood in the womb is called the seed."[121] Although blood represented the body fluid that appeared first in the yet unborn life, this blood was produced by the unilaterally effective male sperm. This made sense in light of the ideology of patrilineality and the assumptions of the primacy of paternity in the Indo-European world view.

Although a woman was perhaps not conceived as an insignificant receptacle or container for the male fluids, she was not regarded as an active partner in the creation process.[122] In Indo-European cosmology, inside blood meant the blood of men, the masculine blood, which granted women membership in social groups. Given the premise of male unilateral creation, wife came to refer to a category of women who contained and were bound by the blood inside the husband's body. Wives were women who gave birth and thereby were conceived as being filled with the procreative blood of men. The ideology of patrilineality placed the wife in juxtaposition to the widow, a term traced to a root *wydh-, denoting empty, inadequate, separate, and set apart.[123] This would suggest that the social status of a woman as wife or accustomed-inside-blood-woman was not durable or permanent: the retention of her identity required perpetual renewal and affirmation by male insemination or impregnation. In the absence of her husband as blood-seed giver, a woman was conceived as barren and infertile, an empty vessel, who once again found herself at the margins of societal identity.

The Management of Reproductive Bodies

The meaning of proto-Indo-European for accustomed-inside-blood-woman not only is congruous with the ideology of patrilineal descent and distant patrilocal residence but also constitutes a distinct paradigm when taken together with the analyses of sister and female affine (see Table 4). My research suggests that the essence of womanhood in proto-Indo-European society was constructed by men. Affiliation was established through male genealogical tracing or male-engendered procreativity. Images of femaleness were thus defined by reference to birth and marriage, as conveyed through idioms of blood and custom. This complementary opposition between organic and rule-bound or learned forms of solidarity (allegiance) finds parallels in contemporary accounts of American conceptions of kinship,[124] which point to the conceptual opposition between relationships in nature (blood and descent) and social order (law and marriage). This dichotomization also corresponds to the linguistic evidence for prehistoric images of manhood:[125] Proto-Indo-European speakers recognized masculinity in terms of gender (male as opposed to female) and sexual function (to impregnate, sire); paternity was similarly defined by the acknowledgment of authority (social, moral, legal) and fatherhood (biological). This seems to suggest that in prehistoric times, social relationships were already embedded in a dual symbolic concept of nature and culture, the juxtaposition of the seemingly immutable and the socially constructed.

Every culture selects particular domains that it attempts to naturalize.[126] Such attempts are products of a cultural mythmaking process that distorts the realities of power. My research indicates that in early Indo-European society women's bodies were singled out for ideological demarcation. This is evident in the appropriation of blood as a male reproductive fluid and the symbolic equation of female menstrual blood with violence and death. The annulment of women's creative potential invokes notions of disembodiment, fragmentation, and loss of control. Such a process of female disempowerment is hardly unique to proto-Indo-European society and is consistent with findings from contemporary cultures as well as historic studies of specific regions or culture areas within the Indo-European domain.[127] My investigation does, however, shed new light on the antiquity of such discursive practices and illuminates the importance of reproductive ideologies focused on blood.

The proto-Indo-European symbolism of the inside and the outside blood constituted a mechanism whereby collective representations of femaleness were constructed and naturalized to reinforce a series of prohibitions, in particular sexual taboos.[128] The concept of blood as a signifier of descent framed assumptions of social reproduction in organic terms. Society was apprehended as a unitary (single) body, in which every descendant, historically or fictively, shared the same blood, flesh, and bones. The loss of blood, equated with the dissipation of social power and death, was regulated by displacing (potentially) bleeding female bodies beyond the communal boundaries. Menstruating girls and virgins, whose production of blood posed a threat, were expelled from inside the social body to minimize the chances of impending lineage "death." These women were forced to take a spouse elsewhere and incorporate the blood of his lineage through exchange and impregnation. Inside the collective body, equated with male procreativity and descent, blood was contained. Correspondingly, women who belonged were culturally typified (by the absence of blood) as nurturing, birth giving, and non-erotic: the widow (postmenopausal), wife (impregnated), sister (premenstrual), and daughter (nurturing).[129] Within the communal body, where men were committed to the containment of power, women could not participate in the normal or regular (socially valued) production of blood through menstruation. The corresponding ideas surrounding exogamous prescriptions were encoded linguistically. The social identity of sister, designated by the marker of inside blood, signified the premenstrual virgin, who was juxtaposed to the woman of the outside blood, the menstruating (death-delivering) female, who was destined to leave her natal community. Thus, in a symbolic sense, proto-Indo-Europeans were preoccupied by a concern with pollution, contamination, and death, which ultimately expressed itself in the exclusion of women from symbolic control of blood and descent.

Chapter 2
Artifacts of Race
Premodern Images of Blood and Ancestry

What happened to the aesthetic of blood in later European history? Did the imagery of family, lineage, and breed endure through the metaphorization and symbolic codification of blood? In a series of remarkable essays, Michel Foucault (1978) claimed that the modern concept of race, that is, the whole thematic of the species, descent, and collective welfare, was endowed with the ancient (but fully maintained) prestige of blood: "The blood relation long remained an important element in the mechanisms of power, its manifestations, and its rituals. For a society in which the systems of alliance, the political form of the sovereign, the differentiation into orders and castes, and the value of descent lines were predominant; for a society in which famine, epidemics, and violence made death imminent, blood constituted one of the fundamental values" (147). Thus, in the modern era, blood remained an important signifier of power and privilege. The ancient regime of blood continued to support ideas of descent, heredity, and genealogy, providing a basis for fundamental social distinctions.[1] Blood endured as a descent ideology that became increasingly racialist. The premodern aesthetic of blood, according to Foucault, served as a foundation upon which a more directly biologist (racist) system of modern heredity could be erected.

But how do we explain this historical preoccupation with and commitment to the symbolic value of blood? Why was blood transformed into a societal fetish? Foucault suggests that this cultural obsession had something to do with the intrinsic qualities of blood. As a liquid, a bodily fluid, blood was always in a state of flux, its containment ever precarious. Blood images could therefore be easily invoked to enhance the drama of violence, suffering, and death: "[Blood] owed its high value at the same time to its instrumental role (the ability to shed blood), to the way it functioned in the order of signs (to have a certain blood, to be of the same blood, to be prepared to risk one's blood), and also its precariousness (easily spilled, subject to drying up, too readily mixed, capable of being quickly corrupted). A society of blood—. . . of 'sanguinity'—where power spoke *through* the blood: the honor of war, the fear of famine, the triumph of death, the sovereign with his sword, executioners, and tortures; blood was *a reality with a symbolic function*" (1978: 147).

Foucault thus presumed that the symbolic valuation of blood was organized not around the management of life but around the menace of death: "Clearly, nothing was more on the side of the law, death, [and] transgression . . . than blood" (1978: 148). The eviscerated body and the body in pain both furnished an image of valued sanguinity, revealing a distinct regime of power and an old preoccupation with blood and the law. According to Foucault, these imageries of blood tended to revitalize a type of political power that was exercised through the devices of the legal order: "the blood of torture and absolute power, the blood of the caste which was respected in itself and which nonetheless was made to flow in the major rituals of parricide and incest, the blood of the people, which was shed unreservedly since the sort that flowed in its veins was not even deserving of a name" (148–49). As Foucault argues, however, such a symbolics of blood gradually gave way to a new order of power: under modernity, the workings of blood and death were replaced by a concern with sexuality and racial proliferation. The propagation of the life of the body, not its blood and death, became a novel object of political struggle.

But the emphasis on bloodshed and death, as I suggested at length in the previous chapter, was never completely dissociated from a metaphorics of sex, vitality, and gender. Even in antiquity, the flow of blood and women's sexuality were closely related in symbolic terms. In early Europe, blood derived its potency and symbolic power from the linkage of reproduction with the female menstrual cycle. Blood and womanhood were thus interconnected in the European premodern. The later historical preoccupation with either the future of the species or the vitality of the social body was likewise implicated in anxieties over female reproductivity.[2] Issues of blood, race, and motherhood converged in a political obsession with the life-giving body of women.[3] My work suggests that the thematic of blood, life, and fertility (which first appeared in proto-Indo-European) was further accentuated in later historical epochs, finding its greatest intensification in German-speaking lands.

In this chapter, I examine how emergent themes of health, progeny, and race, which marked the threshold of European modernity, were prefigured in much earlier blood fantasies. A eugenic ordering of society through a mythic iconography of blood called on, and reified, deeply rooted cultural assumptions about nature, health, fertility, and abundance. My investigation into the European past reveals that metaphoric models of ancestry and blood origin placed the social body into the semantic field of nature. Human fertility and propagation were thus inter-twined with notions of blood loss, bloodshed, and female menstruation as natural processes. I explore these symbolic linkages of blood and nature in north-central Europe, the presumed homeland of the early Germans.

The Early Germans: Historical Constructs

In the absence of mass media or a written standard, people speaking originally the same language, but separated by large distances, are un-likely to maintain parallel changes in their linguistic systems. Similari-ties of speech over a large geographical area normally imply a recent population expansion: the factors of time and distance tend to reduce a single language into a continuum of mutually related but increasingly different vernaculars.[4] Indo-European lost its cohesion through diver-sification into separate speech communities after the third millennium B.C.: Celtic, Slavic, Baltic, Tocharian, Hittite, Sanskrit, Greek, Italic, and Germanic gradually emerged as distinct linguistic systems through geo-graphical dispersion and historical differentiation.[5] The dialect from which proto-Germanic emerged broke off from Indo-European at a rela-tively early date. "In the third millennium B.C. mixed farming was thriv-ing in Northern Europe, practiced by people who spoke only slightly differentiated Indo-European dialects; and with the coming of iron to northern Europe, the Germanic group markedly developed its charac-teristic identity" (Polomé 1987: 237). On the basis of the archaeological record, we can follow the development of Germanic culture and trace the areas of settlement in subsequent centuries.[6] However, little con-crete evidence about Germanic society exists until after the beginning of the northern Iron Age, when German tribes first came in contact with the outposts of an advancing Roman army.

The term *Germanic* is primarily a linguistic designation, referring to a group of languages that are historically related. "How unified [these lan-guages were] is not at all clear, and the enormous geographical spread of its speakers must be recognized. It is probably safer to see proto-Germanic as a linguistic complex rather than a unified language existing at one time" (Todd 1992: 12). The Germanic languages are traditionally divided into three major groups. The western group includes the ances-tral forms of English as well as Frisian, Old Saxon, and High German. The northern group comprises the Scandinavian languages: Danish, Swedish, Norwegian, and Icelandic. Although many of these languages are attested by abundant textual evidence from the medieval period, our earliest substantial documentation exists in Gothic, an extinct east Germanic language. "The Goths had migrated from the north into the

Black Sea region where they ruled until the arrival of the Huns in the fourth century A.D. who pushed most of the Gothic tribes westward into the Balkans. It was here that Wulfilas, Bishop of the West Goths, created a Gothic alphabet (primarily derived from the Greek) and translated portions of the Bible into the Gothic language. Gothic was still spoken up into remarkably recent times, surviving in the Crimea as late as the sixteenth century" (Mallory 1989: 84). In addition to the Gothic source materials, we also have the evidence of runic inscriptions, which appear to have been loosely derived from one of the north Italian or Etruscan alphabets of the first century A.D.[7] Runic inscriptions were widely used in northern Europe until the ninth century.

In combination with the direct textual evidence, we rely on the writings of classical historians:[8] The most important is Tacitus, who described the location and culture of the early Germans in his *Germania* (A.D. 98). During the first century, Tacitus located most of the Germanic peoples in a region bordered by several waterways: on the west by the Rhine, on the east by the Oder, and to the south by the Main. Earlier sources, such as Caesar in the first century B.C., are less reliable but likewise place the Germans east of the Rhine. The earliest historical source, Pytheas, is generally understood to have located the Germanic tribe of the Teutones in present-day Denmark, while locating the tribe of the Gutones in northern Germany.[9] Both the historical and the textual evidence indicate that the earliest Germanic-speaking peoples were largely distributed in an area corresponding to northern Germany and southern Scandinavia.

The area demarcated by the historical and linguistic evidence has provided archaeologists with a relatively reliable geographical marker in their identification of the earliest Germanic region. The northern Bronze Age, which appears to have developed relatively independently until the middle of the first millennium B.C., is commonly regarded as the ancestral civilization of the Germanic peoples. The continuity of the indigenous culture in northwest Germany and the relative homogeneity in ceramics from western Pomerania to the river delta of the Weser have led to the hypothesis that the local population became progressively familiar with the use of iron. The development of iron metallurgy and techniques of smelting had an important socioeconomic impact, which is reflected archaeologically by the emergence of the first characteristically Germanic culture. "[T]he ancestors of the Germans known to our earliest surviving historical accounts can be traced back to the mid-first millennium B.C., the period of the Jastorf culture, on the north German plain between Elbe and Oder, and the Harpstedt culture, in north-west Germany and Holland. To this same period philologists attribute certain sound-changes which were significant in the formation of proto-Germanic" (Todd 1992: 10). Known only through their material and physical remains, these peoples, whose settlements appeared around the fifth century B.C., offer historical evidence for the dominant Iron Age culture of northern Europe.[10] These settlements, which were characterized by a continuity of material culture, covered an area including Schleswig-Holstein, Mecklenburg, Western Pomerania, Brandenburg, and Lower Saxony. These sites formed the "core" of the proto-Germanic territory: from there, German-speaking tribes must have expanded southward at a relatively early date.[11] The continuity of settlements, cemeteries, and demographic distribution in this general area accords well with the historical locations of the earliest known Germanic tribes in the first centuries A.D.

Consequently, the perimeter of the Jastorf site (and probably neighboring locations) provides evidence for a Germanic homeland. This observation is reinforced by the linguistic evidence, which suggests that the changes that transformed a late Indo-European dialect into proto-Germanic probably occurred around 500 B.C.

Blood: Semantic Transfigurations

How did the emergence of Germanic languages affect the existing blood symbolism? Can we discern a transfiguration in the older aesthetic of blood? An initial comparison between the Indo-European and Germanic concepts of blood reveals a dramatic change in terminology. In early Germanic, the former dichotomy between the inside and the outside blood disappears when the proto-Indo-European forms *$\bar{e}s$-$\d{r}$- and *$kreu$- are displaced by one collective noun. With the dissolution of this semantic opposition, Germanic speakers adopt the term *$bl\bar{o}di$-, blossom, blooming flower, as a generic (single) reference for blood. It is precisely this novel use of a linguistic form and its extension into new meanings that concern us in the study of culture change. It is a semantic innovation that is particular to Germanic and cannot be documented in any of the other Indo-European languages.

This premodern change in the meaning of blood has received very little attention. Surprisingly few scholars have acknowledged its significance, and then only in passing. Several commentators, among them historical linguists, attribute the displacement of the Indo-European categories to a superstitious fear of blood and to the subsequent emergence of a word-taboo.[12] According to these scholars, Germanic speakers regarded the verbal recognition of blood loss and bleeding as a dangerous, transgressive act: interpreted as a magical invocation, which threatened to bring about misfortune and death, the conventional (older) vocabulary of blood was prohibited. A new phrase was coined. Lacking the negative connotations of blood loss and death, the meaning and usage of Germanic *blōdi-* "flower" was extended to include the denotation blood: the symbolics of blossom/flower were used to rework the signification of blood.

Other explanations for this semantic equation of blood and flower were proposed. Some scholars suggested that the poetic imagination of Germanic peoples became fixed on the red color of flowers and thereby accomplished the analogical shift from blossom to blood.[13] In other words, philologists assumed that the historical transformation of linguistic categories was triggered not by a fear of blood (as argued by others) but rather by a psychological preoccupation with life and fertility, a preoccupation that resulted in the positive valuation of the color of blood: German speakers appropriated redness and sanguinity for symbolic purposes, turning this color into a focal point and dominant metaphor of kinship and descent.

The linguistic innovation, which we witness in early Germanic, points to a fundamental historical change in the concept of blood. When the meaning of blood merged with the semantics of the blossom, blood assumed a novel cosmological and social significance. Accommodating a newly emerging cultural attitude, blood took on a dual connotation, referring both to the invisible flow within the body and to the emission of blood—its transformation into a visible reality—outside the body. This dual sense of the term blood is attested in all Germanic languages: Old Norse *blóð*, Gothic *bloþ*, German *Blut*, Dutch *bloed*, and English *blood*. Such a linguistic convergence signaled the transformation of a larger semantic field,[14] that is, a change in the complex of meanings that delineated ideas of blood and kin.

Blood and Blossom: The Etymology

During the Germanic era, which dates back to the fifth century B.C., blood became an essential symbol of fertility. The flow of blood signified transformation, in the sense of generation and birth. Blood was equated with life, not death. Germanic speakers assumed a positive cultural attitude toward blood and (as we shall see later) female reproduction. Some documentation for this assertion is offered by the linguistic evidence. According to the standard etymologies, the Germanic form *blōdi-* "blood" can be traced to a set of proto-terms that have been reconstructed with the meaning swollenness, bloatedness, flowering, in full bloom, overflowing with moisture (Table 5). These forms are probable derivations of a primary Indo-European root denoting bloom, bloat, swell, well up, originate from, blaze, shine, flourish, sprout. The multiple meanings of these terms are suggestive of wetness, abundance,

TABLE 5. Blood and Blossom: The Semantics of *blōdi-

Proto-Indo-European	*bhlō-tó-	swollenness, bloatedness, flowering, in full bloom
	*bhelē-	overflow with moisture
	*bhel-	bloom, bloat, swell, well up, originate from, blaze, shine, flourish, sprout
Armenian	bełun	fertile
Greek	phallos	penis
Germanic	*blōdi-	blood/blossom
	*blādu-	flower, harvest, wealth, offspring
	*blestu-	bloom
	*bel-n	penis
Old Norse	bollr	testicle
	blóð	blood
Gothic	blōþ	blood
Old High German	blajan/blāsa	swell, make known, bud, germinate
	bluot	blood, blossom
Danish/Swedish	blod	blood
Dutch	bloed	blood
German	Blut	blood
	Blüte	flower, menstrual blood

References: Klein 1967: 178, 180–81; Kluge 1960: 87; Kelle 1881: 55; Pokorny 1959: 120–122; Ranke 1978: 77; Spalding 1957: 355–56; de Vries 1961: 41–46.

and the generation of plant life, connotations and meanings that were condensed in the metaphorical image of a budding flower in Germanic. Embedded in this semantic pattern, the term *blōdi- assumed a dual reference to blood and flower. Symbolizing both a surplus of moisture and the growth of vegetation, blood came to represent an organic overabundance, a bursting with procreative power.

The image of the blooming flower (through its semantic connection to blood) became a symbolic motif for human reproduction. Cognate terms and derivative forms of Germanic *blōdi- "blood" allude to this conception (see Table 5): examples include flower, harvest, wealth, offspring, bloom, swell, make known, bud, germinate. As a metaphor of procreation, creating offspring, and giving birth, the image of the blooming flower symbolized the generative power of the body. On the one hand, blossom or flower was suggestive of virility and male reproductive potency. This intrinsic connection between blooming, blood, and masculinity is made explicit by the related meanings of such cognate terms as fertile, penis, testicle (see Table 5). The concept of the flower, visualized as blooming to produce seed, became an emblem for the phallic potential of men. On the other hand, the imagery of the flower was appropriated also as a motif for female sexuality: blossom or bloom referred to vulva and menstrual blood in German-speaking lands (see Table 5). Although such a semantic equation between flower and female blood was certainly not limited to Germanic,[15] the imagery of the female flower was associated exclusively with positive connotations in central and northern Europe. The cyclical propagation of floral or vegetative life (with its seasonal patterns of budding, blooming, ripening, and dissemination) was perceived by Germanic-speaking peoples as a natural manifestation of the same sort of generative process that characterized the reproductive cycle of women: that is, menstruation, pregnancy, and birth. Suggestive of both male and female procreative processes, the image of the blooming flower thus became a symbol of androgyny, giving plastic expression to the power of sexual unity.

This same sense of unity is apparent in the Germanic conception of blood. By replacing the two proto-Indo-European categories, the Germanic term *blōdi- came to stand as a collective noun for blood: *blōdi- assumed a dual meaning, including in its field of reference both the visible flow of blood and its bodily containment. The earlier semantic opposition of the "inside" and the "outside" blood was thereby dissolved, foreshadowing a shift in gender categories and a restructuring of the metaphorical connection between blood and femaleness. This emergence of a new way of speaking about blood was a linguistic innovation that signaled a corresponding change in the cultural conception of women. Whereas the proto-Indo-European paradigm enforced the structural exclusion of women from the generative process (defined symbolically as a male prerogative), Germanic speakers began to insist on the inclusion of women as active participants in the creation of offspring. This conceptual shift was expressed through blood. Harnessing the combined reproductive power of man and woman, blood was perceived as a vehicle of immense potency and magical potential. These ideas were conveyed poetically through images of purity, virtue, and health.

Blood Untainted: The Textual Evidence

The unique etymological origins of the category blood and flower seem to have been accomodated grammatically by some Germanic languages. A number of scholars have suggested that the German word for blossom might be an old plural form of blood:[16]

das Blut	*blood*	singular
die Blüte	*flower/blossom*	plural

Others asserted that German blossom could be derived from the genitive or dative of the singular noun blood.[17] All of these suggestions are potentially correct. We find that in Old and Middle High German, the singular noun *bluot* meant blood as well as blossom.[18] Further, the nominative singular and plural of the same word *bluot* was in some instances identical:[19]

bluot	*singular*	blood
bluot	*plural*	blossom

Whereas in Old High German *bluot* may have been used either as a neuter or feminine noun,[20] in Middle High German it is attested in all three genders.[21]

bluot	feminine
bluot	neuter
bluot	masculine

Given this variation in genders, the corresponding declensions are often indistinguishable. As a result of the variability of genders and declensions, in addition to the differences in modern German dialects, the distinction between blood and blossom remains morphologically ambiguous.

Such a duality in reference is evident in a variety of German literary texts and idiomatic expressions. It can be documented in the *Chronica zeitbüch vnnd geschichtbibell* from 1536, written by Sebastian Franck von Wörd. The work consists of the first German treatise of the history of Europe and the Roman Catholic church. Composed as a protest against witchcraft trials and arbitrary murder as an instrument of political power, the book was banned by the church. Its distribution was prohibited by the provincial synod of Cologne in 1549. In a passage describing the persecution of presumed witches, the author concludes: "In this way one commits sheer murder on the innocent bloods/blossoms" (*an den unschuldigen Blüten*).[22] In this instance used as a poetic reference for human beings, the German term *Blüten* denotes blood as well as blossom. As a literary metaphor, the blooming flower is suggestive of life, vigor, and youth. In some contexts, it appears as a symbol of innocence and "freedom from sin or moral wrong."[23] The concept of blood, like that of the blooming flower, stood for the living human being and for life itself. Blood images were correspondingly appropriated as metaphors of "youth" and "innocence."[24] In the text by Franck von Wörd, the semantics of blood and blossom served as an effective means for asserting the perceived opposition between the cruelty of witchcraft trials and the innocent victims of religious persecution.

The semantic proximity of blood and blossom can be documented in other German texts. Persuasive is the evidence offered by a passage from Albrecht Dürer's *Tagebuch der niederländischen Reise*, a personal diary describing the painter's journey through the Netherlands in 1521. In the narrative, perhaps as a result of Dürer's use of a Middle German dialect, the term *Blüten*, blossoms/bloods, is modified to *Blüter*.[25] "Then we shall see the innocent bloods/blossoms [*die unschuldigen Blüter*] who the Pope, priests, and monks have spilled, tried, and condemned."[26] This passage is framed by a discussion about the tactics of power used by the Roman Catholic church and its reliance on capital punishment as a mechanism of political control. Immediately preceding the text, Dürer expresses his grief about the disappearance and supposed death of the Protestant reformer Martin Luther. At the time of Dürer's travels, Luther was arrested for heresy in a small town near the Thuringian Forest—and thereafter vanished from public sight. While in reality Luther's arrest had been staged by some of his followers to bring him to safety, public opinion placed the responsibility for Luther's disappearance with the Inquisition, a general tribunal established by the church for the discovery and suppression of heresy.

The excerpt from Dürer's diary seems to allude to those public executions as they were administered by the Inquisition tribunal. In Germany, as elsewhere in sixteenth-century Europe, these ritual spectacles of punishment had incorporated physical torture and the shedding of blood as the principal elements of penal practice.[27] In fact, the shedding of blood often preceded both the passing of judgment and the execution of the condemned. Especially in witchcraft trials, this sequence of events was maintained by the belief that suspected witches, once captured, could be rendered powerless either by extracting their blood directly or by whipping them to the point of blood effusion:[28] blood was the presumed medium of magical potential.

Dürer framed his reference to these ritual executions with an appeal to the prophetic revelations of the Apocalypse, depicting symbolically the ultimate destruction of evil and the triumph of good. The excerpt from the diary appears to be an adaptation of the religious premonition "souls screaming for revenge, demanding atonement for their spilled blood."[29] Dürer modified the passage to voice his resentment against the political realities of his time. He inserted the term *Blüter* (blossoms/bloods) in the place of souls, thereby alluding to the inner (spiritual) qualities of the victims of ritual punishment. On the one hand, *Blüter* referred to blood, a body fluid whose magical potential had been spilled; on the other hand, it denoted blossom, "a life free of sin," "innocent human being worthy of pity," "unfortunate person,"[30] who was unjustly tried and condemned. This choice of metaphors was based on Dürer's vision of the bloodiness of the ordeal as well as the cruelty of sacrificial death.

The semantics of *Blüte* with its dual reference to blood and flower finds attestation also in other literary texts. The writer Christoph Wirsung, for example, adopted this ambivalent or inclusive sense of the term in his translation of the Spanish tragicomedy *La Celestina*, by Fernando de Rojas,[31] originally published in German in 1520, then entitled *Ain hipsche tragedia*. Act I contains the following example: "She was good friends with students, noblemen's caterers and pages. To these she sold the blood/blossoms [*das Blüte*] of the unfortunate daughters, who all the more dared (to sell it), for all the while she promised them to restore their virginity."[32] This excerpt from the German text contains a descriptive reference to the activities of a woman by the name of Celestina, who was the main character in the Spanish play. The context of the passage informs us that in order to make a living, Celestina had six trades: laundress, perfumeress, maker of faces, professed witch, bawd, and mender of lost virginity. She thought of herself as a sort of physician and helped those women who came to her, "mending their lost maidenhoods, some with little bladders, others she stitched up with a needle, and when the French ambassador came thither, she made sale of one of her wenches three and several times more for a virgin" (Allen 1908: 26–27). The description of Celestina's professional life leaves no doubt about the general meaning of the passage from the German edition of the play. Celestina was the guardian of prostitutes whom she drew into the business on the pretext of restoring their virginity: she at once sold and mended young virgins.

This added bit of information does not, however, completely resolve the dual meaning of the phrase *das Blüte*. It refers in some sense to virginity, for this is what the young women are made to sell. Yet it remains unclear whether Wirsung used it in the sense of blood or blossom. Perhaps some insight might be gained from the Spanish text. There we read that Celestina sold the women's *sangre innocente*, or innocent blood,[33] which probably meant in an extended sense the "untouched" virgin blood. Just like blood, the imagery of blossom conveys a sense of innocence and moral purity: German *Blüte* (like English flower) is a folk metaphor for woman or girl, and as a poetic reference or as a regional colloquialism connotes virginity.[34] The loss of the flower of maidenhood through sexual contact is correspondingly termed defloration: The imagery of deflowering signifies the violation or death of female youth, and innocence.[35] Moreover, *Blüte* or *Blume* (blossom) is attested as a metaphor for female genital blood: German folk speech equates the cyclical flow of menstrual blood with the appearance of a budding flower.[36] The menstrual flow was perceived as the flowering or blooming of womanhood. In Wirsung's translation of the Spanish drama, the meaning of blood merged with the semantics of blossom so that the term *Blüte* became a poetic expression for sexual purity as well as virgin blood.

Blood images, according to the sources discussed so far, were closely linked to images of blooming flowers. The appearance of blood, whether in the context of defloration, sacrificial death, or murder, assumed meaning within the semantic field of blossom. The blooming flower, both perishable and reproductive, was appropriated as a dominant menstrual image. The flower was also a poetic circumlocution for hymen. Since German folk belief associated the onset of the menarche with the breaking of the hymen, these correspondences between blossom, menstruation, and virginity persisted in literary narratives.[37] Blood, suggestive of both sexual potency and victimization, assumed connotations of purity, innocence, and the absence of defilement. In an extended sense, it meant the beginning of life or youth. More specifically, blood came to be defined as procreative and as blooming when it was drawn from the male body for ritual (judicial) purposes or when it emerged naturally, flowing from the female body unmixed with other fluids infused by men: virgin blood.

Menstrual Blood as Symbol: Representations of Inner Self

The metaphorical linkages of blood and blossom are revealed not only by the linguistic and etymological evidence. The semantic fusion between blood loss and flower can be made evident in a wide range of popular cultural materials, including tales, legends, dreams, and folk speech. Northern European tales are characterized by image patterns that rely on blood and flowers as essential components of the narrative plot. Such images appear as organizing motifs in the text of a Danish ballad.[38] According to the text, a recently deceased man returns to his former home in spiritual form and informs his wife that he is tormented by her perpetual feelings of love: every time she is happy, his coffin is filled with red rose petals; when she is sad, it is full of coagulated blood. As a fantastic manifestation of sorrow, grief, and loss, the imagery of blood is juxtaposed to that of the red flower, which represents happiness and the promise of life. Coagulated blood, suggestive of decay or termination, may here be a highly veiled reference to wasted menstrual blood, a symbolic emblem for the death of the womb. The fallen rose petals, blighted buds, correspondingly allude to a menstrual image that hints at female fertility, the return of her season of harvest and birth.

Similar correspondences persist into modern times. The symbolism of menstrual blood as flower can, for instance, be uncovered in the *Interpretation of Dreams*, by Sigmund Freud (1976 [1900]), who documents a dream sequence of flowers that may have had menstrual significance. A Viennese patient dreamed that she was ascending a high place. As she climbed upward, she was carrying *a big branch* in her hand, really like a tree, which was thickly studded with *red flowers*. As she descended, the flowers, which looked like red camellias, began to fall. Freud interpreted both the blossoming branch and the wilting flowers as menstrual images. The patient, in analysis, had associated the blooming branch with lilies and herself with the biblical angel of annunciation, that is, the divine messenger of immaculate conception. The dream, Freud argued, represented therefore both sexual purity, symbolized by the white lily, and sexual guilt, symbolized by the red camellia. The menstruating woman, as conveyed through the imagery of flowers, is both pure and sexual, virgin and temptress.

The generative potency of female blood and its effect on the growth of vegetation emerges as the dominant theme in the German tale *The Juniper Tree*.[39] In the beginning of the narrative, a woman, while standing in the snow under a juniper tree, cuts her finger peeling a red apple. The drops of blood inspire her to wish for a child as red as blood and as white as snow.

And as she said it, it made her feel very happy, as if it was really going to happen. And so she went into her house, and a month went by, the snow was gone; and two months, and everything was green; and three months, and the flowers came up out of the ground; and four months, and all the trees in the woods sprouted and the tree branches grew dense and tangled with one another and the little birds sang so that the woods echoed, and the blossoms fell from the trees; and so five months were gone and she stood under the juniper tree and was beside herself with happiness; and when six months had gone by, the fruit grew round and heavy and she was very still; and seven months and she snatched the juniper berries and ate them so greedily that she became sad and ill; and so the eighth month went by and she called her husband and cried and said, "When I die, bury me under the juniper." And she was comforted and felt happy, but when the nine months were gone, she had a child as white as snow and as red as blood and when she saw it she was so happy that she died.[40]

This allegory of conception, pregnancy, and birth begins with the appearance of female blood. Visualized as drops from the woman's finger, the menstrual flow fertilizes the ground under the tree and causes both the conception of the child and the growth of the tree. The blooming and ripening of the fruit-bearing tree is a metaphor for the ripening of the maternal body. In the final stages of the narrative, the second wife murders the child born of the union between the woman and the tree, and his sister, weeping tears of blood, buries his bones under the juniper. This motif leads to an intensification of the blood/fertility correspondence. The spirit of the true mother now inhabits the tree and receives new vitality from the bones of the child. The repeated equivalence of the reproductive woman and the generative tree is consistent with images of menstruation as flower and of woman as a flowering branch.

Blood and Vegetation: Fertile Nature, Inner Potency

The red flower, on one level a metaphor of menstrual blood, appears in German narratives as a highly allusive reference to defloration, the breaking of a woman's hymen. Examples can be drawn from the *Household Tales*, by Jacob and Wilhelm Grimm (1812–15). Thus, the briar roses that grew around Sleeping Beauty's castle and caused the death of the potential suitors might be suggestive of a fear of defloration. After all, the sleeping maiden was awoken and brought to life by the suitor's sexual advances, which were symbolically marked by a kiss. In the story of *Jorinda and Joringel* a witch changes a maiden into a nightingale, only to have her released from the charm when the lover wields a blood-red flower.[41] Instances of symbolic defloration, in folk belief associated with sexual desire and blood, are here conveyed through images of blooming flowers.

Traces of a more generalized blood-fertility correspondence have been retained in German folkspeech, where blood appears as a metaphorical ascription in several of the names for flowers. Typical are the following examples:[42] *Blutblume* (blood flower or blood lily), *Blutrose* (blood rose), and *Blutröslein* (little blood rose), which develop brilliant red blossoms; *Blutströpfchen* (small drop of blood), that is, the red pimpernel or the burnet saxifrage, and *Blutgarbe* (blood fennel), a knot weed, which can be identified by its scarlet or purplish flowers; *Blutpeterlein* (little blood peter), which is a hemlock, a poisonous garden herb, whose leaf stalks have conspicuous purple spots; *Blutstiel* (blood stalk), a member of the bedstraw and cleavers, a trailing herb, whose roots yield a red or purple dye; and *Blutwurz* or *Blutwurzel* (blood root), *Wundkraut* (wound herb), *Blutkrautwurz* (blood herb root), sometimes referred to simply as *Blutkraut* (blood herb), which is a generic reference for a variety of herbs known for their healing potential, including the red geranium, the sour or yellow docks, the sorrels, the goosefoot, and blites, plants whose calyx becomes pulpy and bright red in fruit, which develop dense clusters of small pink flowers and have a large red root or

stem. These plant names are referential synonyms, designating particular plant species as members of the category "blood flower."[43] Included
in this category are, however, only those herbs or shrubs that characteristically develop red, purple, or pink blossoms, have bright red fruits and
seeds, possess a red root or stem, or ooze a reddish sap. These symbolic
markers are further enhanced by the plants' supposed curative powers:
their dried rhizome and roots serve as a diaphoretic and diuretic; their
sappy essence is taken to thin the "bitter" and "salty" blood, and to
heal inner wounds; their seeds are used to prevent excessive menstrual
bleeding and ease the effects of dysentery; the pulp is applied to expel
menstrual blood and afterbirth matter, and to speed up childbirth.[44]
The German names for such flowers are thus metonymically connected
to their color, and the unique plant properties prescribe the choice of
blood as metaphor. Blood flowers are presumed to harness, and reveal,
the creative properties of life.

The generative power of blood, with its link to vegetation, has remained an important motif in northern European folk narratives. In
German lore, for instance, red flowers are said to sprout from the blood
of gods, heroes, and martyrs, as conveyed by the plants' appearance and
coloration. Traces of this notion have been retained in regional blood
flower names.[45] In northern Germany, the reddish sap of such plants,
which oozes from the stem, roots, and leaves, is called "blood of John"
(*Johannesblut*); elsewhere, it is known as "blood of Christ" (*Christie Blut*).
Another type of flower possesses a red-spotted root, which is named
after the heathen god "Baldur's blood" in some parts of Norway, but in
other regions is known as "blood of John."[46] Presumed to have grown
from the blood of the apostle, this same plant is known as "blood herb"
(*Blutkraut*) in the German city of Augsburg.[47] The leaves' red sap, the
blood of John, is used to ward off the devil.[48] When applied to one's
clothes, the red sap also offers protection against the bite of rabid dogs.[49]
Similar assumptions about the origins and properties of blood flowers
exist in some parts of England.[50] There, the scarlet anemone, the red
wallflower, and the purple marks of the jack-in-the-pulpit are termed
"blood drops of Christ," in reference to the blood of the crucified during his hour of death. According to local legends, such flowers derived
their properties from sacred blood and were thus gifted with miraculous
healing powers.

Northern European folk etymology draws on similar mythological accounts to explain the unusual origins of blood flowers. According to a
German literary narrative, the red rose is said to have grown from the
blood of the Greek god Adonis.[51] Adonis, the lover of Aphrodite, was
killed by a wild boar, which had been summoned to attack him by the
jealous war god Ares. Venus rushed to his aid but could not help him,

and out of the blood of Adonis grew a red rose. According to another German narrative, the red rose received its color from the blood of Venus, who, in her haste to relieve Adonis of his pain, pierced her foot with a thorn. A white rose, growing close by, was stained bright red as Venus's blood fell upon it.[52] A German variant of this myth, first recorded in 1790, explains how the rose derived its red hue from the blood of Amor, the god of love.[53] Amor was searching for an appropriate flower on the occasion of his mother's celebration, but none appeared beautiful enough. Only the silver rose found his approval. When he wanted to pluck it, he cut his finger on its thorns and his blood stained the rose. In German folklore, the red flower, displaying the color of blood, is thus deemed sacred, presumed to be of divine or supernatural origin.

The symbolic proximity of plants and blood is evident not only in the appearance, name, and mythological origin of flowers but also in their presumed medicinal properties. Red herbs are common ingredients in German folk remedies, traditional potions designed to cure the ailments of blood: some flowers are used in attempts to prevent or stop excessive bleeding, while others are used to purge or expel unwanted blood. The antiquity of this belief in the healing potential of blood red flowers can be documented by a passage from the text of Ekkehard's *Waltharius*, a popular German legend originally recorded during the ninth century in Latin.[54] A war ensues between the former allies Walthari, Gunther, and Hagen, and then, in the final battle, they wound each other terribly:[55]

> Two were sitting, the third lay down, and with
> flowers they attempted to quell the flow of blood.
> (Then Walthari called the fearful virgin,
> who came and bandaged all wounds.)

Here, the symbolic correspondence of blood and flower provides a vehicle for magical control. The underlying assumption was that through the manipulation of the concrete object, the herbal substance, the loss of body fluid (blood) could be realistically affected: flowers were applied to injuries in order to prevent excessive bleeding.

Purging the Flow: The Nation's Arterial System

In early modern times (beginning in the seventeenth century), the curative properties of flowers, and the presumed importance of blooming plants in the quelling, purging, and soothing of blood, appeared for the first time in metaphors of social and political change. Such blood and flower correspondences were appropriated as organizing emblems by the German literary societies of the seventeenth century. Initially established as loose confederations of writers and poets, these associations attempted to promote the standard use of German (to the exclusion of French or Latin) as a principal medium of expression in literature, education, and government. The normalization of language, conceptualized through medical metaphors and blood images, was perceived as an effective means for transforming basic social attitudes, thereby abolishing aristocratic privileges and improving the status of the peasantry. The members of these literary societies thus acted ideologically by presenting through prose or poetry their critique of society. As a result of their educational and moralizing efforts, the use of language was politicized: language reforms became a pedagogical tool in a process of national unification.

The most influential among these literary societies was *Die Fruchtbringende Gesellschaft* (The Fruitful Society), founded by Prince Ludwig zu Anhalt in 1617 in Weimar, Prussia. This ever-expanding association consisted of some five hundred politically well-connected writers and literary connoisseurs who had dedicated themselves to the promotion of German literature and language.[56] Their goal was to delete from their verbal repertoire any signs of foreign cultural influence: promoting German nativism took the form of purging everyday language. The explicit aim of the society's members was to create a setting in which they could speak and write "good pure German" in order to elevate their "mother tongue (which was everyone's duty by nature)," and "to preserve standard high German in its correct essence and status, without the inmixing of strange foreign words, and to cultivate the best pronunciation in speech and the purest form in writing and poetic verse."[57] The enhancement of a people's national language became the stated purpose of the German literary society.

According to the code of the society, every initiated individual and everyone intent on joining was required to choose a membership name and emblem. Interestingly, the written statutes of the association limited this choice to vegetative images only: trees, flowers, herbs, and all other things grown from the earth or thereby produced. The cultivation of the German language, which was the society's explicit goal, was thereby equated with the cultivation of plants, and the explicit identification of political society with the natural realm. As suggested by the association's self-proclaimed codex, the writing of German poetry was defined as "fruitful" or "fruit-bearing": a harvest of words.

It is noteworthy that among the selected membership emblems, images of blood flowers prevailed. The stylized image of each flower emblem was etched into a copper plate. These floral representations were framed by a verbal inscription, which described the plant's unique healing potential and properties. Such descriptive references or labels became the emblem owner's name. Examples include "Purger of Heavy Blood," "Engorger of Veins," "The Persistent Blood Stopper," "Cleanser of Polluted Blood," "Purger of Monthly Blood," "The Queller of Blood."[58] The emblematic choice of every flower was justified in poetic form, which was engraved beneath the floral images. In these poetic narratives, the writer commented on the curative attributes of his emblem and thereby documented the selection of his symbolic name. Here follow some examples:

Purger of Heavy Blood
The root "sweet angel" flushes out the body's heavy (thickened) blood. When thus restored, in a state of health and well-being, one can feel happiness, sweet like an angel. Fate has thus granted me the name "purger of blood" . . . Hans Ernst von Freyberg (copperplate engraving no. 140).

Engorger of Veins
This noble herb replenishes the content of our veins with good, pure blood, and it cools down the liver and opens there whatever is congested. I am called the "engorger" and summon the power of the herb . . . Joachim Johann Georg von der Schulenburg (copperplate engraving no. 151).

Cleanser of Polluted Blood
One herb is called "woman's hair." It cleanses polluted blood throughout the human body when it has ceased to function. Therefore I found "cleanser" to be a suitable name for myself . . . Frantz Jeo Freytag (copperplate engraving no. 239).

Purger of Monthly Blood
The mature rose opens her full bouquet once every month to purge the body's blood. This flowering must be well preserved and maintained. Therefore, in this society, "purger" is my name . . . Hans Blume (copperplate engraving no. 394).

Queller of Blood
The black nettle grows from a root that can stop all bleeding, but it must be dug out from the ground in a special, silent manner. Therefore, the "queller of all that bleeds" came to be my name . . . Joachim von Böselager (copperplate engraving no. 400).

In these poetic narratives, the principal aim of the society, its attempt to retrieve the purity of spoken German, was expressed through several organic images: contemporary language, perceived as pathologically degenerate, was equated with polluted, weakened, and congested blood; restoration required the curative aid of special plants. The association members, through their identification with such flowers, defined themselves as language healers: they became quellers, engorgers, purgers, and cleansers not of blood but of words.

The promulgation of such organic/vegetative images of linguistic reform was probably linked to the rise of nationalist ideologies: German

literary societies came into being as a logical extension of nation building, a process in which the normalization of language was deemed essential for the formation of a new political community, that is, the modern
German nation-state.

The Power Within: Concepts of Interiority

When the meaning of blood merged with the semantics of the blossom in early Germanic, blood assumed a novel cosmological and social
significance. Associated with the generative power of nature and the
cyclical rebirth of plant life, blood came to be perceived as a principal source of health. Much of the linguistic evidence implies that the
imagery of blooming plants had long been used as a symbol of fertility
by other Indo-Europeans. The cyclical rebirth and growth of plant life
was generally represented in the image (and through the poetic language) of a blossom. Early Germanic speakers extended this symbolism
of the flower to the idea of blood, thereby drawing the conception of the
body fluid into the realm of vegetative growth and reproduction. The
generative power of nature became an intrinsic quality of blood, and in
the image of a budding flower, blood was transformed into an organic
force. Just as the blooming flower was seen as expressive of the procreative power of nature (and woman), so the health of the body and the
thriving of the clan was attributed to the power of blood. In German-
speaking lands, social relations came to be patterned by blood images.

The societal relevance of such conceptions can ultimately be traced
to the ancient Germanic belief in the charismatic power of the lineage.
The assumption was that the members of a particular kin group derived
supernatural (superior) abilities from their common link in blood, such
as the power to ensure good crops, victory in battle, and the ability
to heal certain diseases.[59] Based on such beliefs, membership in social
groups was explicitly defined by the unity in blood. Even throughout
feudal times, the basic supposition was that there could be no real
friendship save between persons tied to one another by the power of
blood. "Friends" here referred to all members of the immediate family
as well as in-laws; that is, individuals belonged to a social unit by birth
and by marriage.[60] Every new person entering the inner circle of the
clan meant an increase in strength and power for the group:[61] the incorporation of new members into a family was interpreted as a new influx
of blood. In consequence, Germanic peoples tended to focus meaning
on the blood bond generally, and on the unity of blood within a common social body.

Kinship among Germanic tribes followed a cognatic system, based
on a widely extended recognition of kin relations traced through males

as well as females. Each individual had two kinds of relatives, those of the "spear-side" (paternal kin) and those of the "distaff-side" (maternal kin). Men and women were bound, though to different degrees, to the second as well as the first.[62] In this system, a woman, through her marriage, acted as alliance binder. An examination of her status reveals that she enjoyed considerable freedom and a right to be treated with respect.[63] Such a structural pattern differs sharply from the early Indo-European system of patrilineal descent, in which social membership was determined exclusively through men and in which a woman's group affiliation was initially prescribed by birth and later (symbolically) altered by marriage.

Among Germanic-speaking peoples, every person could retain the bond of kinship with both maternal and paternal relatives. This double link had important consequences. Since each generation thus had its own circle of kin, which was not the same as that of the previous generation, the clan boundary continually changed its contours.[64] Such differences in social patterns were also marked in a symbolic sense. On the one hand, proto-Indo-Europeans had relied on patrilineal assertions as a way of determining group membership: blood was a conduit of masculinity, and kin relations were conceptualized through images of motion, the liquid social body, and the competitive exchanges of paternal blood. Proto-Germanic speakers relied on somewhat different images. Although the Germanic kinship system itself allowed for generational discontinuity and shifting alliances, the extended family formed a closed unit, even in a religious sense.[65] This unity of relatives, understood as a merging of power, was symbolized through *organic* metaphors, that is, the single human body, and the actual mingling of blood.

Organic Unity: Adhesion Through Blood

The importance of shared blood suggests that in Germanic cultures strangers could enter the kinship group only through special procedures. Outsiders were incorporated into the community of relatives either by marriage or if, by appropriate genealogical reconstructions, they were found to be related to the dominant kindred.[66] Such alliances were probably thought to result in a mixing of blood that could unite different people organically (and naturally) inside a common social body. Such a notion is made explicit by a passage from an Old Norse prose text, in which kinsmen by marriage are referred to not only as "sib-folk" but also as "minglers of blood."[67] The etymological evidence seems to lend additional support to this observation. Standard terms for kinsfolk in Germanic languages refer to relatives by both marriage and birth.[68] Unlike their Indo-European counterparts, these kinship terms are inclusive of in-laws and blood relatives and make no distinction between maternal and paternal relatives. Such classificatory categories can be derived from a Germanic root *mang, mingle, mix, knead together, and its (non-nasalized) collateral base, *mag, to have power, vitality, might— a word suggestive of a strength or force drawn from inside the earth, an innate power of things grown from the soil.[69] This power of the earth (Old Norse jarðar megin) could be absorbed in distilled form by drinking beer or it could be appropriated directly by contact with the soil, a procedure that conferred health and granted physical endurance.[70] Thus, a person's acceptance by and initiation into the circle of kin might have been conditional on an act of mingling or mixing of blood and earth, a procedure that in some sense bestowed power.

Relations in blood thus became a primary condition for entering a designated social unit: "Suppose that by chance a stranger succeeded in joining the group. Whether it was a question of rustics or a person of higher rank, the act of association was likely to take the form of a fictitious 'fraternity'—as if the only real social contract was one which, if not based on an actual blood relationship, at least imitated its ties" (Bloch 1961: 131). The binding power of blood, or adhesion through blood, emerged as one of the central motifs in German folk culture, where it prevailed in discussions of love magic and in the sealing of contracts, particularly pacts with devils or demons.[71] Blood, conceived as thick and sticky, served as a natural or organic adhesive for social agreements.

Blood and Earth

Social alliances, which emerged as alternatives to kin or sibship, were usually male oriented: the fraternities or "union of men."[72] Every initiated member assumed the classificatory status of a relative, as perhaps suggested by referential terms like Old Norse blóði, blood brother, twin, and *ga-blóðan, companion in blood.[73] Such terms are related in north Germanic languages to words denoting to make bloody, part of a sword, bloodstained (skin), bloody, cutting the skin so that it bleeds.[74] These terms convey images suggestive of aggressive and warlike activities that produce blood, and it seems likely that every initiation into the union of men required an actual display (or shedding) of blood.[75]

Among Germanic tribal units, alliances between men were sometimes cemented by a mutual exchange of blood. The textual evidence suggests that this process of mingling blood was carried out quite literally. We find the most explicit references to such rites in Scandinavian mythology. There exists a brief mention of the ritual in a medieval Icelandic myth. Although first recorded during the early thirteenth century, the text contains much older material that alludes to a pact of blood brotherhood between the gods Loki and Odin. In a short encounter, one reminds the other of their blood brotherhood:[76]

Remember, Othin, in the olden days
That we both our blood have mixed
(*blendom blóði saman*).

There exists no account of any incident in which the two gods swore blood brotherhood, but they were so often allied in various enterprises that the idea is wholly reasonable.[77] Other texts remind us that the actual mingling of blood in one another's footprints may have been part of the ritual of brotherhood. We find this expressed in an Old Norse narrative in which Brynhild reminds her husband of his blood covenant with another man:[78]

Thou hast, Gunnar, the deed forgot,
when blood in your footprints both ye mingled
(*blóði í spor báðir rendot*).

What was the significance of footprints in this ritual context, and why did the participants mix their blood in these earthy impressions? We might speculate that in order to simulate the bond of brotherhood, such rites made use of symbols that allude to birth and descent from a common maternal womb. It has been suggested by some scholars that blood, the medium for binding the contracting parties, represented in a symbolic sense the mother.[79] There is some evidence for this interpretation.[80]

The most elaborate description of the rite exists in *Gísla saga*, an Icelandic manuscript preserved from the beginning of the fifteenth century. According to the text, when two men wanted to conclude a pact of brotherhood, they cut a strip of turf so that it remained fastened with both ends to the ground, then placed a spear under it in the center, thereby lifting up the sod. Then the participants walked under it and each of them stabbed or cut himself in the sole of the foot or the palm of the hand, letting the blood flow together, blending it with the earth. The passage provides the following account:

[The men] go out to the spit of land called Eyrarvalsodi and cut and raise up a long sod in the turf, leaving the two ends fast, and they set a spear with a damascended blade under it, so long-shafted that a man could just reach the rivets of the head with [his] outstretched hand. All four should pass under, Thorgrim, Gisli, Thorkell and Veistein; and now they draw blood and let their blood run together in the earth which was scratched up under the sod, and mix it all together, earth and blood; and then they kneel and swear an oath that they shall avenge the other as his brother, and they call all the gods to witness.[81]

The significance of the ceremony has generally been interpreted as a rebirth from earth, the common mother, symbolized by the passage under the raised sod and the mixing of the participants' blood in the soil. The spear may have had some phallic significance.[82] The rite was discussed in detail by Jan de Vries, who correctly observed that the emphasis on the mixing of blood and earth in connection with the rite of the blood brotherhood is particular to Germanic-speaking peoples.[83] The practice does not exist elsewhere.

The efficacy of the Germanic rite may well be based on the belief in the generative power of blood. The bonds of brotherhood were created specifically by a symbolic rebirth from the bloodstained earth. The fictive kinship tie thereby derived from the assumption of a common origin in blood and soil (*Blut und Boden*). In a metaphorical sense, the ritual participants sprouted or germinated in unison literally from within the earth, growing from the power of the mingled blood like plants.

Metaphors of Human Origin: Tree Trunks, Stems, Genealogies

Vegetative or "natural" images of kinship were closely associated with the concept of descent from plants. In the realm of myth, Germanic ideas of human genesis and birth were conveyed through the symbolic medium of trees. We find several references to such creative events in early Scandinavian texts. According to one Old Norse narrative, the first human beings were born from a piece of driftwood, shaped and brought to life by the gods: "While the sons of Borr were walking along the seashore, they discovered two tree trunks, took them up, and made human beings out of them."[84] Variants of this motif exist in other texts. One myth assimilates the image of the primeval tree to the birth-giving womb and maintains human life without divine intervention: the ancestors of humankind reside inside the tree's wooden core in embryonic form: "In the place called Hoddmímir's Holt [a mythical tree] there shall lie hidden during the Fire of Surt two of mankind, who are called thus: Líf and Lífthrasir, and for food they shall have the morning-dews. From these folk shall come so numerous an offspring that all the world shall be peopled."[85] Safely hidden inside the tree, two beings named "life" (*líf*) and "desiring life" (*lífþrasir*), presumably a man and a woman, escape the final destruction of the known world and there give rise to new human generations.

Trees are associated with fertility and childbirth in other northern European folk narratives. According to the claims of German local legends, children are born from hollow trees. Such trees are correspondingly termed "small children's tree" (*Kleinkinderbaum*).[86] We find an allusion to this notion also in Scandinavian legends. In one such tale, King Volsung built a magnificent hall and designed it in such a way that in its center stood a great tree, the branches with their colorful flowers spreading up to the roof, while the trunk stretched down into a well. This tree was called *barnstokk*, which means "child-trunk" or "racial ancestry of children."[87]

Traces of this connection between human origins and trees is evident in north Germanic languages. Based on the terminological evidence, it seems that members of the same clan or tribe thought of themselves as "descendants of a single tree-trunk," a notion that persists in Old High German *liutstam*, literally "people tree," or lineage. The expression (which conjoins two terms: *liuti* and *stam*)[88] has been reconstructed with the meanings grow, rise, originate, and trunk of a tree, images that hint at the conception of a single family as a natural branch or offshoot from a tree that is firmly rooted in the earth.[89] The social unit of a clan was thus in a symbolic sense perceived as an organic, earth-bound community (whose members shared the same blood). Such concepts persist in modern German terms like *Volksstamm*, literally "folk tree trunk," a reference for nation or tribe, and *Stammbaum*, "ancestral tree," which is suggestive of descent and denotes genealogy or lineage. The verbal allusions to the vegetative origin of people are also evident in Old Norse prose texts, which tell us that "a relation is also called . . . kin-staff, descendant, family-prop, family-stem, kin-branch, family-branch, offshoot, offspring, head tree, plant-shoot."[90]

Up to the early era of the Middle Ages, a clan in the sense of "stem" or "tree trunk" (German *Stamm*) denoted a small, self-governing community whose members spoke a common language and were descendants from the same land or soil.[91] Both the spatial and the temporal origin of a kin group was thereby located within the actuality of the natural world. The clan, like a tree, seemed to emerge, grow, or sprout from the earth.

Mapping Ancestry: Blood, Soil, Tree

The iconography of blood, earth, and tree (as a metaphor of human genesis) survived in modern European depictions of kinship. Diagrammatic representations of consanguinity and kin relations came to rely on the tree metaphor to depict heredity. According to Mary Bouquet (1996: 47), "mapping out ancestry in the form of a tree" provided an iconographic precedent for the genealogical diagram, the modern anthropological device for representing family relations. Drawing on examples from Britain, the Netherlands, and Germany, Bouquet's work suggests that the graphic representation of kinship owed much to prior European use of tree imagery and indeed relied on literalizing the tree metaphor. Modern genealogical diagrams emerged as simulacra or mimetic artifacts that furnished naturalistic images of blood connections. Such a mapping of kin relations relied on the tree as a visual phenomenon: roots, tree trunk, branches, and leaves rendered kinship visibly self-evident.

The choice of the tree to metaphorize relational systems arose from a novel concern with heredity, descent, and genealogy. In nineteenth-century Europe, particularly in the German-speaking realm, such deeply embedded cultural ideas about blood ancestry assumed form within a modern aesthetic of race. But these concerns with descent and the diagrammatic motif of the genealogical tree were prefigured by much older conceptions of blood and power. Perhaps initially inspired by codes of inheritance and succession associated with property,[92] these diagrammatic representations of kinship "emerged in the context of the calculation of prohibited degrees of marriage" (Goody 1983: 276). Degrees of consanguinity were represented in the form of a crucifix as early as the eighth century.[93] "Later documents display the same information in the shape of a tree (*arbor iuris*) or of a man."[94] By the eighteenth century, such graphic images of the genealogical tree were used to retain "control of procreation through keeping written records that enable[d] the careful channelling of 'blood,' as a key to nobility" (Bouquet 1996: 47–48).

The family tree permitted the genealogical mapping of blood by virtue of its symmetrical and bilateral form. This emphasis on (or preference for) visual symmetry and symmetric modeling promoted the scientific appropriation of the tree as a taxonomic device in nineteenth-century Europe. The tree metaphor constituted part of a visual language mined by modern science.[95] But the persistence of these diagrammatic images cannot be explained solely by their usefulness for a scientific imaginary. The tree motif was also a conventional cultural image, a representation of blood and reproduction: it symbolized the integrated social body of man and wife. The genealogical tree, signifying both bloodline and conjugation, was deeply gendered. This is suggested by the frontispiece to a seventeenth-century Dutch example (a genealogy in book form), "which shows Dirk van Dorp and his wife standing beneath their 'tree,' and the score of pages that follow the lateral extensions of that tree."[96] This same emphasis on symmetry, shared blood, and lateral extensions characterizes the iconography of a Dutch "family tree" from the late eighteenth century:

Gerard Schaap's name is shown at the lowest point on the trunk, together with that of his wife Johanna, in a circle—a stylized oak-apple, perhaps—since the leaves are clearly those of an oak. The names of their offspring (two sons and one daughter) are shown, with those of their spouses, on the trunk (Jan and his wife) and two lateral branches . . . [A]esthetics demand a symmetrical layout . . . The bulk of the tree is, indeed, composed of lateral extensions . . . We know nothing of the in-marrying spouses' origins: where does Johanna (Gerard's wife) come from? What does her substance contribute to the solid base of the tree just below her name, where grass and other small plants thrive? . . . The positioning of the name Johanna closest to the earth and the roots of the tree might, however, suggest that she is the ancestral figure. (Bouquet 1996: 47)

In northern Europe, the motif of the genealogical tree reveals a social emphasis on symmetry and lateral extensions. Blood relations, including kin by marriage, appear together in these graphic depictions of ancestry. The tree, in its diagrammatic form, emphasizes the existence of both men and women, husbands and wives, in-laws and offspring. Such an integration and mergence of kin into a common genealogy of blood differs sharply from the proto-Indo-European case, in which the tree stood as a metaphor of patrilineality, that is, a symbolic system of tracing descent and blood connections through men alone. The diagrammatic tree seems to contain vestiges of a different social system, in which kin relations were reckoned bilaterally. In German-speaking lands, as I discussed previously, kinship followed a cognatic system, based on a widely extended recognition of kin traced through males as well as females. In the genealogical tree, traces or vestiges of such a kinship pattern are "embodied in specific graphic conventions, such as the wife's name encircled together with the husband's, in Schaap's family tree, or Maria as an acorn in the tree of Jesse."[97] Unlike the case of Indo-European patrilineality, women were not exorcised from these genealogical diagrams.

Within the conceptual field of the modern ancestral tree, there was an explicit recognition of women and their birth-giving potential. Despite the patronymic emphasis, women (as sisters, mothers, and wives) were identified and named in these genealogical diagrams. Such a recognition of womanhood was also sustained in symbolic terms. The tree appeared to grow from specific female substances: blood and soil. As Bouquet (1996) observed: "If the containers at the base of the tree contain earth . . . this represents a kind of generalized female material" (52). In the northern European tree motif, blood is connected to soil, female matter, mother earth: earth becomes blood, which becomes sap, which nourishes the life of plants, including the tree. Blood wells up from the ground as an ancestral substance. In an eighteenth-century Dutch genealogy (a biblically inspired vision of human genesis), the "tree thus arises from the soil of Mesopotamia, but its foliage represents populations of the entire earth. Blood would appear to be made from the soil, and soil continues to feed the growth of the tree (the whole family of Man), presumably with the sap that flows through the trunk and the branches into the leaves" (52). Here, earth gives rise to blood, and blood is transformed into both arboreal and genealogical essence.

Blood and nature, that is, human bodies and plant life (flowers/trees), are collapsed in such representations of ancestry. Although the diagrammatic image of the tree glosses over the nature of the genealogical substance, the "persuasive fiction underlying [these trees] . . . is that the earth beneath them has been turned into blood, the blood into sap" (Bouquet 1996: 60). In northern European depictions of kinship, the imagery of blood and soil and tree exist as interconnected metaphors of origin.

The genealogical tree thus occupied a certain position in the Germanic etymology of blood: earth became blood, which became sap, which fed the tree. Blood was a symbol of nature, a product of the earth mother. "Genealogical trees would then reflect a (patriarchal) vision of the present projected onto (and struggling with the vestiges of) a (matriarchal) past" (Bouquet 1996: 61). The symbolic linkages of blood, earth, and tree, which placed emphasis on female substance and maternal essence, dislodged the earlier Indo-European model, which posited a homologous relation between the male body and the tree. Modern European genealogical diagrams, including the ancestral tree, belonged to a different metaphorical field. Imagined not as an extension of manhood, a male unilateral channel that arose from a man's seed or corpse, the tree was given life by a different source. In Germanic (northern European) culture, the genealogical tree took root in female substance: blood, earth, and soil.

Such images persist into modern times, taking form in a genealogical mode of thought: the European aesthetics of race. Through blood and tree metaphors—as graphic representations of descent—relational systems like kinship, heredity, and lineage are placed into the semantic field of nature. The "naturalized identity between people and place" (Malkki 1996: 437) is thus not solely based on an innocent botanical metaphor. Taken together, the complex of images (arboreal in form and sanguine in content) is suggestive of origins, ancestries, bloodlines. In later European history, these images were to become structurally embedded in a racial aesthetic, unifying the symbolics of blood, stock, and heredity. The genealogical tree (a prominent symbol of modern German statehood) thus evokes both continuity of essence and territorial rootedness.

Part II
Blood in the
Medieval Imagination

Chapter 3
The Theft of Blood, the Birth of Men
Gender, Sex, and Race in
European Mythology

How were the symbolics of blood and heredity encoded in the medieval imagination? What was the cultural medium through which the indigenous concerns with origin, ancestry, and bloodline could be rendered visible in the European Middle Ages? One of anthropology's contributions to current research on racial aesthetics is an elucidation of the mythic dimensions of power and genealogy: how patterns of social inequality are produced and legitimated through narrative images that focus on pronouncements of descent and pedigree. Such work explores in ethnographic detail the complex relationship between personhood and group identity in the world of myth, ranging from metaphorical depictions of social organization, family, and lineage to representations of heroic figures and the politics of sexuality.[1] In this chapter, I continue in this tradition by attempting to uncover the cultural linkages of gender and race in European mythology. I trace medieval notions of manhood or maleness in relation to femaleness with particular emphasis on the underlying assumptions of blood, sex, and reproduction.

My work is an excursion into the history of ideas and not an exploration of customs or social forms. This chapter investigates how medieval notions of blood and race were encoded in northern European myths. I venture to show how medieval models of difference and otherhood were embedded in mythological images of sex, birth, and creation. More specifically, we will see that competing concepts of creative power (equated with chaos and order, good and evil) were expressed through mythic representations of female eroticism and motherhood, on the one hand, and through the antithetical images of male androgyny and male creativity, on the other. The underlying concerns of the textual material are masked by numerous cosmic stories about the origin of the world: the interplay of fire and ice, a primeval river of venom, the filling up of the cosmic void, the birth of a giant, the creation and annihilation of his offspring, the emergence of a milk-giving cow, the victory of gods over giants and dwarfs and their subsequent creative deeds. While these plots and motifs seem rather commonplace, one can discern the latent content of each myth through an interpretation of narrative details. In other words, the elemental components of creation (fire, water/ice, venom/salt, saliva/blood) and the actions of mythical beings (killing, stealing, copulating, eating, giving birth, nurturing, making blood) provide an arena in which certain social themes are dramatized: incest, murder, birthing, and male sexual usurpation.

In the mythological narratives, these themes and plots are never sharply delineated. They tend to blend one into another, flowing together and diverging, changing from one shape or motif into another. This transformation of symbolic images probably reflects the construction of a systematized body of folklore from the fragments and snippets of a medieval oral tradition: the mythmakers and poets, like *bricoleurs*, pieced their cosmologies together with the cultural scraps that were at hand.[2] The separate yet interwoven themes and images thus correspond to different versions of the myth that were combined into a single text.

Northern European myths about pagan gods and cosmic creation have survived only in the form of medieval Icelandic documents, which were not transcribed until the thirteenth century, several hundred years after the conversion to Christianity had already begun.[3] The resulting uncertainties about chronology and authenticity may have left anthropologists reluctant to explore the cultural and symbolic dimensions of the medieval texts. However, the lack of primary materials is characteristic of studies of this sort[4] and is not generally perceived as an insurmountable problem: "When one tackles mythology . . . it is impossible to reconstruct a skeletal Urtext with any confidence . . . This need not deter us, however, if we are interested in essences rather than origins, in things that survive in many late versions rather than things that may have been present in non-surviving early versions" (O'Flaherty 1980: 166–67). Although there is little likelihood that a prototypical myth was ever told in the form in which it appears in the Old Norse texts, the recurrent elements of Icelandic creation mythology may nevertheless shed light on early historical assumptions about blood and sexuality in northern Europe. Our problem is essentially one of correct decipherment, of how to read the narrative representations of gender.[5] As we shall see, the ideologies and attitudes that govern the social aspects of the reproduction of life are embedded in images of procreative bodies. The differences of form, substance, and bodily function that arise in the process of reproduction supply a steady stream of myth material that "acts as a language" from which are fashioned the messages and explanations for the social inequalities between men and women.[6] Images of blood provide an organizing aesthetic for these emergent visions of violence.

Narrative Images and Events

While Icelandic creation myths often seem inconsistent and contain many contradictions, they are founded on one essential paradigm: the world emerged from a primeval chaos, a state of disorder, in which basic physical distinctions were yet unmade.[7] Composed of formless matter and infinite space, chaos preceded all differentiation. A poetic rendition of such a cosmogonic conception of the early universe is preserved in written form:

> In the olden times
> did Ymir live:
> there was no sand nor sea
> nor ice-cold waves,
> neither earth was there
> nor sky above,
> but a yawning void
> and green things nowhere.[8]

The mythological poem makes comprehensible the primordial chaos by describing that which has not yet been created. Included in the string of negations are water, an essential liquid element, and the ocean shore, which represents its solid counterpart. Absent are also heaven and earth, perhaps thought of as markers of spatial boundaries. While the poem negates the presence of space and matter in either liquid or solid form, it affirms the existence of other elements. During the early state of chaos, there existed a void and a primordial being, Ymir.

In a more extensive prose account of the world's origin, chaos is described in slightly different terms:

> It was in the earliest of times
> when nothing was.[9]

Although here conceived as some sort of void, further elaboration of this statement reveals that chaos was not equated with an empty abyss composed of dead matter. In the myth, it emerges as a primeval gap in space, which was infused with magical potential and power.[10] Furthermore, the text suggests that the outer limits of chaos were defined by a number of mythological worlds. In the southern region surfaced *Múspell*, a land defined as light and hot, glowing and burning, which was protected against foreign intruders by *Surtr* with his flaming sword. In the northern part emerged *Niflheimr*—the nether world— a dark sphere filled with ice and frost. Midmost within this cold world lay a well or fountain named *Hvergelmir*, "roaring cauldron," from which eleven rivers poured forth. These together were called *Élivagar*, or "ice- waves." In contrast to the description of chaos offered by the poetic texts, this narrative does not rely on a string of negations to make comprehensible the unimaginary beginning of the universe. Rather, it assimilates the essence of chaos to known elements.[11] The magically potent center of chaos is here located between the worlds of fire and ice, the hot and the cold, thereby separating nonfluids from tangible liquids, the wet and the dry.

The basic elements of fire, water, and ice assume procreative connotations in the subsequent account of creation, for it is their interaction that produces the first living creature. Following the mythological narratives, the fluids of the primordial rivers solidified under the influence of the northern cold, turning into ice and rime. Upon contact with the heat and sparks from the southern part of chaos, the ice began to melt and produced the giant Ymir. The force of fire acts as a male generative agent in this creative process, anthropomorphized by *Surtr* with his blazing sword.[12] This sword, as the text implies, is the sign of a war god. The image of Surtr as an aggressive god of fire or solar deity is made explicit in the poetic text of the myth:

Surtr fares from the south
with switch-eating flame.
On his sword shines
the sun of the war-gods.[13]

Such a depiction of fire in terms of a masculine and warlike figure alludes, in the context of myth, to the attributes of male creativity. Within the framework of the Norse myth material, the imagery of fire may be interpreted as a metaphor for the generative potential of a primordial male.[14]

In contrast to the masculine force of fire, the elements of water and ice have been consistently interpreted as metaphors for female reproductive power.[15] Even outside northern Europe, mythological fluids and primal liquids, either molten or frozen, tend to be perceived as female in contrast to mineral or organic solids (rock or bone), which are usually regarded as male.[16] It would thus seem plausible that water and ice, like the element of fire, assumed a fundamentally creative role in the genesis of the cosmos. The myth does in fact attribute the initial creation of organic life to the common interaction of these basic elements: according to the narrative, the generative process had its origin in the union of fire and ice. The mythological text describes the creative process in the following way:

The streams called "ice-waves," which come from the fountain-heads, were so long that the yeasty venom upon them had hardened like the slag that runs out of the fire; these then became ice. And when the ice halted and ceased to run, it froze over above. But the drizzling rain that rose from the venom congealed to rime, and the rime increased, frost over frost, each over the other, even into Ginnungagap, the "gaping void" . . . Ginnungagap, which faced toward the northern quarter, became filled with heaviness and masses of ice and rime, and from within, drizzling rain and gusts; but the southern part of the void was lighted by those sparks and glowing masses which flew out of Múspellheimr . . . so also all that which looked toward Múspell became hot and glowing; . . . and when the breath of heat met the rime, so that it melted and dripped, life was quickened from the [poisonous] yeast-drops, by the power of that which sent the heat, and became a man's form. And that man was named Ymir.[17]

In this text, the creation of organic life is expressed in liquid terms and the myth clearly attributes Ymir's birth to the transformation of fluids. The primeval waters of *Élivagar* continuously changed their composition under the combined influence of fire and frost, initially turning into solid ice, then again assuming liquid form. The generative process finally comes to an end within the magic void (perhaps imagined as a macro-cosmic womb), which is filled with procreative fluids that have grown inside it to form the giant's body.

This symbolic emphasis on fire and water/ice in the medieval Ice-landic myth affirms a cultural recognition of the reproductive role of women and articulates an ideology of bilateral descent, that is, a belief in the creative potential of both mother and father, man and woman.[18] Accordingly, in Norse mythology, the creation of life is accomplished through the equal participation of a male and a female element: life begins when fiery semen comes into contact with the icy fluids of the womb.

The Poetics of Female Creation

The generative images contained in Norse mythology can be interpreted as structural or narrative analogues to early north Germanic assump-tions about sexual procreation. Thus the metaphor of "liquid" creation probably alludes to the parallel image of birth and to fantasies about the embryo inside a woman's womb, the world of the unborn perhaps being thought of as wet and fluid. The emergence of a primeval creature from drops of melting ice thereby assumes thematic importance: it symbolizes the process of birth from female uterine waters and placental blood.

These allusions to female sexual creation are dominated by assertions of a *liquid cycle*. According to the Norse myth,[19] moisture from the northern parts of chaos rose to the surface in a fountain or well. Eleven rivers were said to have sprung from this source. As these streams followed their course, flowing toward the primal void, their liquid content froze and became ice. This sequence of events was repeated whenever the drizzling rains, which emerged from the primeval rivers, turned into rime and snow. Such a successive or recurring transformation of elements (from "moisture" to "well" to "river" to "ice" and "snow") assimilates the act of creation to the changing seasons of the year. As suggested by the mythological imagery, the liquid cycle moves from the reviving waters of spring to the frozen waters of winter. These cyclical changes are accompanied by a transition from liquids to solids, from movement to stagnation, and from fertility to temporary latency.

On a cosmological scale, the Icelandic creation myth seems to have been modeled after images of vegetative growth and reproduction. The symbolism of the liquid cycle thus came to represent the earth mother, whose productivity was latent during the cold times of the year, but who was also renewing her procreative potential every spring. By contrast, in an anthropological sense, the seasonal or periodic changes in the composition of creative fluids probably reflected cultural interpretations of female menstruation: rhythmic images, cycles, and seasons belong to a mythopoetic repertoire of sexual metaphors that circumscribe the periodicity of menstrual bleeding.[20] The cyclical renewal of female fertility (typically equated with the rhythmic appearance of blood) is thereby represented in the mythological realm by the transformation of primeval fluids from water to ice.

Such liquid images of sexual reproduction extend beyond the northern European context. Ancient Greek and Vedic texts, for instance, suggest that a woman's menstrual blood periodically retreated to the womb, where it coagulated to become the substance from which the fetus was formed.[21] Human procreation was thereby linked to the stagnation and solidification of female sexual or uterine blood. In northern European mythology, this concept was expressed in cosmic terms through images of frozen fluids: the containment of ice and rime inside the cosmic void reenacted the process of conception in a metaphorical sense. The symbolic representation of female creation in myth is thereby suggestive of winter, the cold time of the year, when the seeds of organic life (produced by the earth mother) lie buried in a seemingly dead world of snow and frost.

The same symbolic associations between blood, snow, and fertility are apparent in German folk narratives, where a barren woman cuts her finger, bleeds on the snowy ground, and wishes for a child "as white as snow and as red as blood."[22] Such formulaic images and utterances reveal the mythological origin of the tales. The colors and substances associated with the (earth) mother can be interpreted as allegories of the female reproductive cycle: blood, suggestive of fertility and menstrual bleeding, turns into ice and snow, a transformation of fluids that symbolizes conception, pregnancy, and the promise of birth.

The primary model of conception in European cosmography was rooted in the liquid rhythms of the female body: while the regular appearance of menstrual blood indicated a woman's ability to bear children, its temporary stoppage during pregnancy suggested a further link between menstruation and the creation of new life.[23] Symbolic equations such as these probably gave rise to the assumption that the fetus was formed from retained menstrual blood, being initially merely thicker blood, that is, uterine blood in a solid or frozen state.[24]

Competing Models of Creation

Despite obvious similarities between medieval Icelandic and other Indo-European concepts of sexual creation, there exist some important differences. Based on textual and linguistic evidence, we know that early Indo-European peoples held that it was men's creative fluids that obstructed and reversed the rhythmic flow of female menstrual blood.[25] The containment of blood inside a woman's womb was thereby accomplished only under the influence of the male "seed." Furthermore, classical (Greek and Vedic) theories proposed that uterine blood (which appeared as the first step in the formation of the fetus) was actually produced by men's semen.[26] Such assertions of male unilateral creation probably made sense in light of the ideology of patrilineality: in early Indo-European communities, a person's membership in social groups was determined exclusively by principles of *male* descent.[27] Given this emphasis on the primacy of paternity in early Indo-European society, it is not surprising that the creation of life became a male prerogative. Correspondingly, the generative symbolism of female sexual blood was appropriated and transformed into a social metaphor of masculinity: blood came to mark relations of descent through men.

It is important to note that these assumptions of male unilineal descent among early Indo-European peoples were accompanied by images of the unilineal motion of creative fluids (see Chapter 1). The procreative masculine fluid, the "blood-seed," was thought to be enclosed in a man's skull and backbone, where it was specifically identified with the generative marrow.[28] In the propagation of new life, this potent fluid presumably moved from the head downward through the spine to the male genital organs. Along this linear axis, the male body was assimilated metaphorically to the image of the tree, whose trunk became the medium for the rising sap from the soil to the branches.[29] According to the early Indo-European iconography of the male body, the linear motion of male fluids was regarded as the ultimate source of creation. It was this concept of the axial channel, the symbolism of the line, that dominated early Indo-European assumptions of male creation and descent.

Northern European concepts of birth and procreation appear to have been radically different. In the mythological narratives of medieval Norse texts, linear images of liquid creation are replaced by cyclical images of reproduction. This difference in symbolic emphasis, from a focus on the line to a focus on the cycle, corresponds to a shift in the reproductive role of women: early Indo-European assertions of exclusive male creativity were antithetically opposed to a belief in bilateral descent by northern European peoples, that is, a belief in the creative potential of both mother and father, man and woman.[30] Thus, correspondingly in Norse mythology, the creation of life was accomplished by the *equal* participation of male and female elements. The first living creature (the primeval giant Ymir) came into existence through the combined power of fire and ice. Hidden beneath this mythopoetic image of cosmic creation one finds allusions to cultural assumptions about human reproduction. In the myth, life began when fiery semen came into contact with the icy fluids of the watery womb. The actual fusion of a male substance and a female substance was thereby defined as the essence of sexual reproduction in medieval (northern) Europe.

Conflicting Images of Motherhood

In the world of Norse mythology, women were envisioned as equal participants in the creative process. Their generative potential, expressed symbolically through liquid metaphors, was explicitly acknowledged. At the same time, however, female sexuality was regarded with feelings of resentment and ambivalence. This is especially apparent in the mythological depiction of the primordial mother, who is impregnated by Surtr (god of fire/sun deity) and subsequently gives birth to the giant Ymir. She is represented in the narratives as a *turbulent river of ice*, a mythopoetic image for menstrual blood. The metaphorical portrayal of the birth-giving female in terms of sexual fluids suggests that the power of the procreative woman was centered upon the vagina: she was defined as carnal and erotic.

The sexually erotic mother was perceived as dangerous and potentially destructive. She was depicted as *liquid venom* in the realm of myth: the primeval river of ice, a metaphor of female sexuality and symbol of her fluids, thus consists of poison. According to the Old Norse texts, the icy stream was neither pure nor fertile: the rivers of Élivagar carried within their waters a poison (*eitrkvika*), and out of this venomous substance the first mythical being was formed.[31] Venom or poison is of course not literally a bodily or sexual fluid. In a symbolic sense, however, it is equated with female genital blood. The anthropological evidence does in fact suggest that menstrual or uterine blood is universally perceived as a pollutant, as a dangerous fluid that causes sickness and death.[32] In a symbolic sense, the sexual blood of women may acquire the destructive propensities of poison: its flow can "cause vegetation to wither and men's legs to swell" (Lévi-Strauss 1978: 503). This negative imagery of female genital blood is translated in the world of myth into a liquid metaphor of venom:

water > female genital blood < venom

The symbolic equation of menstrual blood with poison has prompted several attempts at explanation. Lloyd deMause, for instance, argued that the symbolism of blood pollution may be interpreted as a projective fantasy rooted in fetal memories of the "poisonous placenta," of the polluting and asphyxiating experience in the maternal womb, which produces attitudes of fear and rage toward the murderous mother, serving as a prototype for all later hate relationships (1981: 4–89). Other explanations, focused more narrowly on the qualities of female sexual fluids, point to the symbolic connection between menstrual blood and procreation. The fear and avoidance of women's blood, the taboos and rituals associated with menstruation, are subsequently understood as manifestations of envy, that is, men's feelings of resentment toward female procreative power.[33] Such feelings are typically expressed in the degradation of female sexuality: menstrual blood is transformed into a liquid poison.[34] In Norse mythology, venom came to symbolize the creative power of the primordial mother, because her erotic (sexual) nature was perceived as a threat. The flow of blood, a sign of female fertility and reproduction, was thus denigrated in symbolic terms: it became a poisonous and deadly fluid.

The concept of the erotic mother as a source of danger is equally apparent in other mythical descriptions of her liquid domain. The world of the North, source of the poisonous river and of female procreative power, is demonized, envisioned as both dark and cold. In subsequent accounts of creation, this region is equated with the nether world, the realm of death, which is populated by poisonous snakes and devouring serpents. The demonic mother, who is venom and death, becomes a raging fury: thus, the icy stream (which is her symbolic manifestation), its eleven branches, and their common source bear names denoting violence, turbulence, and danger: roaring cauldron (*Hvergelmir*), stormy sea (*Élivagar*), torture, burning pain, cold (*Svöl* or *Kvöl*), lust for battle (*Gunnþra*), devourer, gluttonous eater (*Sylgr*), the hasteful one (*Fjorm*), mighty subduer (*Fimbulþul*), dangerous, fierce (*Sliðr*), thunderstorm, attack (*Hrid*), she-wolf (*Ylgr*), chain, bondage (Vid), lightning (*Leiptr*), roar (*Gjoll*).[35] These images and circumlocutions of primeval fluids (that is, menstrual blood) as cataclysm, torture, aggressive warrior, or devouring animal seem to reflect a deep emotional ambivalence toward female sexuality. As metaphors of the erotic female, such terms consist of a brutally bald statement of the fantasy of the poisonous or castrating mother,[36] the maternal consort who devours her husband and feeds on his substance. In an extended sense, the demonic, dangerous woman is therefore the wife, the erotic female, whose sexuality is regarded as a threat to her spouse. These same feelings of sexual ambivalence extend toward the parent-child relationship, there revealing a basic oedipal theme. As hypothesized by psychoanalytic theory, a man's lust for his mother, being unacceptable to him, is projected onto her, resulting in the image of the emasculating or life-taking erotic mother. Male fantasies of incest are thereby expressed in myth through themes of female sexual aggression and destruction.

The image of the demonic mother stands in striking contrast to the figure of the loving mother, who suckles her offspring.[37] In the Norse myths, the *nurturing* female appears in the form of a cow, the earth cow *Auðumla*, who feeds the primeval giant with milk from her breasts: "Straightway after the rime dripped, there came into being from it a cow called Auðumla; four rivers of milk ran from her udders, and she nourished Ymir."[38] According to this text, the cow is the image of the mother full of milk, a primary psychological symbol of goodness and love. The earth cow represents the *nurturing mother*, who is culturally defined as non-erotic and made the female ideal. She is the good mother, the white mother, in contrast to the evil, demonic, and dark mother, the venomous and devouring mother, whose sexuality is perceived as a threat.

Thus, in the world of myths, the erotic female becomes a negative force and is replaced by the gentle, milk-producing cow. The transformation occurs through metaphors of procreation: the evil mother, a *venomous river of ice*, is reborn or reproduces herself by liquid means. She gives birth to the good mother in the form of a lactating cow, who comes into existence from drops of melting rime (venom/blood). Here, the most dangerous of substances thus changes into the purest of substances: blood turns to milk, and venom transforms into food. This transmutation of female sexual images suggests that a woman, in northern European society, cannot behave in a manner simultaneously erotic and maternal: she cannot be a mother and a wife, a milk cow and a menstruating spouse. The myth expresses this dilemma by splitting the image of the mother into two: she is either *erotic* (imagined as a poisonous river of ice) or *nurturing* (in the form of a milk-giving cow). As a sexually erotic woman, her power is centered upon the vagina. As a maternal figure, who feeds her offspring, her power is centered upon the breast. Thus, the emphasis is on the pleasure of food rather than the pleasures of sex.

Given this symbolic focus, the dissociation or splitting of the maternal image is equally apparent in the corresponding liquid metaphors: blood stands for the erotic mother, while milk belongs to the cow. Blood is *sexually* productive, and therefore dangerous and life draining. Milk is non-erotic and therefore life giving: it engenders and nurtures. Creation through sexual blood (nature) is negative and demonic, while creation through milk (nurture) is positive and heroic. Whereas blood 'breeds' giants and hostile monsters (Ymir and his kin), the milk-producing cow gives rise to a line of culture heroes and gods (Búri, Oðin, etc.). The mythological depiction of the erotic mother thus amplifies female sexuality through images of blood and violence. The symbolism of the lactating cow negates female sexuality through images of non-erotic benevolence.

The milk-giving cow is a symbol of non-erotic fertility. In the myth, she is named *Auðumla*, the cow "of plenty without horns." This verbal metaphor emphasizes her nonphallic nature: although the cow is fertile, she is not perceived as a threat. Unlike the evil mother, the whore, who procreates sexually, the chaste cow creates offspring unilaterally, without a male agent: "She licked the rime-stones, which were salty; and the first day that she licked the stones, there came forth from the stones in the evening a man's hair; the second day, a man's head; the third day the whole man was there. He is named Búri: he was fair of feature, great and mighty." [39] The chaste cow projects an image of loving benevolence: she is always a mother but never a wife. As a symbol of perpetual plenty, her breasts are full of milk. As a symbol of perpetual fecundity, she bears children. The source of her productive abundance, however, is not erotic or sexual. The cow is androgynous and procreates by herself. As a result, the carnal and erotic circumstances of her reproductive activity are deemphasized and concealed—hidden beneath the mythic imagery.

According to the narrative, the milk cow creates offspring alone with her mouth, a probable euphemism for vagina or womb. She brings into existence a son, a man called Búri, whose birth is represented metaphorically in stages: the appearance of the hair, the crowning of the head, the emergence of the whole body. Búri comes to life from blocks or "stones" (rocks) of frozen rime. The creative substance from which he is made thus consists of solid ice. The cow gives birth to her son by licking (melting/churning) the ice with her tongue. While the tongue, in this context, is probably a phallic and life-creating symbol, ice and rime are symbols of female blood. These mythological images seem to suggest that procreation occurs *outside* the body of the cow: they are images of disembodied and non-erotic creativity.

In the text, the sexual nature of female creation is veiled by a string of highly illusive body metaphors: mouth (*vagina*); licking (*sex*); tongue (*phallus*); ice (*uterine blood/placenta*). The erotic qualities of the nurturing mother, the androgynous cow, are here negated. Genital and sexual references are replaced by visions of food. This point is made even more explicit by the fact that the cow gives birth by licking the ice blocks. This implies that she ingests them. And whatever she eats apparently tastes "salty." Thus, inside the body of the cow, the raw essence of sexual blood is transformed or distilled into food: *venom* turns into *salt*. Once filtered by the body of the cow, even a dangerous and deadly substance may be safely ingested.

Northern European mythology appears to be rife with incestuous fantasies that can be expressed precisely because they are masked by animal and food symbolism. Venom is the symbolic manifestation, in an *inedible* form, of female sexuality, of which the other manifestation, salt, represents the *edible* aspect. From a male perspective, the milk-producing cow is sexually accessible, while the erotic woman is not. Venom stands for the "castrating" mother, who is a *taker* of male essence: she devours her husband and lusts after her son. This image of female sexual aggression is opposed to an image of loving (passive) endurance, which is equated with salt. Salt belongs to the gentle, nurturing cow, who is a *giver* of food: she feeds the primeval giant with milk from her breasts, and he in turn "eats" her. Here, female sexuality is negated, while male dominance is affirmed. Articulated through fantasies of oral aggression, the erotic qualities of the devouring mother are transformed into food, which can in this manifestation be eaten and conquered. Consequently, the symbolic opposition between venom and salt, blood and milk, inedible and edible substances, or poison and food, becomes an expression of the corresponding contrast between *negative eroticism* initiated by the mother and *positive eroticism* initiated by the son: incestuous relationships may be tolerated in the Old Norse texts if they are initiated by the male. However, by displacing the role of the erotic mother onto a non-erotic (domesticated) female animal, the cow, incestuous encounters are deflected into the non-human world so that any attempt to decode them, to read these encounters in anthropomorphic terms, results in distortions and confusions.

The dissociation of the defining qualities of a mother, the ascription of her responsibilities to either a sexually erotic or a nurturing maternal role, seems to be a dramatic expression of a social pattern that was once common throughout the northern European world: women were forbidden to have sexual intercourse while nursing their infants. In order to circumvent this taboo, mothers sometimes placed their children in the care of wet nurses. One of the earliest accounts of this practice can be found in *The Ecclesiastical History of the English Church and People*, written by the Northumbrian monk Bede (A.D. 673–735). The manuscript explains how Augustine, the first archbishop of Canterbury, asked Pope Gregory for advice on questions concerning sexual practices and marriage. Bede's commentary includes the citation of a postpartum sex taboo and a discussion of its effects on nursing practices: "Her husband should not approach his bedfellow until her infant is weaned. But an evil custom has arisen among married people that women scorn to suckle the children they have born, but hand them over to other women to be suckled; and this presumably has arisen solely as a result of incontinence because, as they will not be continent, they are unwilling to suckle their infants." [40] According to Bede, a mother's desire to resume sexual relations after the birth of a child gave rise to the practice of wet nursing, a custom that successfully circumvented the application of a cultural taboo. The contents of this papal document circulated throughout the German lands:[41] in its separate manifestations, the manuscript appeared in Switzerland, Germany, Denmark, and England, where it was used as a point of reference and where its terms were seen as a concession to the practices of the local inhabitants.

Both the northern European taboo on sex and the practices designed to circumvent it tended to reinforce the conceptual dichotomy of womanhood, the separation of the *good mother*, who cared for her children by giving them food, from the *evil mother*, who abandoned her offspring by denying them food. A woman's domestic role was thus apparently subject to conflicting social expectations: she could not be both a nursing mother and a sexually desirable spouse, a giver of food and a taker of male essence. Norse mythology expresses this dilemma by splitting the image of the mother into two: she appears either as a venomous river of ice or as a milk-producing cow. In the social realm, the taboo on sex further supported this dichotomy by dividing a woman's reproductive cycle into phases or stages, during which she was to be either sexually active, and therefore dangerous, or non-erotic and chaste. Ironically, the development of wet nursing, a practice designed to circumvent the taboo, promoted the underlying schism even more dramatically: the tasks of female eroticism and maternal care were not only divided into separate roles, but the respective responsibilities were assumed by different individuals, the biological mother and the wet nurse. It was the church that would have it otherwise and attempted to impose another model of mother-child and husband-wife relations.[42]

Male Androgyny

In Norse mythology, the symbolism of female procreation and child-bearing is sharply opposed to the mythic images of male creation. This is especially apparent in the myth about the primeval giant, which begins with a description of his birth. When the primeval fluids had been transformed into a creative substance under the combined influence of fire and frost, the first mythological creature was born in the form of a giant man. After his birth, he assumed the name Ymir. Based on the etymology of this term, there has been some speculation that Ymir may have come into existence as a male androgyne, a being capable of producing offspring by himself: Old Norse *Ymir* has been derived from terms denoting twin, hermaphrodite, double fruit.[43] The etymological meaning of the name *Ymir* possibly hints at bisexuality, thereby alluding to the giant's androgynous form, his body being half male and half female.

In a mythic sense, male androgyny is an element of chaos within creation. It promotes the symbolic restoration of a primordial condition during which basic sexual and physical distinctions were not yet made.[44] This state of disorder was anthropomorphized by the androgynous figure of Ymir.[45] Interestingly, such a fusion of male and female sexual characteristics is associated with a destructive substance in the mythological narrative: the Norse myth states explicitly that the hermaphroditic giant was born from *venom* or *poison*.[46] This image is made explicit once again in a poetic verse about his birth:

> Out of Élivagar
> spurted venom drops,
> then they grew until a giant emerged therefrom.[47]

Thus, if symbolized by *poison*, male androgyny was charged with negative connotations in Norse mythology, perhaps despised as an anomaly, an undesirable blurring of sexual categories. In this context it is important to note that poison is a liquid symbol of the erotic mother: the primeval giant was born from the carnal female, who in the myth is represented as a *venomous river of ice*. Creatures born by her are said to be excessively evil and lustful: the male androgyne is thereby explicitly denigrated in symbolic terms.

As an anthropomorphic androgyne, embodied in human form, Ymir was fertile and had the ability to generate life unilaterally. By implication, he was therefore perceived as a complete being who could create from within himself: his children were born from his armpits and from contact between his feet.

Initially, Ymir gave birth to a set of fraternal twins, a boy and a girl. Through the making of these twins, the mythical giant reproduced his androgynous identity in an unambiguous, physically separate form. A fragment of the Old Norse prose text tells us how the act of creation took place: "and it is said that when he was asleep, a sweat came upon him, and there grew under his left arm a man-child and a maid." [48] This nocturnal event of creation might be expressive of male pregnancy envy. Giving birth in a dreamlike state alludes to the subconscious desire of men to procreate like women. Such a collective fantasy is here projected into the text of the myth, where the primeval giant comes into existence as a male hermaphrodite. This fantasy (which in the wider Indo-European context was concretized through the idea and practice of patrilineal descent) is treated as a perverse and immoral manifestation in the Old Norse narratives. The figures of the androgynous giant and his offspring are rejected by the Norse text as contemptible: "he was evil and all his descendants." [49]

The giant's physical or bodily attempts at creation resemble natural childbirth. Ymir, as a primordial male, creates offspring unilaterally from his left *armpit*, a probable circumlocution for a displaced "vagina" (imagined as a "hairy cavity"). At the same time, the giant gives birth by producing generative fluids: his body emits "sweat," a salty substance, which is implicated in the act of creation (just as are the salty rime stones churned by the earth cow Auðumla, when she creates the god Búri). In Norse mythology, as in the context of Indo-European folklore generally, sweat, when produced by the body of men, may serve as a "seed" (semen) substitute, the symbol of male procreative power. [50] Yet the discharge of this liquid results in demonic and perverse creations, because sweat is also regarded as an inferior, negative form of male seed: [51] it is the fluid of involuntary emissions and uncontrolled emotion. Given these connotations, it only makes sense to find that sweat is a common blood metaphor in Old Norse poetry and prose narratives: sweat appears as a circumlocution for "blood from a wound," "blood lost through injury." [52] In such instances, both sweat and blood are perceived as negative discharges.

After the initial creation of the (incestuous) twin-siblings, the primeval giant produces a single male descendant by rubbing his feet together. A poetic verse renders the event in the following way:

And foot with foot
did the frost giant fashion
A son that six heads bore.[53]

The metaphor of "rubbing" projects the latent image of creating off-spring by masturbation.[54] In the myth, it is a gesture or motif of male sexual reproduction. Again, however, this creative effort appears to have been negatively charged: it brings to life a demonic creature, a monstrous being with six heads.

In the medieval texts, the male androgyne's creative efforts are thus judged to be perverse. The giant's offspring are described as monstrous beings and abnormal creatures, who restore and populate a world of chaos. Androcentric and more fundamentally *male-unilateral* procreation is thereby explicitly rejected as a *negative* cultural model by the mythological text. This negation of male unilateral creation results ultimately in the death and dismemberment of the primeval giant. The Norse myth, in subsequent cosmogonic accounts, describes how Ymir and his descendants were killed by the gods.

In a cosmological sense, the death of the giant may reflect the need to dispel chaos (here regarded as noncreative) and to establish order. Chaos is something that must be transcended or overcome before life can begin.[55] In cultural terms, the giant's murder has been understood by some as a variant of sacrificial dismemberment: "So close are the analogies between the splitting of the androgyne and the dismemberment and sacrifice of the primeval deity that at least one scholar has advanced the suggestion that the basic Indo-European myth of creation was in fact a combination of these two themes: the sacrifice and dismemberment of an androgyne (this hypothesis is not, however, generally accepted)" (O'Flaherty 1980: 295). Others have argued that the death of the primeval giant evokes images of cannibalism: such an imagery usually includes not only visions of torture and mutilation but also the tearing apart of the sacrificial body.[56] There is, however, little evidence to support either one of these interpretations with the mythological material at hand.

From an anthropological point of view, it seems plausible that the murder of the primeval androgyne reflects a symbolic attempt to displace an earlier or competing model of creation: male androgyny embodies the principles of patrilineal descent and male unilateral creation. Such conceptual images are necessarily negated by a society that favors women as equal participants in the creative process, and whose patterns of social organization are based on principles of bilateral descent.

It is significant that in Norse mythology *male* androgyny is rejected and denigrated in favor of *female* androgyny: the Icelandic image of the androgyne is morally positive if female, but negative if male. As in the case of the primeval giant, the androgynous figure may be primarily male: Ymir plays male social roles (son/father), has male physical characteristics (large body, emits sweat or semen), and manifests basic male sexual patterns (nocturnal emissions, masturbation, procreation through genital substitutes). In the myth, the figure of the male androgyne and his desire to create by himself is regarded as morally contemptible by what appears to have been a female centered or matricentric society.[57] The male androgyne plays a perverted and culturally unacceptable role, in this instance, controlling women through unilateral creation, which is depicted as an antisocial and hostile act.

The figure of the primeval giant thus stands in striking contrast to another type of androgyne, the earth cow Auðumla, who is female, maternal, and good. The androgynous cow plays a nurturing and motherly role, has basic female physical characteristics (breasts), and manifests female sexual patterns (produces milk, gives birth, nurtures). Unlike the male giant, the maternal cow is regarded as a symbol of loving benevolence. In the realm of Norse mythology, female androgyny thus assumes a positive social role by affirming culturally validated concepts of the relationship between the sexes: the good mother is both nurturing and procreative, but *not* erotic. Her creative abilities are therefore not experienced as a sexual threat (by men): she gives birth "outside" her body. Her reproductive potential issues from her head and mouth. This image of the earth cow is antithetically opposed to the male hermaphrodite, the giver of life from "inside" the body, whose erotic actions violate northern European cultural ideas about sexual creativity, social order, and descent.

Male Creation

While Norse creation myths clearly oppose the idea of men's appropriation of female procreative power, the narratives hint at the emergence of other forms of male sexual domination. This becomes apparent in the mythological descriptions of the giant's murder and dismemberment by the gods. The Icelandic texts reveal that the deities, after having torn Ymir apart, also murder all but one of his descendants by drowning them in a deluge of blood: "The sons of Bor slew Ymir the giant; lo, where he fell there gushed forth so much blood out of his wounds that with it they drowned all the race of the rime giants."[58] Here, the primeval androgyne is killed by several gods, "the sons of Bor," who are identified in one of the texts as *Oðinn* and his brothers *Vilji* and *Vé*.[59] These deities are the descendants of *Búri* (literally, progenitor), who was born from the earth cow Auðumla.[60] The non-erotic, nurturing mother is thereby defined as the "totemic" ancestor of the gods. By contrast, the giant and his offspring trace their ancestry to a primeval *river of venom,* the emblem of the dangerous and sexual mother. According to the text of the myth, the giants and gods, who are mutually antagonistic, derive their respective existences from separate mothers or primogenitors. This difference in mythopoetic origins suggests that the hostility between giants and gods mirrors the tension between opposing images of femininity: erotic sexuality and motherliness. The gods, as children of the good mother, the chaste cow, act as culture (or epic) heroes, who protect the ordered universe from forces of destruction.[61] The giants, as children of the evil mother, the whore, represent the realms of moral chaos, which are conquered by the gods. This conquest may perhaps be viewed as yet another kind of male dominance: female sexuality is negated in symbolic terms through the death of Ymir, onto whom the destructive or demonic (and subhuman) qualities of the erotic mother have been projected or displaced. We find here an interesting reversal of the oedipal theme as proposed by psychoanalytic theory: in the guise of a divine hero, the male offspring seek to control their mother's erotic desires and to overcome her incestuous lure by killing the androgynous giant in place of her.

Further allusions to the disempowerment of the erotic mother may be found in subsequent mythological accounts, hidden beneath images that make void or negate female creation. According to the Old Norse texts, the death of the androgyne is marked by a great surge of blood, a deluge, with which the gods drown all but one of Ymir's descendants.[62] In narrative terms, the giant's blood hints at a return to liquid chaos, the realm of the erotic mother, which in the myth is described as a turbulent river of icy venom. When the gods thus submerge the existing universe in blood, they emulate (in macrocosmic dimensions) a carnal state that (in anthropomorphic terms) is linked to the reproductive cycle of women: here, the controlled appearance of blood serves as an instrument for *annulling* the creative potential of women. This male conquest of the erotic female is expressed in a symbolic sense not only through liquid images of dissolution, and the reduction to the inorganic, but also through the very death of the giants. As such, the gods' creation of a deluge of blood appears to be an expression of male procreative competition: men, as divine actors, reproduce symbolically the important carnal or erotic element that women have naturally.[63] Such an appropriation of female procreative power through the manipulation of blood is apparent in ceremonial episodes throughout Europe and elsewhere: the dramatic attempt to simulate menstruation through male circumcision, genital mutilations, bloodletting (phlebotomy, venesection, cupping, leeching), the drawing of blood from the nose, and other forms of bleeding during rites of male initiation.[64] Implicit in this imagery is the male fantasy that ritual or symbolic control of blood provides men with the power to create life.

Having thus annihilated the universe as made by the erotic mother, the gods proceed to take possession of her procreative potential. After murdering Ymir in a state of ritual frenzy, the deities take hold of his body and hurl it into *Ginnungagap*, the primordial void, which in the myth is envisioned as a maternal womb. It is the realm of liquid chaos from which the giant was originally born: "They took Ymir and flung him into the middle of the cosmic void."[65] The gods then appropriate his physical substance (flesh, blood, and bones) to make the earth. Male creation is here revealed through the "filling up" of the void by the divine heroes.[66] In this process, the primeval mother does not seem to play an active role: she is mentioned only as a passive receptacle or container for the male "input." While such images of femininity and motherhood stand in opposition to the northern European model of bilateral creation, they are compatible with the broader Indo-European concepts of patrilineal descent through the exclusive focus on the primacy of paternity and male creativity.

This interpretation is consistent with the final steps of the creative process, in which the gods establish their dominion over a benign and non-erotic universe. They accomplish this task through an act of sexual abduction: after returning the primeval giant to his "prenatal" liquid realm, the divine heroes steal his body's essence from the maternal womb and then make the world out of his *flesh, blood,* and *bones.*[67] A description of this event exists in prose narrative form:

They took Ymir and bore him into the middle of the cosmic void, and made of him the earth: out of his blood the sea and the waters; the land was made of his flesh, and the mountains out of his bones; gravel and stones they fashioned from his teeth and grinders and from those bones that were broken. They also took his skull and made of it the sky and placed it up over the earth.[68]

When the gods thus create the distinct parts of the universe from the elements of the primeval giant, in each instance, the matching parts or elements have been so codified that nearly identical versions can be found in several other medieval Icelandic poems. Here is an example of a poetic verse:

Out of Ymir's flesh
was fashioned the earth,
and the mountain's were made of his bones;
The sky from the frost-giant's skull,
and the ocean out of his blood.[69]

Another version suggests a similar sequence of events:

> Out of Ymir's flesh
> was fashioned the earth,
> and the ocean out of his blood.
> Of his bones the hills,
> of his hair the trees,
> of his skull the heavens high.[70]

During these acts of male creation, the organic elements of the giant's body are (alchemically) transformed: the earth is made from the giant's flesh, the ocean from his blood, the mountains from his bones, and the sky from his skull. Thereby, the significant carnal parts of the giant's androgynous body are transposed or changed into seemingly indifferent (nonorganic) elements: the *earth*, the *ocean*, and the *sky*.

The birth of the non-erotic universe may be seen as a male creative event, which seeks to negate female sexuality and reproduction. As we have seen, this feat was accomplished through a series of nullifying acts: the murder of Ymir, the deluge of blood, the death of the giants, and, finally, the appropriation of female creativity. The male quest for power, both in a sexual and political sense, culminates in the gods' construction of a sexless world[71] in which the earth mother, in her erotic and dangerous manifestation, is rendered impotent.

Sexual Domination

An analysis of northern European origin myths reveals a succession of opposing models of creation, from female reproduction to birth by androgynes to male creation. It is significant that the initial set of mythological episodes contains images drawn from pre-Christian ideas of femininity and motherhood, while the final episodes reflect a medieval androcentric emphasis on the primacy of paternity and male descent.

In the first model, the beginnings of organic life are attributed to the union of fire (semen) and ice (blood), symbols of the generative potential of the sky father and the earth mother. The fusion of male and female substances is thereby defined as the essence of sexual reproduction in Norse mythology. This focus on the equality of man and woman in the propagation of life is sharply opposed to the mythic images of male creation: the figure of the androgynous giant and his birth-giving efforts were regarded as morally contemptible by a society that favored women as equal participants in the creative process, and whose patterns of social organization were based on principles of bilateral descent. The giant Ymir, through his desire to create by himself, played a perverted and socially unacceptable role, ultimately resulting in his death and dismemberment. Male unilateral creation was thus explicitly rejected as a negative cultural model by the mythological text. The early episodes of Norse mythology can thus be interpreted as a symbolic affirmation of a characteristically pre-medieval (perhaps Germanic) model of creation.

In the world of the Norse myth, women were envisioned as equal participants in the creative process. Their generative potential was consistently acknowledged: through metaphors of "liquid" creation, symbolizing birth from uterine waters and placental blood; through the assertion of a liquid cycle, reflecting cultural interpretations of menstruation; and through images of the solidification and containment of primeval fluids, expressing assumptions about the beginnings of fetal life in the maternal womb. This affirmation of female reproductive power, which typifies the initial (and probably older) model of creation, was, however, framed by feelings of resentment and ambivalence: images of the birth-giving mother were paired with her image as death giver. Male procreative envy surfaces in the denigration of female sexuality. This is especially apparent in the portrayal of the reproductive female as a potentially destructive force. Depicted in the realm of myth as "liquid venom" (i.e., blood), her sexual nature was associated with death, violence, and animality.

In the Norse myth, this image of the emasculating or life-taking erotic woman is opposed to the figure of the loving mother, who suckles her offspring. She appears in the form of a cow, who feeds her children with milk from her breasts. The symbolism of the lactating earth cow negates female sexuality through images of non-erotic benevolence: providing food for her children; creating offspring without a male agent; giving birth outside her own body; and procreating through oral rather than vaginal means. By concealing the carnal circumstances of her reproductive activity, the erotic mother is not perceived as a threat. Masked by animal and food symbolism, male fantasies of incest can thus be safely expressed: incestuous encounters are deflected into the nonhuman world, conveyed through images of oral aggression.

The representation of female sexuality in Norse mythology is rooted in a set of psychological themes: procreative envy and oedipal longing. The affirmation of female creation in myth is thus accompanied by male projective fantasies that find articulation in the symbolic opposition of erotic femininity and motherhood. Accordingly, the mythological model implies that the northern European woman, while she is creative, cannot behave in a manner simultaneously erotic and maternal. She cannot be a mother and a wife, a milk cow and a menstruating spouse. Norse mythology expresses this dilemma by splitting the image of the mother into two: she is either erotic, imagined as a poisonous river of ice, or nurturing, in the form of a milk-giving cow.

A very different model of creation surfaces in the final set of events: images of female reproduction are replaced by episodes of male creation. It is significant that this second model draws on competing medieval ideas of patrilineal descent. The succession of creative models is marked by the disempowerment of the erotic mother and the conquest of her domain. The male usurpation of power begins with an act of genocide: the gods kill Ymir, the giant, and drown his descendants in a deluge of blood. These acts of murder may have been motivated by feelings of competition or rivalry: the sons of the gentle earth cow (the good mother) destroy the male offspring of the erotic female (the evil mother). Framed by the tension between the opposing images of femininity (erotic sexuality and motherliness), the gods' extermination of the giants can be interpreted as a symbolic negation of female sexual creation. The disempowerment of the erotic female is thereby expressed through images of death and dissolution: the dismemberment of Ymir; the submergence of the universe in blood; the destruction of the giants by drowning. Having thus annihilated the world of the primeval mother, the gods proceed to appropriate her creative potential. They hurl the giant's body back into the maternal womb, then retrieve his physical substance (flesh, blood, bones) to shape a new world. In this creative process, the primeval mother does not play an active role: she is reduced to a mere receptacle for the male "input." The male quest for power comes to an end when the gods establish their dominion over a benign and non-erotic universe.

The mythological evidence suggests that the Nordic emphasis on bilateral creativity and female reproduction was replaced by an emphasis on male creation. This shift in procreative models may have been triggered by a process of societal change: the male conquest of the erotic female, the destruction of her children, and the appropriation of her domain may be mythopoetic allusions to a drama of political conquest and domination. In the realm of myth, this act of political subjugation was conveyed through the acquisition of female sexual power by men.

The politicization of sexual images and metaphors has been documented in our more recent history for the period of German fascism.[72] The promotion of glorified hypermasculine values and an emphasis on proficiency in physically aggressive activities like sports and warfare were intertwined with a fear of pollution from "bad" blood: fascism in Germany became obsessively concerned with controlling both women and reproduction. Politically effective images were drawn from fantastic fabrications about female carnality and animality and from visions of the destructive power of the vulva and its fluids. Society's energies were subsequently directed inward, toward "containing" the penetration of the political body by elements of reproductive impurity. The Norse narratives suggest in much the same way that the destructive power of the erotic mother could be subdued or neutralized by negating her creative potential and by killing her offspring. Similarly, territorial conquest and cultural domination in the medieval era was conveyed through mythical images of blood pollution, and in terms of male sexual victory.

Male Creativity Through Magical Means

As we have seen, the thematic focus of the Norse myth material reveals a preoccupation with the transference of reproductive power from women to men. The narratives present a succession of models, beginning with female reproduction, followed by birth from androgynes, and ending with male creation. It is significant that the initial set of mythological episodes concentrates on images of femininity and motherhood, while the final episodes dramatize the primacy of paternity and male descent. In the initial model, women are envisioned as equal participants in the creative process. Their generative potential is consistently acknowledged. This affirmation of female reproductive power, although framed by feelings of resentment and ambivalence, is further enforced by the negative depiction of the male androgyne. The figure of the androgynous giant and his birth-giving efforts are presented as morally contemptible by matricentric society. The giant Ymir, through his desire to create by himself, plays a perverted and culturally unacceptable role — in this instance, controlling women through unilateral creation, which utimately results in his death and dismemberment. Male unilateral creation is thus explictly rejected as a negative cultural model by the Icelandic texts. Nevertheless, in the final set of events, images of female reproduction are replaced by episodes of male creation. As we have seen, the male usurpation of power begins with an act of genocide and ends with the gods' universe making. While the historically earlier mythological narratives clearly oppose the idea of men's appropriation of female reproductive power, later medieval texts hint at the emergence of alternate, culturally celebrated forms of male domination. I now explore this transformation of creative models. I show how the meaning and intent of male procreativity is reinterpreted, how it is dissociated from female generative power and focused instead on the production of knowledge. Such a shift in creative purpose encodes a denigration of carnality, a privileging of the mind over the body.

The sequence of procreative models, from life-giving mother to world-creating male, is characterized by a unifying theme: the progressive dissociation of creative action from female corporality. Thus, in the myth about the making of the world, the gods complete their usurpation by an act of magic: the transformation of organic substances into geophysical (natural) elements. This imagery marks a shift in focus from the creative potential of the body to that of the mind. Other myths, such as the creation of dwarfs and the creation of people, contain a similar motif: the gods' transformation of organic substances into other life forms. While here male creative action has been dissociated from the physiological model of female procreativity, and the power to bestow life resides within the male gods, nevertheless this process is channeled through flesh. And furthermore, despite the exclusion of reproductive female figures from the texts, control of blood continues to signify, in a symbolic sense, the possession of creative power. For instance, the gods' production of a deluge of blood (by an act of murder) precedes their universe making. In subsequent narratives, this theme is further accentuated. Male creativity, while perpetually contested and explicitly linked to the possession of blood, is equated with mental power, which issues from the head rather than the body and engenders wisdom, insight, and knowledge.

The connection between reproductivity and carnality is made most explicit by the myth of dwarfs: the origin of dwarfs is linked to the primeval giant's flesh. From the myth text, we learn the following:

Then the gods seated themselves on their thrones and held counsel, and remembered how dwarfs had quickened in the earth and under the soil like maggots in flesh. The dwarfs had first emerged and come to life in the flesh of Ymir, and at that time were maggots. But by the decree of the gods they acquired human understanding and the appearance of men, although they lived in the earth and in rocks.[73]

The dwarfs come into existence as maggots, eating the flesh of the murdered giant Ymir. They are therefore equated with mortality, death, and decomposition or rot. Whereas the maggots reduce the giant's body to food (which becomes a source of life through oral incorporation), the gods magically transform the carrion eaters into dwarfs. Similarly, the dwarfs are consistently linked to the earth and its tangible substance. They are said to live beneath the earth's surface and in rocks or mountains.[74] The dwarfs thus continue to inhabit the very domain that was made from the giant's flesh and bones. And although dwarfs are said to lack the magic wisdom of the gods, they are known as artisans and master craftsmen who make miraculous objects, sources of plenty and life renewal. Thus the dwarfs, like the androgynous giants, are creative through their physical labor. The power of their productive activity is located in the body, and so is possibly a concealed manifestation of female creativity.

The symbolic connection between creation and carnal substances persists in other versions of the myth.[75] A poetic account renders the birth of dwarfs in the following way:

> Then sought the gods
> their assembly seats,
> The holy ones,
> and council held,
> To find who should raise
> the race of dwarfs
> Out of Brimir's blood
> and the bones of Bláinn.[76]

In the poem, the gods magically create the dwarfs from two elements: blood, a liquid (perhaps female) ingredient, and bones, a skeletal (perhaps male) ingredient.[77] Here, as in the previous myth, it seems that the gods take both blood and bones from the primeval giant's body: *brimir* (sea, surge of waves, bloody moisture) and *blain* (black, dark, pale) are presumed to be metonymic attributes of his mythic identity.[78] In their universe making, the gods kill Ymir and use his blood to make the salty ocean waters. The dark-colored giant is thereby associated with death and loss of vital fluids. His genealogical (maternal) origin marks him and his descendants as evil, a conception symbolized by the semantics of color.[79] In accordance with his ancestry, the giant is equated with blackness or darkness. The dwarfs (made by the gods from the giant's body) assume similar characteristics. The connection is affirmed by the meaning of their names: "Most seem to refer to the nether world of death, cold, [and] dissolution."[80] The dwarfs are thus equated with the negative connotations of the corporal substance from which they were made.

This relation of male creative action with corporality is increasingly deemphasized in other narratives. For instance, in the myth of human creation, we read:

> Out of that group then came,
> kind and mighty,
> From the gathered gods
> three great Æsir;
> On the land they found,
> Askr and Embla,
> Two without fate,
> empty of strength.
>
> Breath they had not,
> mind they had not,

Blood nor manners
nor sallow hues;
Breath gave Oðinn,
mind gave Hoenir,
Blood gave Lóðurr
and a fair complexion.[81]

The gods endow the human ancestors with physical and spiritual characteristics: blood and external appearance confer their status as "full fledged members of the ethnic community," transforming them into "people" (Polomé 1969: 288–89). Breath and mind are the attributes of life and, like human thought and mental ability, are qualities localized in the upper torso and the head.

A different, although structurally similar, version of human creation also exists in prose form. Although an elaboration upon the same theme,[82] here the first human beings are made from pieces of wood:

While the sons of Bor [Oðinn, Vilji, and Vé] were walking along the sea shore, they discovered two tree trunks, took them up, and made human beings out of them; the first gave them breath and life, the second wit [inspired mental activity] and movement, the third appearance, speech, hearing and vision. Then they gave them names Askr and Embla, clothed them and set them in Midgard where they and their descendants were to dwell.[83]

Here, male creativity is completely dissociated from female physiology. The creative process is presented as a true act of magic: the gods transform a natural substance (wood) into a corporeal one (flesh, blood, bone).

The Origin of Poetry

The progressive disembodiment of the creative process culminates in the myth of the origin of poetry.[84] The narrative begins with an attempt at male unilateral creation. In order to end their warfare, the gods conclude a truce, which is consecrated by the members of each faction (*Æsir* and *Vanir*) spitting into a vat. From this substance, the gods then make a man, unequaled in wisdom and knowledge.

The gods had a dispute with the folk which are called Vanir, and they appointed a peace-meeting between them and established peace in this way: they each went to a vat and spat their spittle therein. Then at parting the gods took that peacetoken and would not let it perish, but shaped thereof a man. This man was called Kvasir.[85]

As in the preceding mythological texts, male unilateral productivity, when posed in physiological terms, is treated as a negative cultural model. Due to an unfortunate sequence of events, Kvasir, the divine son, is killed and his blood is transformed into a drink. Through this motif of murder and reduction, male procreative action is contested and annulled. "[Kvasir] travelled widely through the world teaching people knowledge, and when he arrived as a guest to some dwarfs, Fialar and Galar, they called him to a private discussion with them and killed him." [86] The murder of the gods' offspring, Kvasir, is motivated by a quest for blood: the dwarfs, who commit the killing, take the body and drain its blood into two vats and a kettle. [87] After thus containing the blood, the dwarfs mix it with honey, transforming it, by a process of fermentation, into mead: whoever drinks it (we are told) becomes a skald or scholar. [88] Through their act of containment and transformation, the dwarfs become the repositories of poetic knowledge. Hearing of this, the mighty giant Suttung threatens the dwarfs and takes possession of the blood; he hides it in a cave, to be guarded by his daughter. In the myth, the control of blood, and thereby control of creative power, passes from the gods to the dwarfs to the giants. These events constitute a reversal or inversion of the initial sequence of creation. [89] Generative power, previously originating with the sexually creative mother, now stems from a pantheon of male gods; the murder of her son, the primeval giant, is replaced by the murder of the god's offspring; the act of murder, previously carried out by the gods, is now committed by creatures (the dwarfs) who trace their origins to the carnal manifestation of the primeval mother (the giant's body); the gods, who in the making of the world take possession of her creative power by killing the primeval giant and by drowning his descendants in a deluge of blood, are here dispossessed of this power; the blood of murder, which previously engendered a deluge, is now contained; this blood, previously identified as maternal and venomous, is now identified as a substance of manhood, which can be consumed. The message of these contrasting or oppositional images is twofold: while attesting to the shift of creative models, from birth-giving mother to generative males, they also convey a challenge or contestation to this appropriation of creative power by men. Control of blood/power is temporarily regained by female progeny, but only after its destructive propensity is vitiated through containment and fermentation.

Thus, in the final passage of this myth, (female) procreativity is envisioned as a "vat of blood," guarded by a female giant. The culture hero and god Oðinn gains access to the liquid by sexual seduction: he swallows the blood and escapes. Taking the shape of an eagle, he flies away. In flight, he vomits this fluid and thereby imparts to the gods the gift of poetry. "And when the Æsir saw Oðinn flying they put their containers out in the courtyard, and when Oðinn came over Asgard he spat out the mead into the containers."[90] These images stress analogy and imitation of female reproductive processes while acknowledging the failure to retain stolen power permanently. In the mythic realm, this dilemma between possession and loss is resolved by a focus on mental creativity: the birth of poetic thought is attributed to men.

The medieval myth material thus hints at the emergence of an alternative order of male creation: from the production of offspring to the production of knowledge. The "natural" (or biological) female model, that is, procreation through the body, is rejected as unsuitable for the purposes of male creativity.[91] Instead, male procreation is redefined in terms of mental labor: the generation of poetic insight, wisdom, inspiration.

The assertion that wisdom and knowledge originated with men rather than women is thus crucial to the cycle of Icelandic myths. The initial source of spiritual creativity, however, is the female body: it is killed, reduced to blood, transformed into a drink, and reborn through men. Poetic creativity is thereby still linked to the ownership of blood: men gain possession of a ritual substance, which contains or harbors the power that was originally controlled by women.[92] This imagery of blood renders cosmic and natural the competition for creative power. Poetry or oral productivity similarly relies on a physiological metaphor: the motif of swallowing and regurgitation;[93] the recognition that the mouth, like the vagina, can both admit and expel productive substances; the circumscription of poetry in terms of saliva, drink, vomit. Yet, creation from the mouth, being an organ of the mind or spirit rather than the body,[94] connotes control and intentionality: the regurgitation (vomiting) of blood constitutes a reversal of the natural course of events, which is opposed to female genital bleeding. The swallowing and regurgitation of blood displaces the locus of productive power from the body to the head. Consequently, "an important opposition exists between the body and the head. The body is associated with mortality in alimentary and sexual symbolism, while the head is associated with wisdom and immortality" (Oosten 1985: 66).[95] This shift in focus from body to mind, the privileging of the spirit over the flesh, promotes an antithetical model of male control: what men create is a "cultural" order, while women reproduce the "natural" order.

Gender in Medieval Europe

The mythological evidence suggests that the initial (and possibly historically earlier) Icelandic emphasis on bilateral creativity and female reproduction was superseded by a characteristically medieval concern with male creativity. This shift in procreative models may have been triggered by a process of societal change: the male conquest of the erotic female, the destruction of her children, and the appropriation of her domain might be mythopoetic allusions to a contemporary drama of conquest and domination. Iceland was settled in the late ninth century by men and women from southwest Norway, who were later called "landtakers." The society that they constructed in this uncultivated and uninhabited terrain was based on a system of decentralized self-government, which endured until 1262, when the Icelandic polity lost its autonomy to Norway. In Iceland, as in Christian Europe, king and church grew in authority while the power of women declined. In the realm of myth, this act of political subjugation was conveyed through the control of the female body by male deities.[96] Similarly, the territorial conquest of Iceland by Continental Europe may have been conveyed through mythical images of blood pollution, and in terms of male sexual victory.

The directional change in creative models also hints at the radical transformation of gender roles that occurred throughout medieval Europe. Norbert Elias (1982), in an analysis of the dynamics of medieval feudalism, documented that changes in cultural attitudes toward women can be linked to the beginnings of a "civilizing" process: the emergence of courtly society and its concern with manners and codes of conduct. Until the ninth century, according to Elias, a man's social position was defined by his control of territory: political power and land were inextricably linked in feudal Europe. The eventual collapse of this land-based economy was triggered by a multitude of factors, such as the scarcity of land, the hereditary control of property, and new transportation technologies. New sources of wealth through business and trade radically altered the social structure of feudal society. Money displaced land as a medium of transaction, giving rise to novel forms of prestige and status display.

Initially, change was gradual: local lords were not yet fully integrated into the money economy and continued to rely on military conquests to enhance their power and wealth. These rulers, lacking the "refined pleasure" known to those of greater wealth, were characterized by their mistrust and brutalization of women, by their delight in plundering and rape. The richest and most powerful knights began to invest economic resources in symbolic forms of display: their courts gradually assumed more cultural significance than the medieval towns and became, in effect, the great cultural centers of their time. It was these courts of the feudal lord that began to sponsor poets, singers, and performers, and from which the ideals of courtly love emerged.

While far from egalitarian, the great courts allowed women room for intellectual development, promoting their literacy and learning. These women were in a position to attract poets, singers, and learned clerics. This led to "courtoisie," or the polishing of conduct in the feudal courts. The relationship between these high-ranking women and socially inferior men (not husband and wife) became a characteristic of troubador poetry: *Minnesang* (medieval court poetry) articulated a man's desire for an unattainable woman. For men of low rank, court poetry became a means for upward mobility by "expressing the interests and political opinions of the Lord and the beauty of the Lady" (Elias 1982: 86). This same relation of unequal rank led men to the restraint, renunciation, and transformation of aggressive conduct, resulting in more "civil" forms of behavior. Yet while *Minnesang* and courtly forms of conduct attest to the changing behavior and attitudes accompanying the social transformation of feudal society, such new forms of conduct also attest to the simultaneous disempowerment of women: the Lady became a mere ornament, a decorum, of male power. And the term *Minnesang* itself suggests that the female voice was muted:[97] language had become politicized. Oratory and verbal art came to be defined as exclusive male prerogatives.

This pattern persists well into the modern era. Ruth Bottigheimer (1987), for instance, documents the portrayal of women in early modern German texts. Her analysis, focused on a discursive representation of gender, reveals that female characters are increasingly silenced: women are dispossessed of their power of speech. Female silence occurs on several levels: heroines are not authors; they are condemned to muteness as part of the plot; they speak more passively; they speak illicitly; and their speech evokes a negative response by other characters in the tale text. In the older set of manuscripts, women have control over magical power, which they may invoke by reciting formulaic incantations. Although the world in these earlier tales seems to be populated by conjuring witches, it is actually beautiful young girls who call forth natural forces with their words and spells. Such images, Bottigheimer suggests, are constituted by a world view in which magical and natural processes are the domain of women. As the folk tales were rewritten by the German romantics (i.e., the Grimms), women's powers were reduced: magical power becomes tied to magical artifacts, which are appropriated by men. The silencing of women can therefore be interpreted as a political act. Speech patterns, the presence of "voice" or "silence," the ability to cast spells, to control events with words, can be linked to the possession (or absence) of power and authority.

Finally, the dissociation of male creative action from corporeality or physicality, as suggested by the Norse myths, articulates a change in European religious ideology: flesh and the mortal body (equated with woman—"Eve") were rejected in favor of spiritual immortality (a symbol of manhood). The cultural construction of gender in medieval Europe was deeply rooted in early Christian teachings. "Menstrual blood ceases in the female after conception so that the child in her womb will be nourished by it. And this blood is reckoned so detestable and impure that on contact with it fruits will fail to sprout, orchards go dry, herbs wither, the very trees let go their fruit; if a dog eats of it, he goes mad. When a child is conceived, he contacts the defect of the seed, so that lepers and monsters are born of this corruption" (Pope Innocent III, *On the Misery of the Human Condition*, 9). Women, in medieval Christian theology, were the prototype of the human condition—bound by flesh, by lust—the mortal body: "Man was formed of dust, slime, and ashes, what is even more vile, of the filthiest seed. He was conceived from the itch of the flesh, in the heat of passion and the stench of lust, and worse yet, with the stain of sin" (Innocent III, 6). Such views came to dominate ecclesiastical writing, letters, sermons, theological tracts, and canon law.[98] The topic of womanhood and physical reproductivity, through its dissemination in church scriptures, was probably identified with questions of language, literature, and poetry in late medieval Europe. Sacred knowledge was sought in written texts, which consistently equated women with the carnal body and men with spiritual creativity.

A very explicit depiction of such views of the body and gender appears in European religious paintings of the twelfth and thirteenth centuries. In an analysis of medieval and Renaissance art, Leo Steinberg (1983) discusses the visual representations of early Christian doctrine. The significant theological motifs were based on the assumption of "incarnation" (God becoming flesh), which declared "God's descent into manhood" (8), the "humanation" of Christ, who was mortal, sexual, and reproductive. According to Steinberg, these themes can be seen in the depiction of devotional imagery: the nursing Christ child (signifying his mortality); the circumcision of the infant (the shedding of blood attesting to his humanity); the Madonna's hand shielding the child's genitals (attesting to the vulnerability of Christ's humanity); the child's erect penis (symbolizing his capacity for sex and lust, which he rejects and denies); the dead Christ's erect penis, or "flesh enlivened" (a manifestation of power over death). In contrast to the associations of "humanation" with the lower body, the genital or sexual domain, Renaissance painters located spiritual transcendence in the upper torso and head, representing it by a halo or gestures of benediction.

Steinberg suggests that the symbolism of the unclothed and "naturalistic" body of Christ, accompanied by different types of genital displays, served as a visual affirmation of mortality. The exposure of Christ's sexuality signified power, particularly the power to procreate. Yet through his chastity, Christ triumphed over the sins of the flesh, and ultimately death, thereby abolishing the need for physical procreativity. This is much the same theme as articulated by the medieval Icelandic myths: the production of offspring or creation through the flesh/body is rejected as an appropriate model for the construction of manhood. The mythic symbolism of male power celebrates disembodied creativity and the production of ritual (poetic) knowledge.

Chapter 4
Sanguine Visions, Sacred Blood
The Cult of the Body in Late Medieval Europe

What happened to the mythic models, images, and representations of blood in medieval Christianity? Did the mythological emphasis on blood, male power, and genealogy persist in later European history? How were metaphors and allegories of the fecund male body reconfigured within a medieval aesthetic of blood? During the late Middle Ages, particularly after the eleventh and twelfth centuries, the motif of blood was codified as a male generative (salvific) symbol. Blood, in medieval Christianity, became a sacred substance, a medium through which God's power was focused. Blood assumed a polysemous, fertile, and paradoxical quality, an attribution that was made evident by the oneiric exaltation of a superior blood: the sacred body and blood of Christ.

In an early essay focused on blood and the sacred, the French sociologist Emile Durkheim (1897) echoed several preoccupations of late medieval doctrine: the law of alliance, tabooed consanguinity, and the Sovereign-Father. Intrigued by the religious significance of blood, Durkheim sought to uncover the sanguine nature of premodern social systems. Society, he argued, began as a "community of blood," a powerful alliance of individuals connected through the bond of consanguinity: blood contained "that . . . common principle, which [was] the soul of the group and each of its members" (1963: 88–89). The physiological unity of premodern society was thus based on a blood covenant: ancestral and genealogical linkages were "propagated and dispersed across the lives of [all] descendants" through this medium of blood (89). In Durkheim's view, the archaic preponderance of blood was connected to its symbolism as a vital fluid. To the ancient observer, "life ended when blood spilled out; therefore it had to be the vehicle of life" (89). From the equation of blood with life, Durkheim argued that sanguine flows and emissions were deemed sacred. Blood was treated with reverence and even fear, as indicated by the strict prohibitions against contact. In Durkheim's words, "blood is taboo in a general way, and it taboos all that enters into contact with it. It repulses any contact and creates a vacuum, in a larger or smaller area around the points where it appears" (85). Yet such prohibitions also revealed the special nature of blood: "[T]aboo is the mark placed on all that is divine: it is therefore natural that the blood and whoever it concerns should be equally tabooed, that is to say, retired from vulgar commerce and from circulation" (85).

In Durkheim's view, the magical or sacred properties of blood derived from a premodern religious system centered on the figure of a common (totemic) ancestor: "The totemic being is immanent to the clan; it is incarnate in each individual, and it is in the blood that it resides. It is the very blood itself. [Thus] members of the clan, having been descended from this unique being, are made of the same substance"— the same blood. They "consider themselves as forming a single flesh, 'a single meat,' a single blood, and this flesh is that of the mythical being from whom they have all descended" (89, 86–87, 88). Durkheim insisted that the unity of premodern social systems was physiological or organic,[1] based on blood. Such an archaic regime of blood derived its power and genealogical potency from a sacred source: the clan ancestor. But this totemic being, Durkheim proposed, was not merely an ancestral figure but also a god, a deity. "As a result, there is god in each individual organism (for he is complete in each), and it is in the blood that this god resides; from which follows that blood is a divine thing. When it runs out, the god is spilling over" (89).

Indeed, such motifs of blood and the sacred were closely linked in late medieval Christianity: blood, ancestry, and godhood were juxtaposed in religious representations of the divine. But while Durkheim saw bloodletting as a negation of life, a loss that depleted the body of its vital substance, late medieval theology attributed a different function to blood. Beginning in the eleventh century, normative religious culture treated bloodshed as sacrifice, as a means of redemption. The wounded body of Christ and its mortal suffering had become important symbols of God's promise to save the world. In late medieval Europe, Christianity began to establish a new covenant of blood by encouraging a ritual partaking of the blood of Christ: God's sacred blood was made ritually accessible during the celebration of mass, in the eucharist or holy communion, which permitted a *feasting on the body and blood of Christ.* Such a participation in divine sanguinity was not, however, limited to assumptions of descent from a Sovereign-Father (as had been implied by Durkheim). Late medieval Catholicism encouraged devotional practices that recapitulated Christ's suffering and bleeding. Blood thus became an extraordinarily complex and potent symbol in the late Middle Ages: "As the letters of Catherine of Siena [d. 1380] suggest, blood was life itself, coursing through Christ's veins, leaping forward from his violated side. It was food, both because blood itself feeds flesh and because blood (processed into milk, according to medieval physiological theory) feeds the young. It was a purging bath. It was bloodshed, the palpable sign of attack on God" (Bynum 1987: 65).

During the eleventh and twelfth centuries, Western Christianity promoted forms of piety that established the blood motif at the center of religious worship. Insistent on the recapitulation of God's broken body, "later medieval theologians and visionaries saw in Christ as bleeding flesh not only the redemption of humankind but also an entity under attack" (Bynum 1987: 65). The religious iconography of blood was thus closely connected to late medieval fears of violation, of being rent and broken, by potential enemies. Deeply concerned with Christ's wounded body, medieval Catholicism projected the threat of corporeal violence onto outsiders: women, heretics, and Jews. Charged with violating the integrity of the body of God, a great number of Jews were murdered in the years before 1350. We see in these fearful visions a conflation of premodern notions of gender, race, and anti-Semitism.

What were the specific sanguine properties that enabled the symbolic fusion of Jewish and female bodies? And why were the iconographic displays of Christ's blood so suggestive of a gendered physicality? The blood that poured from the broken body of a male deity fed and cleansed the individual Christian. The blood of the man/God was thus perceived as extraordinary, as nurturing and healing. But religious attitudes toward women's menstrual emissions remained at best ambivalent. How were different forms of female bleeding subsumed within the Christian cult of sacred blood? And how were menstrual flows symbolically configured by such a sanguine aesthetic?

In his discussion of the sacred, Durkheim (1897) acknowledged that religious attitudes toward blood were firmly connected to normative cultural conceptions of femaleness. Thus, when discussing the phenomenon of taboo, Durkheim tried to explain fears of menstrual bleeding by reference to blood's function as a sacred genealogical substance. "The religious respect that blood inspires proscribes any idea of contact, and since the woman, so to speak, passes a part of her life in blood, this same feeling involves her, marks her with its imprint, and isolates her. . . . Thus the woman, in a rather chronic manner, is the theater of these blood demonstrations. The feelings that the blood evokes are carried within her" (1963: 90, 85). Menstrual blood, in Durkheim's words, produced "a more or less conscious anxiety, a certain religious fear" of contact; this prohibition served "to prevent the dangerous effluvia which [came] out of [the female body] from reaching the surrounding environment" (86). Endowed with a mysterious and undefined potency, women's bodies needed to be cared for and protected from the many dangers of contact, to be isolated from others so that their blood would retain its differential value. The menstrual manifestations of taboo were, in Durkheim's opinion, merely a heightened expression of the sacred (totemic/divine) properties of blood.

In late medieval Europe, the religious symbolism of blood was configured by similar preoccupations with the sacred male body: Christ's suffering, death, and redemption. The blood of the son of God, the Sovereign-Father, stood at the center of religious practice. Woman's natural bleeding, her menstrual flow, was regarded as unimportant or was altogether repressed. Late medieval women, as I document in this chapter, showed their piety by recapitulating, on their own bodies, Christ's bleeding wounds. Self-mutilation and extraordinary bloodletting (in contrast to natural menstruation) were characteristic of female religiosity after the eleventh century. Sacrificial blood (not natural bleeding) was perceived as having sacred properties. In Durkheim's words: "That is why it is forbidden to eat it [blood], to touch it, and why the bloodstained soil becomes taboo" (1963: 90). Ironically, however, late medieval religiosity created a new covenant by the literal partaking of the sacred blood: normative culture insisted on the sensual experience (eating, touching, seeing, reenacting) of Christ's suffering and bleeding. Accusations of transgression or taboo violation were leveled against "outsiders" and were used as powerful weapons in the violent persecution of heretics, women, and Jews. In this chapter, I explore the late medieval cult of blood, underlining the connection between sanguine devotion, misogyny, and anti-Semitism. Blood, while a symbol of unity, also served to demarcate and exclude.

Corpus Christi

In late medieval theology, religious doctrine proclaimed two miraculous deeds: God's act of creation, and God's descent into human form: his becoming flesh and dwelling on earth, where his carnal body suffered hunger, pain, and even death. In normative Christian culture, the motif of blood thus assumed an essential symbolic function. Images of blood, especially depictions of Christ's wounded body, proclaimed God's humanity and affirmed that godhood had vested itself in the infirmity of the flesh. "The rendering of the incarnate Christ ever more unmistakably flesh and blood [was] a religious enterprise because it testifie[d] to god's greatest achievement" (Steinberg 1983: 10). It was through these visions of blood that medieval Christians began to see and comprehend the promise of their redemption. Medieval historians observed that the "theology of the Western Church ha[d] generally tended to pinpoint the redemptive act in Christ's death on the cross, or in the conjunction of his suffering, death, and resurrection" (O'Malley 1979: 138–39). But late medieval realism insisted on the depiction of, and symbolic emphasis on, the *humanation* of God's divine power. In the Catholic West, blood images were used and displayed as palpable proof of Christ's descent into flesh and into manhood.

Once embodied in human form, the figure of Christ (the incarnated god) became mortal and sexual. His emission of blood was taken as a demonstrative sign that "he had assumed true human flesh" and had not "taken on a phantasmal . . . not a true body": "for a body phantastic shall shed no blood."[2] Such bloodshed attested to the leasing of God's humanity to mortal suffering. But the motif of blood also intimated a tragic, anatomically localized vulnerability, as revealed by the flow of blood in circumcision and, later, in the crucifixion.[3] According to medieval theologians, Christ gave his blood in an act of sacrifice. His was the gift of blood, promising renewal, regeneration, and (as phrased by the Venerable Bede in the sixth century) a "healing against the wound of original sin."[4] Five centuries later, Pope Innocent III decreed that this divine bloodshed had redemptive value, permitting entry "to the kingdom of heaven, whose gate the blood of Christ [had] mercifully opened for his faithful."[5] In a work of naive sentimental piety by the Pseudo-Bonaventure, composed shortly before 1300 and aimed at the common reader, the bleeding body of Christ was elevated as a redemptive sacrifice, commemorating the circumcision of Jesus: "Today our Lord Jesus Christ began to shed His consecrated blood for us . . . began to suffer pain for us, and for our sins He bore torment . . . Today His precious blood flowed. His flesh was cut."[6]

The wounding of Christ's mortal body inaugurated the redemption of humankind. As the Dominican Archbishop of Genoa, Jacopo da Voragine, phrased it in the late thirteenth century: "On this day he began to shed his blood for us . . . and this was the beginning of our redemption . . . [Elaborating on additional effusions of the precious blood, the Archbishop then comes to the last shedding] . . . when his side was opened [with a lance] and this was the sacrament of our redemption, for then out of his side issued blood."[7]

In fifteenth-century sermons, this same message was affirmed: "What shall be said about this first holy shedding of blood, which pertains to the salvation of mankind and your immortality," inquires a Ciceronian humanist (who died in 1431, and whose undated oration was composed for delivery by a Franciscan friar): "What shall be said about this first holy shedding of blood . . . this most precious of blood which today our Lord spills for the first time."[8] By the voluntary gift of his blood, we are told, Christ has prevailed over the devil, and "the oration congratulates him as a victor, whose triumph is compared with the military triumphs of ancient Rome" (Steinberg 1983: 61). The visible presence of blood was understood as a sign of divine mercy, as the pledge and commencement of human salvation. Thus, in a published sermon, delivered c. 1460 by Giovanni Antonio Campano, blood is equated with redemption: "Today he began to open for us the door and to make accessible the entry to life . . . the weapons for our salvation appeared for the first time in the blood of that infant . . . It would not have been enough for Christ to be born for us had he not begun to shed that divine blood in which our salvation reposes." [9] So again in Antonio Lollio's oration of 1485: "Here issues the first blood of our redemption . . . Today we begin to be saved, Holy Father, for we have Jesus . . . who today has chosen to spill his blood for the sake of man whom He created." [10]

After the eleventh century, blood took on material significance as a sign or symbol of Christ's mortal body: the body enfleshed, sexed, circumcised, sacrificed, and restored to grace by suffering on the cross. According to Leo Steinberg, "without proof of blood, the flesh assumed by the godhead might have been thought merely simulated, phantom, deceptive" (1983: 63). In late medieval Europe, blood was celebrated for its signifying power. In art and religious iconography, as in the early textual sources, the wounding of Christ's body was recalled in a copious effusion of blood: streaming from the chest, the groin, the hands and feet, blood became visible proof of the mortal body—Christ's sacrifice and ultimate triumph over death. In late medieval hymns, poems, and paintings, the visual emphasis was on "the flesh of Christ, ripped open and spilling pulsating streams of insistent, scarlet blood, to wash and feed the individual hungry soul." [11] Artists found a variety of ways of emphasizing this all-healing and saving blood, in particular through the motif of Christ as bleeding victim:[12] Christ points with his bleeding hand to the wound on his side; Christ bleeds into a eucharistic chalice; Christ displays and offers the bleeding wound on his right side; Christ's wounds emit a stream of blood that is received by a female figure representing humanity; Christ pours forth his own blood from palm and breast into a chalice in order to feed humankind. Late medieval art abounds with such devotional images of God's fecund blood: Christ's gift of healing and redemption was rendered tangible through these iconographies of bloodshed.[13]

This preoccupation with the blood and body of Christ attests to the growing importance of physicality in late medieval Catholic theology. After the twelfth century, the treatment of the body had become a central issue in religious thought. Social historian Caroline Walker Bynum (1987) argues that behind these shifts in image and metaphor lay a heightened concern with physical (earthly) substance, with corporeality, and with sensual experience. Thus the role of blood in late medieval spirituality was framed by the need to come to terms with (rather than merely to deny) the body, with its pain and suffering. In a religiosity "where wounds [were] the source of a mother's milk, fatal disease [was] a bridal chamber, pain or insanity clings to the breast like perfume, physicality [was] hardly rejected or transcended. Rather, it [was] explored and embraced" (250). In the Catholic West, the notion of redemption was made plausible by Christ's descent into flesh. It was therefore the image of a suffering god (with his wounds, his blood, and his pain rendered visible) that had moved into the center of religious piety. For by assuming mortal form, by becoming truly flesh and blood, Christ took on humanity and then saved the world by being broken. It was only by bleeding, by being torn and rent, by dying, that God's body redeemed humanity. Such visions of a god, who saved and healed through his physical human agony, introduced into medieval Christianity a new sense of the power of the body.

The particular implications that late medieval theology gave to the body were themselves, however, historically conditioned. By carefully tracing the fundamental shifts in devotion that transpired in the long span between antiquity and the late medieval period, we see indications of a new acceptance of the body by the twelfth and thirteenth centuries: "Indeed, wherever we turn in the later Middle Ages, we seem to find the theme of the body—and of body in all its aspects, pleasure as well as pain" (Bynum 1987: 253). Although deeply rooted in the religious reverence for Christ's body and blood during the later Middle Ages, it was the emergent cult of saints that best attests to this changed perception of the body.[14] Christian culture of the later Middle Ages revered death and bodily mutilation: "Beginning in a Roman world that feared the dead as polluting and legislated against their removal or dismemberment, a Christian enthusiasm for bodies, especially mutilated dead bodies, as loci of divine power made steady headway throughout the early Middle Ages. Indeed, those (such as Guibert of Nogent in the twelfth century) who opposed the cult understood precisely what was at stake: the cult of relics not only abolished a distinction between spirit and matter; in giving terrifying power to bone and sinew, it forced a new look at what it meant for every human to be a body" (Bynum 1987:255). Spiritual power, argued common Catholics, could be sedimented in the body and preserved in a person's fleshly remains.[15]

By the thirteenth century, this sense of the body as locus of the divine had become so powerful that the consecrated bread (used in mass to symbolize the presence of God) was frequently compared to the bodies of saints and revered as a relic of Christ. Religious devotions involving the consecrated host (*corpus Christi*) spread rapidly, especially after the church's enthusiastic endorsement of miracles in which the eucharistic sacrament turned to flesh and blood.[16] After 1200, the host was displayed in tabernacles, partially transparent monstrances, or reliquaries, often positioned alongside other relics and saintly remains, which were illuminated with burning candles. Indeed, some vessels were used both for the display of saints' relics and for the exposition of the host.[17] The treatment of the consecrated sacrament was clearly borrowed from the manner in which relics were handled and viewed. A particularly vivid example of this parallelism of eucharist and relics is provided in the behavior of Hugh, Bishop of Lincoln, who chewed off a piece of Magdalen's arm while visiting her shrine and defended himself to the horrified onlookers by replying that if he could touch the body of Christ in the mass, he could certainly apply his teeth to a saint's bones.[18] Divine power resided in those bodily or material remains that were taken as signifiers of God's presence.

The emphasis on Christ's body as flesh and blood led to an increasingly literal sense of religious piety. During the late Middle Ages, Christian practitioners began to reject spiritual meditation and displays of compassion as insufficiently devout religious performances. Western Catholics began instead to embrace practices that were focused on *the corporal enactment* of Christ's suffering and death. By 1200, Mary of Oignies actually received in her body the wounds of Christ (while a seraph looked on); she bled from wounds in the form of Christ's wounds; she mutilated her flesh, and often she ate only coarse black bread that tore her throat and made it bleed.[19] About 1275, hagiographers described a recluse, Elizabeth of Spalbeek, who acted out the persecution of Christ every twenty-four hours, dragging herself about, beating herself, and bleeding from stigmatic wounds and from under her fingernails.[20] Intensely literal in their imitation of Christ, desiring to fuse with the physical body of Christ, these women provide some of the earliest examples of the novel phenomenon of stigmata, the sudden (or miraculous) manifestation of wounds, injuries, or marks resembling those on Christ's body.[21] Thus Elizabeth of Spalbeek supposedly received in her body "very clearly . . . without any simulation or fraud" the five stigmata of Christ as recent wounds, "which frequently, and especially on Fridays, emitted a stream of blood."[22] Another woman, Gertrude van Oosten, supposedly received all five stigmata in 1340 when she prayed before a crucifix: the wounds bled seven times a day. She later asked God to take away the bleeding, but the scars remained.[23] During the late fourteenth century, Julian of Norwich asked for and received the grace of sickness and death in literal imitation of Christ. In her thirtieth year, she "died" and returned to life while receiving a vision of the crucifixion with "the red blood running down . . . hot and flowing freely and copiously, a living stream."[24]

Blood effusion through self-mutilation and systematic attacks on the flesh had become an important element of women's piety during the late Middle Ages. The author of the *Nuns' Book* of Unterlinden in the Alsace thus wrote:[25] "In Advent and Lent, all the sisters . . . hack at themselves cruelly, hostilely lacerating their bodies until the blood flows."[26] The results of such discipline, called stigmata, appeared on the bodies of many female saints in the thirteenth, fourteenth, and fifteenth centuries. And women's wounds often appeared or bled on the day and hour of the crucifixion. Even after death, the bodies of saintly women were discovered to have been marked in strange ways: intestines and stomachs were found to be empty, hearts were discovered to be etched with the signs of Christ.[27] For example, Clare of Montefalco's spiritual sisters came to believe so intensely that Christ had planted his cross in her heart that at her death in 1308 they threw themselves upon her body, tore out her heart, and found incised upon it the insignia of the crucifixion.[28] Three precious stones, with images of the Holy Family on them, were supposedly found in the heart of another holy woman after autopsy.[29] These wounds or marks that women bore within their bodies were perceived as signs of the presence of Christ, internal manifestations of God's divine power. The suffering female body—the body of a woman in pain— thus emerged in late medieval Catholicism as a plausible vehicle of redemption.

Between the late twelfth and the sixteenth centuries, many women were reported to have experienced the bleeding wounds of Christ on their bodies, "a miracle never before reported" (Thurston 1952: 81). Francis of Assisi and, in modern times, Padre Pio "are the only males who are believed to have possessed all five of Christ's wounds in visible stigmata; and they are not said to have displayed periodic bleeding. But many cases were reported in the late Middle Ages of women who displayed full stigmata which bled in a rhythmic pattern—most frequently, on Fridays [the day of Christ's crucifixion]" (Bynum 1987: 200–201). To late medieval women themselves, what appears to our modern eyes as self-punishment was *imitatio Christi*: the means of becoming Christ— of imitating the incarnate god whose suffering was assumed to save the world. Bleeding from imaginary or inflicted wounds was a way for late medieval women to achieve a physical union with Christ's agony on the cross. This preoccupation with blood shed from women's bodies emerged out of the late medieval concern with matter and physicality and from a general sense of the body as necessary for salvation.

The emphasis on female suffering, and its expression through the blood of Christ, coincided with the growing importance of women in medieval Christianity. According to Bynum, "[t]he late Middle Ages, especially from the twelfth to the early fourteenth century, witnessed a significant proliferation of opportunities for women to participate in specialized religious roles and of the type of roles available. The number of female saints, including married women saints, increased" (1987: 13). For the first time in Christian history, women's piety took on distinctive characteristics. Over the course of the twelfth and thirteenth centuries, especially in the Rhineland, Flanders, and other German-speaking regions (Holland, Belgium, and Luxembourg), there was a significant increase in female monasteries, wandering woman preachers, female convents, and nuns. Seeking new ways to give religious significance to ordinary lives, women were powerfully drawn to such callings (17). In northern Europe (especially the Low Countries, Switzerland, and the Rhineland), we find women living chaste lives in which charitable service and manual labor were joined to worship.

From the thirteenth century on, women's prophetic alternatives and the forms and themes of women's religiosity were centered on the iconography of bloodshed. Women used self-mutilation in an effort to become, metaphorically speaking, Christ. The somatic manipulations that accompanied the desired abrogation, even complete negation, of physical sensation and need were an almost exclusively female phenomenon. Wounds imitating those on Christ's body appeared on the bodies of many female saints after the thirteenth century. And the bodies of these holy women were frequently seen by medieval people as exuding miraculous fluids, substances, or odors. Religious chroniclers, deeply concerned about women's effusion of extraordinary effluvia, frequently pointed out that holy women did not excrete or menstruate. Late medieval hagiographers explicitly emphasized that the menstruation of their saintly heroines had ceased. Albert the Great, for instance, noted that holy women ceased to menstruate because of their fasts and austerities.[30] Women's failure to excrete ordinary menstrual fluids was, however, explicitly associated with the emission of extraordinary sanguine liquids. "Unusual bleeding (in contrast with the ordinary bleeding of menstruation) was a sign of holiness in many of these Low Country *vitae* [biographies of Dutch and Flemish saints]. Ida of Louvain, Ida of Léau, Mary of Oignies, Lutgard, and Beatrice of Nazareth all suffered violent nosebleeds during eucharistic ecstasies, and their hagiographers saw the bleeding as a sign of mystical favors. Lutgard's various biographers report that even her hair dripped with blood when cut. [T]hey also claim, in the cases of Elizabeth of Spalbeek and Gertrude van Oosten, that the wounds bled in a periodic pattern."[31]

The popular preoccupation with miraculous fluids was directly implicated in the assertion that holy women did not excrete or menstruate. Female saints were said to exude extraordinary effluvia but to repress normal physical functions (like eating and menstrual bleeding). Such notions attest to a growing concern with the closure or "closing off" of female bodies in late medieval Europe. An account published in 1603 of Jane Balam states explicitly that this fasting girl excreted neither feces nor urine, did not menstruate, never sweated except from the armpits, discharged no filth or dandruff from her hair, and only occasionally gave forth spittle from her mouth or tears from her eyes.[32] Another case describes the unusual blood effusions of a Flemish holy woman, Lidwina of Schiedam. Like the bodies of many other women saints, Lidwina's body was closed to ordinary intake and excretion but produced extraordinary effluvia: "From mouth, ears, and nose she poured blood. And she stopped eating."[33] The fasting saint, Columba of Rieti, who died in 1501, was rumored to subsist on the eucharist alone, taking only water and bread or unripe fruit. "Attempting to prove that Columba was kept healthy by the eucharist and that her body gave no evidence that she had eaten 'heavy' food, especially meat, the biographer details her lovely smell, her failure to sweat, the purity of her fingernails, the strength of her limbs and teeth, and the beauty of her countenance."[34] As in the case of other Flemish or German holy women, Columba's asceticism was accompanied by extraordinary closure. Her hagiographer, Sebastian Perusinus, reports that she did not menstruate; he also claimed that water ran right through her when she drank and that she only occasionally eliminated a tiny bit of yellow fecal matter.[35] But no matter how closed and controlled her body was, the investigators who opened her chest five days after her death discovered around her dry heart "a stream of pure living blood."[36]

Thus in Columba's life, as in many other female lives from all over Europe, eucharistic devotion, abstinence, and self-starvation were major themes. The stories of such medieval saints were woven around the central motif of bodies: the closure and drying up of the flesh and the unusual exuding of blood. Jane Mary of Maillé, who fasted and punished her body, found blood in her mouth when she prayed for a drink from the chalice.[37] Lukardis of Oberweimar, fasting and suffering, received Christ's wounds inwardly in a vision, and afterward she induced visible stigmata by compulsively digging her fingers into her own flesh: "she drove the middle finger of each hand, hard as a nail, through the palm of the opposite hand," until the wounds bled.[38] The Flemish holy woman Beatrice of Nazareth tortured her body in extreme asceticism and ate only dry bread; but during cycles of intense prayer, "rivers of copious blood frequently poured from her mouth and nostrils."[39] Elsbet Achler, who died in 1420, received miraculous stigmata after three years of total fasting: she was unable to keep food in her stomach, and as she became sick and bedridden, her body broke out in sores that paralleled Christ's wounds; the wounds oozed blood every Friday.[40] Colette of

Corbie began to fast as a child, and imitating Christ's macerated flesh in her own body, she beat and starved herself and sometimes briefly displayed on her body the marks of Christ's crucifixion. Colette's biographer stressed that she never menstruated, "a special grace not heard of in others."[41] Although these medieval women experienced "abnormal" bleeding from nose, mouth, or stigmatic wounds, they also tried to induce the cessation of that more ordinary female bleeding that their religion regarded with contempt, and at best with ambivalence.

Thus the female body was seen as powerful in its holy or miraculous exuding of blood. Such extraordinary flowing out was predicated upon extraordinary closure: holy women were said neither to eat nor to excrete. Stigmatics were often miraculous fasters, and theologians underlined the fact that those who bled or exuded unusual fluids did not excrete in ordinary ways.[42] Women's devotional practices were not just meant to control but also to attack and punish the body. To be sure, a rejection and a negative sense of the female body clearly underlay behaviors that were directed toward shutting off menstruation, excretion, and other ordinary physical functions. But in medieval religiosity, such transfigurations were ways of fusing with a Christ whose suffering would save the world. Women's bodily changes and miraculous effusions of blood were attempts at shaping oneself to Christ and of becoming or being the suffering body on the cross. "Closing herself off to ordinary food yet consuming God in the eucharist, the holy woman became God's body. And that body flowed out, not in the involuntary effluvia of urine or menstrual blood or dandruff, but in a chosen suffering, a chosen excreting, that washed, fed, and saved the world."[43] The theology and culture of late medieval Europe taught that the redemption of all humanity lay in the fact that Christ was flesh and blood. In western Europe, during the late Middle Ages, religious women thus offered their bodies for the salvation of others in this image of Christ. Their blood became a healing effluvium that recapitulated the wounded body of Christ.

Blood as a Religious Sacrament

Religiosity in the late Middle Ages was marked by an extreme interest in physicality: the body, mortality, and flesh. This preoccupation with bodies emerged out of the late medieval concern with matter and substance and from the general sense of the body as necessary for salvation. In western Europe, Catholic doctrine proclaimed God's descent into human form, into flesh, to be a divine act of redemption: the incarnation of God's miraculous power was to save the world. The body, blood, and pain were perceived by late medieval Christians as crucial signifiers of God's mortal suffering. After the twelfth century, devotional practices were thus directed toward the recapitulation of Christ's crucifixion by immersion in experiences of the flesh: fasting, bleeding, and physical agony were used to achieve a mystical union with the suffering deity. Religious women tormented and manipulated their bodies to become the wounded man/God on the cross, their torn and broken flesh offered for the salvation of others.[44]

Late medieval asceticism was thus a profound expression of the doctrine of incarnation: the doctrine that Christ by becoming human redeemed all humankind. It arose in a religious world whose central ritual was the coming of God into physical form. In the Christian Middle Ages, divine descent into mortal flesh was a drama reenacted at every altar, during every mass, in the rite of the eucharist.[45] Medieval theologians argued that Christ's essence, through the operation of the priest's words, entered the eucharistic elements to become blood and macerated flesh. As the monk Paschasius Radbert put it in his *De corpore et sanguine domini*, in 831: "Imagine, then . . . that following the consecration [by the priest] Christ's real flesh and blood is truly created."[46] The rite of the eucharist, formerly a sacrifice of praise and a memorial of redemption, rose to prominence throughout medieval Europe. In its early form, the eucharist, this central act of the church, consisted of a single meal, a simple feast. Its basic elements, bread and wine, were not just expressions of abundance and fertility: "The central meal, the central liturgical act, was a frugal repast, evoking less the luxurious, proliferating richness of the natural world than the human life it supported. Indeed, Christ had said it *was* human life, was [his] body and blood. From the very beginning the eucharistic elements stood primarily not for nature, for grain and grape, but for human beings bound into community by commensality" (Bynum 1987: 48). From the very beginning, the elements of the eucharistic feast, bread and wine, were identified with the "body of the Lord": the suffering Christ and his redemptive sacrifice. The eucharist was understood as a commemorative ritual that required participants to feast on God's physical presence, his flesh and blood. Indeed, eating Christ's body was an inclusive act, one that created community. An early Easter hymn (fourth to sixth century) expresses this:

[We are] looking forward to the supper of the lamb . . . whose sacred body is roasted on the altar of the cross. By drinking his rosy blood, we live with God . . . Now Christ is our passover, our sacrificial lamb; His flesh, the unleavened bread of sincerity, is offered up.[47]

Or, as a slightly later Irish hymn put it:

Come, holy people, eat the body of Christ, drinking the holy blood by which you are redeemed. We have been saved by Christ's body and blood; having feasted on it, let us give thanks to God. All have been rescued from the jaws of hell by this sacrament of body and blood . . . The Lord, offered as sacrifice for us all, was both priest and victim . . . He gives the celestial bread to the hungry and offers drink from the living fountain to the thirsty.[48]

Catholic theologians saw the eucharist as a central liturgical act, a crucial feast, whose ritual focus was centered on receiving God's body in the form of bread and wine during the celebration of mass; exactly how Christ was present in the bread and wine was not a question that animated early theologians. Between the ninth and twelfth centuries, however, it became such a question. Preachers and schoolmen argued over what sorts of metaphors were acceptable for expressing the nature of God's presence. The majority clearly favored language that was frankly literal and physical. Thus when the Fourth Lateran Council (1215) stated that Christ was present in substance on the altar at the consecration, it was merely making explicit what theologians and layfolk had assumed for centuries: "There is one universal church of the faithful, outside which no one at all is saved. In this church, Jesus Christ himself is both priest and sacrifice, and his body and blood are truly contained under the appearance of bread and wine, the bread being transubstantiated into the body and the wine into the blood by the power of God."[49] In the central Christian ritual, the eucharist, God became a physical presence: when the priest celebrated mass and consecrated the elements, divinity became flesh, assumed a body.

Eleventh- and twelfth-century theologians repeatedly emphasized their conviction that God was present in the eucharist, that his entire body was present in every particle, and that both the body and the blood of Christ were present in each element. Late medieval hymns associated with Thomas Aquinas (d. 1274) reiterated this belief in the physical manifestation of Christ's presence: "The word made flesh by a word changes true bread into flesh, and wine becomes the blood of Christ."[50] "(To his disciples) he gave, under [the guise of] two consecrated elements, his flesh and blood, so that it might feed the whole man, who is of twofold substance."[51] "[Beneath the sacraments] lie hidden wonderful things. The flesh is food, the blood is drink, and yet the whole Christ remains under each offering."[52] Priests and people alike began to adore the consecrated elements. After all, one could meet Christ at the moment of his descent into the elements—a descent that paralleled and recapitulated God's incarnation: Christ appeared, substantially and totally, in the wafer (or wine) when the consecrating words were spoken.

Again and again, theologians stressed the coming of the whole Christ to the individual Christian: he or she would *see by faith* God's body and blood in the consecrated elements, in the fragment of bread or the draught of wine. Given this focus on physical experience, and in their devotion to God's body, celebrants on occasion encountered Christ's flesh and blood through private visions. Contemplating the new devotional object, the crucifix, in dim and dark churches, pious people sometimes thought it dripped blood because of their own sins.[53] During the celebration of mass, religious women often "saw" Christ himself, with his wounds exposed, all bleeding.[54] Hildegard of Bingen, a German holy woman, reported a vision in which the "image of woman"— that is, humanity—stood below the cross and received Christ's blood.[55] Catherine of Siena, like many of her holy predecessors, repeatedly received a sensation of blood in her mouth when she took communion.[56] The Flemish mystic Hadewijch had a vision in which she received, and drank, a chalice full of blood.[57] Another Flemish holy woman, Jane Mary of Maillé, was granted a vision in which Christ appeared as a young child: he displayed five wounds gushing with blood.[58] Later, while attending mass, she found blood in her mouth when she prayed for a drink from the chalice.[59] Christ offered himself to the senses of the faithful with astonishing familiarity, through visions of blood.

The perception of the consecrated bread, the host, as blood has been reported by others: John of Alverna, while celebrating mass, saw a wounded Christ appear and bleed into the chalice; when the apparition faded, John saw instead the form of the bread.[60] An English priest reported a similar occurrence: during his celebration of mass, he saw the consecrated bread, the host, turn into flesh and blood.[61] In northern Europe, Colette of Corbie, a fifteenth-century holy woman, frequently had visions of Christ before taking communion. On one occasion, she saw the Christ child on a dish, carved up like a piece of meat; afterward, as she brooded over the horrifying apparition, she knew that it represented Christ's reparation for our sins.[62] In these private visions, the physical presence of Christ insistently forced itself upon the senses of believers, experienced by them not as a phantasm but as a tangible reality (with firm boundaries), a mortal body of flesh and blood.[63]

Of Flesh and Blood

Late medieval theology was centrally concerned with the notion of "incarnation," that is, God's descent into human form and his suffering on earth. Christ had become flesh, a flesh that—by bleeding and dying— was to save the world. The eucharist (the central rite of the church) not only commemorated but also recapitulated this miraculous deed. Beginning in the late Middle Ages, Catholic doctrine insisted that Christ could be summoned into the sacrament, to take on physical substance through the act of consecration. The proliferation of eucharistic miracles of the twelfth and thirteenth centuries—in which the host, lying there on the paten, shut away in the tabernacle, or raised on high in the priest's hands, turned visibly into Christ—were not (as some have argued) the result of this doctrine of transubstantiation. Rather, as Bynum put it, "they were expressions of the sort of piety that made such doctrinal definition seem obviously true" (1987: 51). Late medieval realism insisted on the depiction of, and symbolic emphasis on, the humanation of God's divine power.[64] In the Catholic West, blood images were used and displayed as palpable proof of Christ's descent into flesh and into manhood. Such notions were recapitulated by iconographic representations (and popular visions) of the eucharist.

The conviction that God was present in the eucharist more literally than in any other sacrament is well attested by the religious raptures of a thirteenth-century Dutch recluse, Beatrice of Nazareth. In Beatrice's visions, the "eucharist becomes a cascade of blood, with which the woman's body [her own body] unites itself."[65] Such sanguine flows signified suffering but also healing and restoration. Attempting to achieve union with Christ through pain, Beatrice tortured her body "to pour out in blood" for her sisters and for humanity. Images of Christ's agonized and wounded flesh were central to Beatrice's eucharistic devotion. Indeed, throughout her monastic life, the motif of blood appeared as an important metaphor of her passion for the suffering man/God. She frequently saw visions of blood at mass. Once, when she received the sacrament and meditated on Christ's wounds, she "saw that all the blood which flowed from those wounds flooded into her heart . . . so that she was washed perfectly clean."[66] In another written piece, a meditation on the mysteries of the incarnation, her basic metaphor is drinking Christ, as rivulets, as streams, or as a mighty river. According to Beatrice: "Those who drink rivulets are those who strive for virtues; those who drink streams are those whose compassion grows in memory of the passion [crucifixion]. But highest are those who imitate and fuse with the cross, for they drink Christ himself."[67] Thus, to Beatrice, drinking Jesus' blood was both a metaphor for *imitatio Christi* and a ritual act (the reception of communion) that lay at the heart of religious practice. The female recluse, as suggested by her visions, language, and devotional practices, proceeded to divinity through a humanity that was intensely physical: inundated with the blood of Christ and her own sanguinity, she strove to fuse with the suffering god on the cross.

Eucharistic piety was at the core of medieval religious practice, and blood (as sacred sacrament) was the central metaphor. The visions of bodily encounters with Christ (conjuring up blood, wounds, bodies, flesh, mouths, and drink) reveal how much God was perceived as humanity, a humanity that suffered, nurtured, and healed. The eucharist, the central ritual with its iconography of bread and blood, provided crucial images for describing personal encounters with the physical presence of God.

Given such graphic images of divine incarnation, many pious people in the late Middle Ages developed, along with a frenzied hunger for the blood/host, an intense fear of receiving it. The notion of "eating God" (i.e., consuming/ingesting the "body of the Lord") seemed more and more audacious. But some of the devout women found that their hunger, seasoned and impelled by fear, merely intensified. In their visions, the eucharist served as a marvelously sustaining food, replacing all other nurture. For instance, the Flemish recluse Jane Mary of Maillé (d. 1414), who fasted and punished her body as part of her eucharistic devotion until she was pale and skeletal, was said to look rosy, well fed, and happy after communion, because Christ had offered himself as food.[68] Margaret, a nun from girlhood, avoided eating but craved the eucharist; her body was so "emaciated and pale" from fasting that all marveled: she went into ecstasy at communion, remaining for hours afterwards in the church and refusing ordinary food.[69] The German recluse Lukardis of Oberweimar (d. 1309) found ordinary nourishment unnecessary after she was miraculously fed by Christ during mass.[70]

Another holy woman, Alpaïs of Cudot, perceived the eucharist as nourishing and sustaining blood: unable to eat normally, she lived forty years on the eucharist alone.[71] Her Cistercian hagiographer underlined the interdependence in her life of eucharistic feast and bodily fast, of a closed and shriveled earthly body and the "fattening" ecstasies sent from heaven.[72] In his chronicle account for the year 1180, Robert of Auxerre observed that her body was "withered and thin," "but she was still fat and beautiful in her face"—not emaciated because she was truly fed by the eucharist.[73] The laywoman Dorothy of Montau (or Prussia), whose food asceticism began early, developed nausea at the sight or smell of food; she ate so little she ceased excreting and would have gone without food entirely. She was passionately devoted to the eucharist, around which her most elaborate visions and images clustered, and she developed a kind of mystical pregnancy or swelling in preparation for communion.[74] Her descriptions of eucharistic trances, written down by her confessor, John Marienwerder, not only mention sensible effects such as visions of Christ bleeding on the cross or offering a heavenly banquet; they also make it clear that she saw the agony of actual hunger for the host as a necessary preparation for the proper reception of communion and as the extension, in this life, of the pains of purgatory.[75] Despite her craving for the eucharist, she experienced overwhelming sensations of unworthiness and had to be reassured repeatedly that Christ desired her to partake of the precious food of his body. In these excruciating visions, the sacrament of "the Lord's body" was blood/flesh that nurtured as it was consumed.

Sanguine Visions

Once a communal meal that bound Christians together and fed them with the comfort of heaven, the eucharist had become an object of adoration by the thirteenth century. The physical appearance of food on the altar was in fact a veil through which holy flesh was spiritually or mystically seen. "In sermon and song, theology and story, of the high Middle Ages, . . . the food on the altar was the God who became man; it was bleeding and broken flesh. Hunger was unquenchable desire; it was suffering. To eat God, therefore, was finally to become suffering flesh with his suffering flesh; it was to imitate the cross" (Bynum 1987: 54). Exactly because the eucharist became so insistently Christ's body, his very flesh and blood, it emerged as a powerful symbol of redemption, and with it the conviction that seeing the host had spiritual value—that it was a "second sacrament," along with the receiving of communion.

Indeed, in late medieval culture, beginning in the twelfth century, the eucharist was designed by the church as the foremost sacrament: a central liturgical act, a crucial feast. It was set apart from a group of sacraments that included baptism, confirmation, and marriage. Although all sacraments issued from divine reality and were granted by the grace of God, the eucharistic feast was distinguished by virtue of Christ's presence. According to thirteenth-century theologians, "in all other sacraments Christ's power is spiritual, but in this one [the eucharist]—Christ exists corporeally . . . [as] a physical entity."[76] This unambiguous assumption of Christ's physical presence had several important consequences. As discussed earlier, given the graphic realism of God's descent into flesh, many believers both desired and feared receiving the blood/host. The reception of God as food between one's lips implied not only a promise but also a threat of physical contact with divinity. Through the consumption of the eucharistic sacrament, God could be experienced directly, in a bodily sense, and assimilated into one's own body.[77] On occasion, participation in the eucharist was accompanied by overwhelming sensations of terror and unworthiness. Margaret of Cortona, for example, pled frantically with her confessor for frequent communion but, when given the privilege, abstained out of horror at her wretchedness.[78] Gertrude the Great expressed a sense of Christ and sacrament as truly dreadful; an intense desire for the eucharist and obsessive fear of receiving it were themes throughout her writings.[79] But for all the terror the eucharist inspired, it remained a uniquely important mode of spiritual encounter. Late medieval saints, especially women,[80] frequently received from confessors, or even the pope himself, the privilege of daily communion as an almost official recognition of their sanctity. The deathbeds of pious women sometimes became the settings for bitter struggle over how the holy food could be taken. Religious superiors, bishops, and canon lawyers legislated against communal reception during ecstasy, in an effort to control the waves of frenzy for the eucharist that shook religious houses.

The claim that this ritual brought into presence Christ's own body and offered it to believers placed enormous significance on the act of consecration: one could "meet" Christ and "see" God at the instant of his descent into physical substance. Indeed, the very practice of consecration became increasingly fraught with meaning. Since Christ arrived at the moment of consecration, not of communion, he arrived in the hands of the priest before he appeared on the tongue of the individual believer.[81] Whether or not one held or tasted the wafer, one could meet Christ at the moment of his descent into the elements—a descent that paralleled the incarnation. But this conviction that God was present in the eucharist more literally than in any other sacrament, that behind the veil of grape or grain lay the substance of the body of God, raised certain problems for theologians: "How could the *totus Christus* be presented in physical elements so distressingly fluid or breakable? Would not the pious draw the conclusion (as they unquestionably did on occasion) that little bits of Jesus fell off if crumbs were spilled or that one hurt God by chewing the host?"[82] Desiring to avoid the implication that the faithful did eat little pieces of God's flesh, theologians like Thomas Aquinas affirmed that Christ's entire body was present in every particle.[83] Thus God's body could not be physically broken during the celebration of mass, even if the host was accidentally fractured. Medieval theologians also elaborated the doctrine of "concomitance," the assertion that both the flesh and blood of Christ were present in each element and in every bit of sacramental matter.[84] The whole of God's body was said to reside in the bread or in the wine as a single entity of flesh and blood. Faced with growing devotion to the sacrament iteself, exactly because the crumbs of bread and drops of wine masked the bodily substance of Christ, theologians struggled to retain a firm emphasis on "Christ's body as one, because one church and one humanity were saved in it."[85] The eucharist, a metaphor for "the sight and presence of God," retained its ritual significance as a celebration of divine incarnation.

Late medieval theologians stressed again and again the coming of the whole Christ to the eucharist: individual believers could "see" by faith the body of the Lord in the consecrated matter.[86] Early theological tractates associated with Thomas Aquinas proclaimed: "The flesh is food, the blood is drink, and yet the whole Christ remains under each species . . . Finally, when the sacrament is broken, do not doubt, but remember: there is as much hidden in a fragment as in the whole."[87] Twelfth-century theologians like Peter of Poitiers, who died in 1205, stressed that Christ was present beneath the veil of the sacrament like "a hand under a coat."[88] And Peter the Chanter went so far as to ask: "If we concede, without reservation, that the body of Christ is eaten, as Augustine says, why not say absolutely that one sees God?"[89] But he did not quite dare to answer, "yes, the faithful do literally *see* God through the elements as through a transparent veil."[90]

Many changes in piety, some coming as early as the ninth century, foreshadowed this shift in devotion toward a new focus on "seeing" and on consecration (rather than communion). Early medieval Christians had sometimes reserved the sacrament on the altar in a pyx (for carrying to the sick) and had combined it with or substituted it for relics in the consecration of churches.[91] Perhaps as early as the eleventh century, at Bec and at Canterbury, they venerated it with genuflection, incense, and procession.[92] But the cult of the sacrament, of devotion to the consecrated host itself, did not really begin until the twelfth century, although it then developed rapidly. The containers, pyxes, and reliquaries in which the host was reserved became more and more elaborate, both to protect God's body from profanation and to allow the faithful to adore it outside the mass.[93] Lamps and candles were burned before it.[94] The performance of the eucharist was not to be witnessed in darkness: "The essence of the rite lay in seeing the host and so candles were part of any scheme of veneration; bearing warmth and illumination into the dark chancels of medieval European churches, they were essential at the moment when the holiest appeared. Lighting was provided for illumination as long as consecrated hosts were kept in the church, as well as for the duration of the mass, and additional lights were required during the elevation" (Rubin 1991: 53–63). Small, usually circular openings (*oculi*) were placed in the exterior wall of the apse, so that the pious could look directly into the eucharist chest and venerate the host from outside the church.[95] Late medieval chroniclers described scenes of people trying to gain a glimpse of the host through holes in church walls, on occasion even breaking a window to improve their view.[96] Perhaps as early as the ninth century, recluses had their cells in churches positioned so they could adore the host each day.[97] Visits to the host began in the twelfth century, and some theologians suggested that such visits might substitute for going on a crusade.[98] After the twelfth century, the issue of visual access to the host became even more pressing than that of communion, which in any case was experienced far less frequently.

In the mass itself, communion and consecration were increasingly separated, and the elements were treated with heightened awe. Communion was given before, after, or completely apart from mass. Monks and nuns might go to the high altar; layfolk usually received at the side altar, where the sacrament was sometimes placed beforehand. Women had been prohibited since the days of the early church from receiving in their bare hands.[99] From the ninth century, women and laymen usually received communion directly on the tongue. By the eleventh century, only priests could take God in their hands.[100] The rhythm of the service and the liturgical practices surrounding it rendered the eucharist more awesome, magical, and remote.

As the physical encounter or union with God's body became increasingly problematic, pious people insisted on "seeing" the host. A gesture of elevation came to mark the moment of consecration: after the priest had uttered the necessary words, he raised the consecrated element so that the host/body could be adored. This ritual gesture provided a sort of substitute "sacramental viewing," which (like communion) was taught to confer general well-being.[101] The sight of the host, marking the moment of God's descent into flesh, became a source of health, prosperity, and power.

The first evidence for the elevation of the host after consecration comes from about 1200.[102] In his synodal statues, Odo of Sully, bishop of Paris from 1196 to 1208, required his priests to elevate the host; this requirement existed in the Cistercian order before 1210.[103] The practice spread rapidly, and with it the conviction that seeing the host had great spiritual value. Prayers were composed for the moment of "seeing," honored by the ringing of bells, genuflection, and incense.[104] By the thirteenth century, we find stories of people attending mass only for the moment of elevation, racing from church to church to see as many consecrations as possible and shouting at the priest to hold the host up higher.[105] An account even survives of guild members bringing charges against a priest for assigning them places in church from which they could not see the elevated host.[106] When John Marienwerder, Dorothy of Montau's confessor, wrote his account of her visions and teachings, he especially emphasized the saint's devotion to "seeing" Christ: "And if she managed to view it a hundred times in one day, as sometimes happened, she still retained the desire to view it more often."[107]

The cult of the eucharist was fully established by the late thirteenth century, with the institution in 1264 of the feast of Corpus Christi.[108] "The feast made little headway at first, in part because some argued that a special festival for Christ's body might imply less reverence for it at every mass. But after . . . 1317, it spread rapidly. In the fourteenth century, 'showing' was separated entirely from the mass, with the introduction of the monstrance, a special vessel for displaying the consecrated wafer. The host was now carried uncovered in procession on Corpus

Christi and left exposed on the altar for adoration . . . By the fifteenth century certain feasts ended with the exposition and benediction of the blessed sacrament" (Bynum 1987: 55). The cult of the host/body was promoted with particular intensity in central Europe. There, after 1400, eucharistic processions became so common that legislation was established to bring the eucharist back into church. German and Bohemian councils ordered that the eucharist be shown only on Corpus Christi and for the duration of the festival.[109] In 1451, the council of Mainz criticized the custom as detracting from the reverence owed to the divine sacrament of Christ, and "lets the people's devotion cool down due to frequent viewing . . . from [now] on that sacrament shall not be carried visibly in monstrances except on the octave of Corpus Christi, and even then only during the divine office of that octave."[110] The council of Cologne in 1452 decreed: "And for the sake of the great honour of the holy sacrament we ordain that from now on that holy sacrament will never be put or carried visibly in any monstrances, except on the feast of Corpus Christi . . . once a year in every city or town."[111]

Such explicit legislation emerged in areas where the showing of God's body had become most frequent. In Germany, for instance, we witness a nearly permanent exposition of the host in processions and on the altar.[112] Despite attempts to curb the frenzy of devotion, pious people persisted in their demand that Christ's body be shown in every parish and every neighborhood. In the Low Countries, Bohemia, and Germany, where this practice of exposition was especially lively, a particularly flamboyant type of church architecture was developed, the *Sakramentenhaus*:[113] an elaborate gothic tower, a gabled structure, complete with steps and railings, in which the eucharist was kept but also exposed.

Display of the chalice, which contained the sacred blood, emerged more slowly. The showing or elevation of a vessel full of Christ's blood posed a danger: it was open to spillage, accidental loss, and profanation. The precious blood was deemed more fragile, more easily corruptible, than the solid body (wafer), the fleshly host. Indeed, by the late thirteenth century, the drink of God's blood was permanently withdrawn; its consumption became the exclusive privilege of priests.[114] The desire to protect the sacred blood limited its integration into the ritual of the mass. Eucharistic devotion to Christ's blood surfaced elsewhere, in the Low Countries and Germany, among woman mystics and female saints. The feasts of the Sacred Heart and Precious Blood were established only in modern times. But the roots of these festivals go back to the intense devotion to Christ's blood found among the Saxon nuns and Flemish holy women of the thirteenth century.[115] And, as we will see, late medieval texts were awash in references to "the blood of the lamb," a eucharistic metaphor. It is not surprising, therefore, that blood became an

ever more common and insistent symbol, both of salvation and of violation, during the later Middle Ages.

Blood, Body, Wounds

Thirteenth-century preoccupations with "seeing" the sacrament (God's
blood and body) were closely related to a fascination with the redemptive promise of the suffering Christ: his sacrifice on the cross (signified
by wounds, blood, and pain) and his becoming food on the altar. Such
a fusion of eucharistic metaphors surfaced in late medieval Germany,
where vernacular references to the feast of Corpus Christi relied on
visions of blood: "Day of the holy blood" (*der heilige Blutstag*; *des hilghen
blodes daghe*; *des hl. pluets tag*) and "The feast of the body and blood of the
Son of God, Jesus Christ" (*festum* [*dies*] *corporis et sanguinis D.N.J. Chr*).[116]
The suffering that Christ endured was recapitulated, and rendered tangible, through images of blood effusion. Such a focus on the blood motif
suggests an insertion of eucharistic symbolism into the iconography of
divine humanation: Christ's wounded flesh was offered up on the altar
to redeem the world.[117]

The exposition of Christ's bleeding wounds had symbolic significance.
The man/God revealed his wounds to chosen holy women—Ida of Louvain, Catherine of Siena, and Julian of Norwich in 1373—just as he
offered them his body in private communion.[118] This theme was captured in a thirteenth-century painting in which Christ shows his wounds
while offering a consecrated host to a group of nuns.[119] In these visions,
the eucharist becomes the suffering Christ, the man/God on the cross,
who bleeds and offers himself, "who beckons through identification,
who opens his body to the rising mystic" (Rubin 1991: 317). The interest
in Christ's wounds thus operated in a variety of ways. For late medieval men and women, the wounds were literally an entry into Christ,
with whom they wished to be united. According to Thomas à Kempis, a fourteenth-century mystic (and hagiographer), the wounds were
a "refuge," a point of escape into redemption: "Rest in Christ's passion,
and live willingly in His holy wounds. If indeed you escape into Jesus'
precious wounds and stigmata, you will sense great comfort in your
tribulation."[120]

In late medieval iconography, blood and wounds became a source of
"immersion in God," a joining with Christ that could be achieved by
taking communion—by eating the eucharist. The eucharist, the sacred
food on the altar, was God's blood and broken flesh. It was the suffering Christ who died on the cross. As Richard Poore put it in 1217, "that
which [we] receive under the species of bread, is without doubt that
which hung on the cross for us, and what [we] receive in the chalice,

that which flowed from Christ's side." [121] Late medieval theologians, like Peter of Poitiers, clearly expressed the view that after the priest's consecration, the "body [of Christ] was full in flesh and blood, *the historic body* which suffered on the cross." [122] To eat God, therefore, was finally to become suffering flesh with his suffering flesh; taking communion was to imitate the cross. And "seeing" the host—the wounded Christ—was clearly experienced as a source of healing and restoration.

According to late medieval theology, exposition of the eucharist offered a "spiritual communion" that was achieved through a fervent viewing, even without tasting, of Christ. [123] As early as 1222, the Franciscan monk Alexander of Hales proposed that a visual contemplation of the eucharist, although not a "tasting" or *smackyng* of the host—the body of God—was clearly an "eating by sight." [124] Sight, as a sense experience, permitted the interiorization of Christ. Fourteenth-century theologians echoed similar notions. In his work on Christ, the preacher Ludolf of Saxony (d. 1377) explicitly assimilated "eating" to "seeing": "Nonetheless, you shall come daily to see Jesus in the spiritual fold [i.e., the host], which is on the altar, so that you may be replenished with the nourishment (grain) of his flesh by the holy spirit." [125] A merging or joining into God's wounded body could thus be effected through a pious viewing of the eucharist, the consecrated host, on the altar.

In Western Christian culture, the motif of blood thus assumed an essential symbolic function. Images of blood, especially depictions of Christ's wounded body, proclaimed God's humanity and affirmed that godhood had vested itself in the infirmity of the flesh. Christ's wounds were adored in formal liturgy, with prayer, devotion, and appropriate indulgences. [126] Often uttered after consecration, at the moment of the host's elevation, the salutations were directed at Christ's physical presence: "You noble, blessed, precious, rose-colored blood, . . . You untainted, powerful blood, . . . You invigorating, warming, beatifying blood, . . . dear blood, sweet blood, . . . You blood full of mercy, have pity on us." [127] In this fifteenth-century invocation, as in other German liturgical prayers, the blood streaming from Christ's wounds was praised as a source of all that was good:

O holy blood of our hope/ sustain us.
O holy blood: a true salvation for the sick/ heal us.
O holy blood: an alleviation for hearts of stone/ soften us.
O holy blood: a well of grace/ moisten us.
O holy blood: a source of love/ give us warmth.
O holy blood: an ocean of mercy/ pour over us.
O holy blood: a remedy for the spiritual composition/ purify us.
O holy blood: a payment for sin and guilt/ settle us.
O holy blood: a eulogy for the aged and weak/ refresh us.

O holy blood: a life for the dead/ awaken us.
O holy blood: a salvation for the prisoners/ redeem us.
O holy blood: a refuge for sinners/ help us.
O holy blood: strength and perfection of the blood-sacrifice/ renew us.
O holy blood, sweet blood:
O precious blood of Christ/ remain with us forever.[128]

Such visions of the suffering Christ and his descent into flesh and blood were experienced by pious people as a source of renewal or healing. In Germany, as elsewhere in northern Europe, these devotional salutations found their way into private books of prayer.[129] There, such written meditations on Christ's wounds were often accompanied by appropriate pictures of open gashes and effusions of blood. Popular interest in these wounds thus produced iconographic visions that were as explicit as those of theology: both derived from a preoccupation with the redemptive meanings of the suffering Christ.[130]

Masses dedicated to the wounds first appear in the fourteenth century, when the interest in Christ's wounded flesh developed into a special devotion and, further, a feast.[131] This feast was encouraged by papal bulls in the fifteenth century with the grant of a seven years' indulgence to those gazing at, wearing, or kissing a representation of the wound, the *mensura vulneris*: King Henry VI had such a picture of Christ's wounds at his bedside.[132] Once established in formal liturgy and prayer, the eucharistic meanings of blood began to thrive within a wide range of devotional practices that placed increasing emphasis on experience — on tasting, seeing, and meeting God.

After the twelfth century, blood became an altogether more complex and ambivalent symbol. Blood was life itself, coursing through Christ's veins, leaping forth from his violated side. It was a purging bath. It was bloodshed, the palpable sign of attack on God. Association with blood, a powerful symbol of salvation as well as of violation, was therefore fraught with much significance. Devotion to Christ's wounds drew attention to the violence done to Christ's body; yet graphic visions of his tortured flesh served to promote health and general well-being. Throughout the fifteenth century, in crudely drawn diagrams on amulets, pictures of the wounds were represented in every possible way: five wounds in a semicircle, or the single wound of each limb depicted separately and uniquely side by side.[133] Particularly privileged in its eucharistic and sacrificial overtones was the side wound, the gash made by the lance, which was usually shown gushing with blood.[134] The wounds were recorded and incorporated in acts of writing, measuring, wearing, and eating.[135] Pious people began to carry images of the wounds on a piece of parchment hanging from their necks, as amulets and as remedies.[136] An amulet containing a "measure" of Christ's wounds was expected to stop the flow of blood by appealing to Longinus, the Roman soldier: "Longinus: who pierced the side and had blood flow—I dare you—in the name of Jesus Christ, so that the blood of Margery will stop flowing."[137] A little parchment roll, traced to the fifteenth century, served as an amulet by virtue of a drawing of the cross and nails and wounds; it bore an inscription of the name of Jesus to which appeal was made for protection.[138] The drawing not only symbolized but also reproduced the scene of crucifixion, a sort of sacramental gesture. In a fifteenth-century amulet roll, the cross was drawn to scale, protecting its wearer from "sudden death" and "injury by weapons."[139] During the fifteenth century, even the blood drops oozing from Christ's wounds became subject to speculation, attention, and scrutiny.[140] Metaphors, images, and similes of Christ's bleeding flesh, although treated with devotion and pity, were tested for efficacy by people in search of protection. Christ's body became a sought-after property, whose approximate dimensions, measurements, and representation to scale could be used in late medieval efforts at healing.

Such attempts to harness, in a symbolic sense (and with iconographic means), the miraculous power of God's humanation were coupled with the treatment of blood as a relic. After the eleventh century, Catholic doctrine encouraged the search for remnants of Christ's physical body. There was some speculation that the blood of Christ's crucifixion had been preserved by those who had witnessed his death: Mary (his mother), Mary Magdalene (sister of Martha and Lazarus), Joseph of Arimathaea, Nicodemus, even Longinus, the Roman soldier.[141] In the twelfth century, bits of God's blood were miraculously discovered in small vials or reliquaries like a bottle or a cross. These pieces of the incarnate Christ, according to various tales, had been brought from Palestine to Europe, where they were cared for by pious people.[142] Adored in shrines and at popular sites of pilgrimage, or worn in amulets and medallions, the sacred blood effected the recovery of the sick and offered protection.[143] These blood relics, which were found to have medicinal value, functioned as curatives and inhibitors of disease.

The act of God's descent into human form held a promise of restoration: from Christ's suffering body issued salvation; from his blood issued redemption. It was body as flesh that God became most graphically on the altar. And it was through suffering in human form that Christ restored the world. The blood motif essentialized these notions in powerful ways by conflating the incarnation (and God's crucified body) with the symbolism of the eucharist. The recluse Columba of Rieti (d. 1501) took comfort from such a vision: she saw Jesus hanging on the cross above a chalice (which brimmed with his blood).[144] At the very end of the Middle Ages we find another fitting representation in an emblem of a Corpus Christi fraternity, showing an inscribed host above a chalice framed by two wounded hands and two wounded feet.[145] The theme of the eucharist as suffering Christ, as broken flesh, had become a common iconographic motif of late medieval piety.

Christ's Broken Flesh

During the later Middle Ages, in the twelfth and thirteenth centuries, the emphasis of devotion in hymn, sermon, and story was less on the "bread of heaven" than on flesh, meat, and blood. To eat (or see) God was to take into one's self the suffering body on the cross. Christ's crucifixion, and his limitless pain, were acts of redemption that would save humanity. God's incarnation, his descent into agonized (mortal) flesh, was a miraculous deed that promised to heal the world. Not surprisingly, Western Christianity promoted forms of eucharistic piety that established the blood (wound) motif at the center of religious worship. As Bynum (1987) observed, "exactly because the host became so insistently Christ's body—whose firm outlines had been violated by Roman (or Jewish) spears and nails—it remained a powerful corporate symbol, a symbol of humankind, of Christendom, and of the church" (61–62). Twelfth-century theologians explained that the body on the altar was Christ interceding for us; it was the physical body, born of Mary; it was also the mystical body, representing the church.[146] Indeed, late medieval eucharistic devotion, paralleling the theological discussions of Christ's physical presence in the sacrament, "came to express an almost frantic sense of the wholeness, the inviolability, of Christ's body, and a tremendous fear of rending and breaking" (Bynum 1987: 63). An index of exempla in medieval religious tales lists fifty-three miracles having to do with the host and only three concerning the chalice.[147] It is hard to avoid the conclusion that this emphasis on the inviolability of the host—the body of Christ—reflected a fear that the mystical (religious) body, the church, would be rent by its enemies.

Late medieval theologians and visionaries came to see in Christ as bleeding flesh not only the redemption of humankind but also an entity under attack. Twelfth- and thirteenth-century iconographies of Christ's blood, wounds, and pain were thus closely linked and often fused with fears of violation. The many miracles of consecrated wafers oozing or streaming drops of blood were understood to be announcing not just the sins of individual Christians but also attacks by outsiders, especially heretics and Jews.[148] The corporeal implications of late medieval eucharistic symbolism were thus at least in part defensive.

Miracles of bleeding Hosts, which proliferate from the twelfth century on, often had sinister overtones: the host became flesh to announce its violation; the bleeding was an accusation.[149] When the nun Wilburgis took the host to her enclosure to help her avoid sexual temptation, it revealed itself, in a quite common miracle, as a beautiful baby who spoke the words of the Song of Songs.[150] But when another nun hid a host that she dared not swallow because she was in mortal sin, it turned into flesh.[151] The second miracle sounds a threatening note not present in the first. In a comparable case, a sinful woman "kept the Lord's body in her mouth" for use of magic and found that it had turned into flesh that stuck to her palate.[152] Similarly, Peter Damian tells of a host that protested its abuse when used superstitiously: a woman who tried to conjure with it found that half of it had turned into flesh.[153] In the fourteenth century, Caesarius of Heisterbach reports that when another woman tried to use the consecrated wafer as a love charm and then guiltily hid it in a church wall, it turned to flesh and bled.[154]

The eucharist announced its presence, when profaned or secreted away, by leaving a trail of blood. When the nun from Sent (in the German Alps) received communion with doubts in her heart, she could not swallow the host and hid it under her veil:[155] after taking the host to her cell at the convent, she saw that this consecrated sacrament had turned into flesh and blood. Horrified, she revealed her observations to a local priest. Surprised by the miraculous vision, he secretly took the sacrament to his church, pledging to devote his life to the bleeding host. But after the host had been transported to the church, it transformed itself again, appearing first as a bloody hand, then in turn an arm, a man's bleeding face, a lamb, and, last, a piece of bloody flesh. When these visions were made known to the abbess of the order, she requested that the bleeding host be returned to the convent. There it was revered until the eighteenth century.

In these miraculous visions, the appearance of blood was an accusation that announced a breach or transgression. The priest of Herckenrode (Limburg), offering last communion to a dying man, witnessed how the host began to bleed profusely when touched by a layperson.[156] After a fire destroyed the church of Wilsnack (c. 1383), the local priest assumed that the three consecrated hosts, which he had hidden inside the altar, had been consumed by the flames. Yet when he searched the premises, he found the wafers unharmed, although tinted with blood.[157] The three miraculous hosts, which were discovered intact but bleeding, were kept in a crystal and shown to pilgrims who streamed to the site as to the site of any other great relic.[158]

Unusual visions of blood not only exposed a ritual breach or violation but also attested to the presence of Christ in the eucharist. The message was clear: the host was God's body and blood; its fracture or profanation also wounded the body of Christ. The tale of the miraculous blood of Walldürn, dating back to the early fourteenth century, offers explicit documentation.[159] According to the legend, a priest, while celebrating mass, accidentally tipped over the chalice, spilling its consecrated contents. The wine/blood poured out over the white corporal and stained it bright red. With dismay the priest noticed how the image of the crucified Christ, surrounded by eleven additional heads of Jesus, gradually took form in the middle of the cloth. The terrified priest at first tried to hide the cloth but then revealed his vision.

The church of Walldürn became a popular site of pilgrimage during the fourteenth, fifteenth, and sixteenth centuries, and an assortment of devotional images recapitulated the blood miracle. A German reproduction of the bloodstained cloth showed the image of the crucified Christ in its center. A representation of eleven heads of Jesus appeared below the sides of the cross, each crowned by a pelican. An inscription stated: *Abbildung des / H. Blutes von Waldthurn / im Reich* ("Representation of / the holy blood of Walldürn / in the empire"). A prayer devoted to the blood of Christ appeared in print on the right side: "O merciful pelican. Lord Jesus / Christ; cleanse my impure / heart with your blood."[160] Another famous reproduction appeared in the seventeenth century, patterned after an image released in 1674 by Andreas Eisenhut, a local priest from Walldürn. It shows the corporal with the chalice and Christ's spilled blood: the cloth is held up by four angels. Above hovers a dove, a symbol of the Holy Spirit. The bottom half of the picture shows pious people with rosaries and two angels carrying devotional flags. These are depictions of pilgrims making their way toward the city, which is shown on the right of the painting.

In Europe, during the late Middle Ages, eucharistic miracles were explicitly seen as vindications of orthodox doctrine and as evidence that Christ was truly present in the elements. After the eleventh century, preachers embellished their sermons with stories of bleeding hosts.[161] Several thirteenth-century theologians, including the hagiographer James of Vitry, supported the increasing frenzy of women's eucharistic piety as a counter to the heretical denial that God could be present in matter.[162] The proliferation of eucharistic miracles in the late Middle Ages, in which the host turned visibly into Christ, were expressions of the sort of piety that made such doctrinal definitions seem obviously true.[163] A thirteenth-century German mystic, Christina of Stommeln, doubted that consecration transformed the host truly into the very body and blood of Christ until she saw a child in the celebrant's hands.[164] When Gregory the Great was conducting mass, a woman in the congregation chuckled before the reception of communion. When he asked her how dare she laugh, she answered that she herself had baked the bread: how could she believe that God resided in it? Gregory prayed for a sign, and this came in the form of a bleeding finger.[165] In another, somewhat threatening blood miracle, a priest recounted to his bishop, Hugh of Lincoln, how, when he celebrated mass after committing a mortal sin, the host turned into flesh and blood, freezing him with fear. When the priest broke the host in three before consuming it, "[i]mmediately blood began to flow copiously through the break, and the middle part of the host which I held in my hand suddenly took on the appearance of flesh and became blood-red."[166] He dared not communicate but was moved to confess his sin, do penance, and receive absolution.

The sudden effusion of blood from the sacrament offered uncontestable evidence of God's bodiliness and physical presence. When an honest German priest (while doubting the reality of the eucharist) celebrated mass, he saw the consecrated bread as true flesh, inundated with blood: drops of this blood fused to form the bleeding face of Christ on the chalice.[167] Another priest was conducting mass when doubts began to stir in his heart: doubting in this way, he completed the consecration and saw blood rising in the chalice.[168] Similarly a tale from the fifteenth century tells of a priest who celebrated mass in spite of his lack of faith; during his act of consecration, blood began to foam over the edge of the chalice onto the paten, thereby reforming the skeptic.[169] When Hieronymus Wild visited the site of the holy blood in 1609, Christ revealed himself through a series of visions: a bloodstained child, an infant exposing his wounds, and a blood-drenched male torso.[170] Despite the aura of awe or majesty that surrounded the eucharist in the later Middle Ages, it seemed to the faithful to offer itself to their senses with astonishing familiarity. It rang with the music of song, glowed with light, dissolved on the tongue into flesh, and announced its presence by sanguine visions. Christ appeared again and again in the host and the chalice, as a baby, a glorious youth, or a bleeding and dying man (i.e., the various manifestations of the incarnate God).

Jews appear in these stories in their traditional role as witnesses to the faith: they are confronted with a miracle and thus compelled to accept conversion, sometimes in groups. A classic story is that of the mass of St. Basil in which a Jew enters a church and sees, instead of the host, a child torn asunder: the Jew was convinced of the truth of Christianity and converted.[171] But Jews were increasingly associated with vicious and willful attacks against the host.[172] These accusations of sacramental violation surfaced just when the theological interpretation of Jewish culpability in the crucifixion of Jesus was being rethought by late medieval thinkers.

After the doctrine of transubstantiation had been promulgated the wafers of the host assumed a far more awesome power. They were synonymous with the body of Christ, and it was easy to endow them with fleshly attributes . . . Theft of the wafers became sacrilegious, even demonic. When some of them were seen to bleed . . . the conclusion that they had been tortured was almost inevitable . . . Christians lept to the conclusion that the Jews, who had hated Christ and cruci-fied him, were responsible . . . [L]ess than forty years after the council of 1215, there . . . [began] an epidemic hysteria that was to last well over two centuries. (Tannahill 1975: 60–61)

Such stories of abuse (which proliferated in the thirteenth century) tell of a Jew or a group of Jews who procured a host, often through a Christian maid or a debtor, and attacked it with knives, axes, and fire: "The host bled, and survived all manner of attack; finally, the Jew was led to execution, the miraculous host was revered, a chapel built in its honour, and processions, hymns and memorials created for it" (Rubin 1991: 126). In a 1293 variant, several Jews talked a Christian servant girl into bringing them a consecrated wafer.[173] After they received it, they began to torture it, eventually throwing the host into boiling water. In-stantly, the water became blood red, rising up in the kettle, flooding the kitchen and the well. The red stream poured into the hallway and, after inundating it completely, burst into the street, revealing the attack on the host/body of Christ. The act of defilement was punished severely: the young maid was decapitated, and the Jews were burned. From the late thirteenth century on, Jews were frequently charged with violating the host, which announced the abuse by miraculous bleeding. Lionel Rothkrug (1979) has emphasized this connection between eucharistic devotion and anti-Semitism. In the years before 1350, many Jews were murdered for the alleged desecration of the host.[174]

The Fractured Body

Frightful images of carnage and wounding were an integral part of late medieval religiosity. The eucharist was the suffering flesh of the man/God who had died on the cross. This violated body, God's gift of re-demption, was offered up as food on the altar. Fearful visions of God's macerated flesh were thus implicit in the belief that godhood was em-bodied in the eucharist. Eating the consecrated bread during commu-nion was a potential assault on the integrity of Christ's physical form.

God's body was broken and fractured by chewing the host, a notion made explicit by the following oath from 1056: "[T]he bread and wine . . . on the altar are after the consecration . . . the true body of our Lord Jesus Christ, and they are physically taken up and broken in the hands of the priest and crushed by the teeth of the faithful."[175] As suggested by this oath, which was forced upon the (quasi) heretic Berengar of Tour, the belief in God's physical presence raised critical concerns for late medieval theologians: how to prevent the breakage, spillage, and profanation of the "body of the Lord"?

The consecrated host, this special food—Christ's very body—was a small and fragile object: round, white, and thin, it was often inscribed with a cross, a crucifixion scene, or the lamb of God.[176] In the early twelfth century, the host began to be stamped with pictures of Christ rather than the simple monograms common earlier.[177] White, shimmering, made of unleavened bread (because it adhered more easily to the tongue), and embossed with the image of Christ, the host seemed magical but also vulnerable and frail. Exacting protection from abuse, fracture, and decay, every aspect of the host's appearance was deemed important. The bishop of Sodor in the Isle of Man, William Russell, explained the symbolism of the host's features in 1350: "The wheaten host should be round and whole and without blemish, like the lamb . . . who has not had a bone removed from it. Hence the verse: Christ's host should be clean, wheaten, thin, not large, round, unleavened. It is inscribed, not cooked in water but baked in fire." [178] By the thirteenth century, a whole set of regulations emerged to control the making, keeping, and disposal of the sacraments.[179] English synods, for example, like the Canterbury Council of 1213, explained how the sacramental matter was to be processed: "[We stipulate] that the eucharist be reserved in a clean pyx, and consecrated hosts be kept for seven days, and renewed every week on Sunday, so that after the reception of the newly consecrated host and before the reception of the Lord's blood, the reserved [old] hosts [can] be consumed by the celebrant." [180]

Concerns about mishandling the body of God were intensified by fears of the physical functions whereby the eucharist was consumed. Indeed, twelfth-century theologians like Thomas Aquinas proposed that perhaps Christ's body was not really eaten by believers: "Whatever is eaten as under its natural form, is broken and chewed as under its natural form. But the body of Christ is not eaten under its natural form, but under the guise of the sacramental species [i.e., bread or wine]." [181] Moreover, the question of digestion was related to the process of eating the host: chewing, digestion, and excretion were perceived as degradations that should not be allowed to work on the holy substance.[182] The taking of communion, receiving God as food between one's lips, inspired awe as well as apprehension. There was the perpetual danger of spilling crumbs of his flesh, of swallowing him in little pieces, or of hurting him by chewing the host.

This terror of the accidental fracture of the body of Jesus is well documented among pious women and late medieval Christians generally: to eat was to consume, to take in, to become God; and to eat was also to rend and tear God. Yet it was only by bleeding, by being torn and broken, by dying, that God's body redeemed humanity. The food on the altar was thus for all Christians a symbol of suffering and maceration, of a flesh that healed by being broken. But blood (and bleeding flesh) was also bloodshed, the palpable sign of attack on God.

Whereas earlier theological doctrines had seen the eucharist (the bread of heaven) as a symbol of Christ's church precisely because the grains of wheat were gathered into a whole, later medieval visionaries saw in Christ as bleeding flesh the redeemer or healer *and* an entity under attack. And however powerfully that entity sometimes suggested the Christian commmunity, either united in love or violated by enemies, it was basically not a corporate symbol at all. The bread on the altar was the suffering flesh of the man/God who died; the blood that poured from the broken body fed and cleansed the individual Christian. And although themes of violation and bodily harm (the rending and breaking of God's body) were sometimes reconstituted to function as metaphors for larger social bodies—that is, humanity, the church, the community of faithful—such images did not work to unify or assemble.

God's broken body, offered up as food in the eucharist, came to mark identities and boundaries precisely because late medieval eucharistic piety had become increasingly individualistic—focused on personal suffering and experience. Thus when Gertrude the Great made the eucharistic host into many crumbs in her mouth, thinking that each particle stood for a soul in the flames of purgatory, she seemed to be equating the crumbliness of bread not with the unity of Christians (as did earlier theologians) but with their individualness, their separateness, their suffering.[183] Gertrude, who often feared to take communion, was aware of the audacity of thus violating the integrity of the body of God.[184] A similar note of warning appeared in a vision of crumbs received by Francis of Assisi. When he was ordered to gather up the crumbs and make them into one host for the brethren, he also saw in a vision that those brothers who did not receive the gift devoutly were afflicted with leprosy.[185] The joining of "fine crumbs" into one host here symbolized unity, but the host stood for an interior state of faith, and those who experienced it improperly were made ill by it.[186] Since the requirement of worthy reception could rarely be tested by external signs, it was difficult to enforce. Stories proliferated, therefore, about the consequences of undeserving reception, reflecting the fear that God's body might be breached by unworthiness or heresy.

Illness, leprosy, and even death were the punishments imposed upon those who received God's body in a state of sin. The German recluse Hildegard of Bingen, who died in 1179, had a vision in which the communicants approaching the altar were transformed into five categories: those shining in purity and with souls of fire; those with pale bodies and dark souls; those with rough and hairy bodies and dirty souls; others who looked as if surrounded by thorns with souls emaciated by leprosy; and, finally, those dripping blood with souls that smelled like decaying corpses.[187] The broken body of Christ, the bleeding host, while a symbol of unity, also served to demarcate and exclude.

Female Hunger for Blood

In late medieval Europe, the blood/flesh/body motif became an ever more common and insistent symbol of power and privilege. This was made evident by the growing number of restrictions that governed access to the eucharist. As noted earlier, by the eleventh century, only priests could take God in their hands: both women and laymen usually received the host directly on the tongue.[188] There seems to have been a tacit acceptance that menstruating women should abstain from communion.[189] It was understood that the reception of communion must follow confession and be "taken in purity." The enormity of undeserving reception of Christ's body was thus made increasingly clear.[190] In the twelfth and thirteenth centuries, the drink of Christ's blood was withheld entirely.[191] Thomas Aquinas justified the withholding of the cup (chalice), the "blood of the Lord," by pointing out that the priest received both elements, for the sake of the laity.[192] The theory that the priest received for the people was elaborated gradually: "Otto of Bamberg said that the converted Pomeranians should communicate through their priest if they could not receive themselves. Berthold of Regensburg explained that the communicating priest "nourishes us all," for he is the mouth and we are the body. William Durandus the Elder suggested that the faithful receive three times a year "because of sinfulness" but "priests [receive] daily for us all." Ludolf of Saxony argued that the eucharist is called "our daily bread because ministers receive it daily for the whole community." [193] Not only was the priest the channel through which God descended, he was also seen as assimilated to Christ (or the Virgin Mary) in the act of consecration. He was seen as "deified" at the moment in which God arrived between his hands, when he touched or held the precious flesh/blood/body. An often-cited twelfth-century text thus reads: "Oh revered dignity of priests, in whose hands the Son of God is incarnated as in the Virgin's womb." [194] The priest became the spiritual "womb" that "birthed" the incarnate God during the rite of the eucharist. Francis of Assisi expressed the same awe of priests in the early thirteenth century: "If it is right to honour the Blessed Virgin Mary because she bore him in her most holy womb; if St. John the Baptist trembled and was afraid even to touch Christ's sacred head; if the tomb where he lay for only a short time is so venerated; how holy, and virtuous, and worthy should not a priest be; he touches Christ with his own hands . . . A priest receives him into his heart and mouth and offers him to others to be received."[195] Contact with Christ's blood (and body) was thus seen as a sanctifying act, clearly perceived by medieval theologians as a clerical prerogative.

The increased determination by the Western church to withhold the cup (the blood) from the laity thus may have had a deeper reason than the one usually cited, fear of profanation through spillage. According to Bynum (1987), the direct association of the laity with such a powerful symbol of violation as well as of salvation may have carried too much significance. The push, and demand, by some thirteenth-century theologians for communion in both elements (i.e., God's body and blood) was probably deemed to be a dangerous (and threatening) democratization of an extraordinarily potent and complex metaphor: blood.

As the role of the clergy became exalted, the gap between priest and people widened. By the late Middle Ages in northern Europe, elaborate screens were constructed to hide the priest and the altar.[196] Thus, at the pivotal moment of his coming, Christ was separated and hidden from the congregation in a sanctuary that enclosed together priest and God. In a certain way, the priest (not the eucharist) was the powerful corporate symbol of late medieval Christendom: he was the "mouth" of the church. But he also was the "body" of the church by consuming Christ's blood: he received for all. Certain twelfth-century texts suggested that insofar as the priest was the "womb" within which Christ was consecrated, he stood for all humanity.

In such an atmosphere, marked by an increasing awe of blood, body, and priest, a deep ambivalence developed about the reception of communion. On the one hand, theologians and canon lawyers encouraged frequent communion. The requirement of at least yearly confession and communion, established at the Fourth Lateran Council (1215), was intended to set forth a minimum of observance. And a number of new monastic orders required frequent communion. But on the other hand, theologians feared that frequent reception might lead to loss of reverence, to carelessness, even to profanation of the elements. Albert the Great, for example, who supported the practice of daily communion, argued against it for women, fearing frequent reception would trivialize their response.[197] Faced with such ambiguous advice, many pious people (particularly women) in the later Middle Ages developed, along with an intense fear of receiving the host, a frenzied hunger or thirst for Christ's blood, a desire "felt in mind, soul, and entrails."[198] Indeed, as the moment of consecration became increasingly burdened with meaning, as the power of priests grew ever more awesome, as the notion of eating God seemed more and more audacious and the drink of Christ's blood was permanently withdrawn, some of the devout found that their hunger, seasoned and impelled by fear, merely intensified. Descriptions of the eucharistic piety of Mary of Oignies attest to these experiences: "The holy bread strengthened her heart; the holy wine inebriated her, rejoicing her mind; the holy body fattened her; the vitalizing blood purified her by washing. And she could not bear to abstain from such solace for long. For it was the same to her . . . [as] to die, to be separated from the sacrament by having for a long time to abstain . . . she was not able to bear any longer her thirst for the vivifying blood."[199]

In the sermons, theology, and visions of the Middle Ages, the food on the altar was the God who became man; it was bleeding and broken flesh. Hunger was unquenchable desire; it was suffering. To eat God, therefore, was to become suffering flesh, to fuse with Christ on the cross. Hunger prepared the way for consuming (i.e., becoming) Christ in the eucharist and in mystical union. It was identification with the cross. Filled with Christ as bleeding flesh, recipients were simultaneously crucified with his agony. Desiring to fuse with the physical body of Christ that they chewed and consumed, medieval women often claimed the cup (or chalice), the blood of Christ, as their own in visions.

When religious superiors forbade the faithful to partake of the wounds/blood/flesh, Christ fed them directly. For example, Ida of Léau was denied the chalice because of frenzy and Alice because of leprosy; Ida of Louvain was denied the cup because of frequent nosebleeds: in consequence, all were comforted, fed, and vindicated by Christ.[200] "The more church architecture, liturgical practice, and priestly power contrived to make the elements seem distant, the more some people luxuriated in them in private, ecstatic experiences" (Bynum 1987: 59). The visionary meetings with God that medieval women received were often eatings, tastings, and savorings. Such metaphors of bodily encounters, conjuring up lips, teeth, mouths, bowels, and breasts, flesh chewed and swallowed, reveal how much God was perceived as humanity, a humanity that suffered and fed.

The southern European recluse Angela of Foligno had eucharistic visions in which Christ appeared to her all bleeding and gave her his wound to suck; she prayed to be allowed to drink his suffering and death but knew she was not worthy to die a martyr.[201] Blood and drinking were her dominant images for encounters with God. Alda of Siena, in one of her eucharistic visions, tasted a drop of blood from Christ's side; on another occasion, the drop fell onto her girdle and she sucked it out with her mouth.[202] Other medieval women showed a similar concern with the eucharist as nurturing blood. In their visions, Christ appeared at the moment of consecration, sometimes bleeding graphically into the chalice to provide food and drink for Christians.[203] The German mystic Lutgard had vivid experiences of nursing from Christ's breast. When she stood before the crucifix during one of her illnesses, she suddenly "saw Christ with his wounds all bleeding. And then she sucked such sweetness with her mouth at his breast that she could feel no tribulation."[204] The Flemish holy woman Jane Mary of Maillé, in a vision, entered the tabernacle to "taste" Christ's sweetness: Christ himself summoned her to the eucharist, appeared in visions with his wounds all bleeding, and kept her rosy and beautiful with himself as food.[205] Such interior visions and fantasies were not just intended for solace but provided a means of rebellion against clerical control, a bypassing or defiance of (male) authority at moments of crisis.

A most vivid example of women's hunger for Christ's blood exists in the writings and visions of Catherine of Siena, a fourteenth-century holy woman from southern Europe. After a life of service and fasting, she died in 1380. Frequently, in Catherine's usage, the soul "eats" liquids: milk, wine, or blood. And blood was Catherine's central image. Almost all of her letters begin with greetings in the sacred blood, and she screamed out "Blood! blood!" on her deathbed.[206] Such a preoccupation with blood was unusual for the Mediterranean world during the late Middle Ages; Catherine's views more closely approximate the German or Flemish notions of sanguinity in the twelfth or thirteenth centuries.[207] Although devotion to the blood of Christ had a long history in late medieval Italy, and Christ's blood was, to earlier devotees, most fundamentally a symbol of the washing away of sin, blood to Catherine was food or life.[208] Blood "feeds" or is "eaten" in her letters almost as frequently as it "cleanses" or "washes."[209] As in the northern parts of Europe, two aspects of the religious world of the fourteenth century (as Catherine experienced it) help explain why blood as food was central to her thought: her reverence for the clergy and her devotion to the humanity of Christ.

Catherine revered priests as "little christs"; her awe centered on their control of the eucharist, which she craved.[210] But in Catherine's day the cup of blood was denied to the laity altogether, and Catherine's respect for priests' authority thus focused on their control of and access to the awesome and taboo chalice. It is significant that she repeatedly referred to clergy as "ministers of the blood" (not "of the body"): they drink blood; serve up blood; shepherd souls by administering the blood; and they have the "ministry of blood."[211] She called the pope "vicar of Christ's blood" and said that he held "the keys of the blood."[212] In eucharistic miracles, it was blood that remained in her mouth or poured from it, although what she actually received was bread.[213]

Blood may also have had, to Catherine, other associations with an authority and power she wielded only indirectly, through prayer or persuasion. Blood was in general a more public and social symbol than bread, as well as a more ambivalent symbol. Bread (flesh) symbolized household and charity and support of life, but blood symbolized war, civil strife, and executions. Moreover, it was the support of life even more basically than bread, because it coursed through the veins as life itself.[214] In a famous incident in which Catherine stood beneath the scaffold to receive the head of a young man executed for a political crime,[215] the blood that covered her and smelled so sweet was clearly a symbol of politics and the public arena, of suffering and injustice, and of life itself— all of which could be redeemed only by assimilation to Christ's innocent blood, on which pious women fed in suffering and service.

Catherine's craving for blood was not merely a craving for encounter in Christ with all that was denied her socially and politically: the chalice, the power of the clergy, the public arena. She also craved blood because she craved identification with the humanity of Christ, and she saw this humanity as physicality. To her, physicality was the foreskin of the circumscision—flesh that bleeds.[216] Catherine understood union with Christ not as an erotic fusion with a male figure but as a taking in and taking on—a becoming—of Christ's flesh itself.

Women, Blood, and Motherhood

Eating, and the consumption of blood, became a central metaphor not merely because the eucharist was the place in Christian ritual in which God was most intimately received but also because *to eat* and *to be eaten* expressed that interpenetration and mutual engulfing, that fusion of Christ's flesh with fleshly humanness that medieval women saw as necessary for uniting with God. Eating or being fed was to the Flemish holy woman Hadewijch not merely a union in which God took the initiative, a swallowing or devouring of the soul by God. Her own soul too gave food: blood. It "suckled" with blood what it loved. And it reached out to taste and masticate the body of Christ in the eucharist. In a poem, Hadewijch spoke of her own loving as a kind of feeding:[217]

> I greet what I love
> With my heart's blood . . .
> I long, I keep vigil, I taste . . .
> I suffer, I strive after the height,
> I suckle with my blood [*bloede*];
> I greet the sweetness that can
> Alleviate my madness of Love.

At this historical juncture, in southern Europe, Catherine of Siena said of herself and other women that "they were all children, drawing the milk of suffering from the breast of Christ's humanity . . . Thus the soul was a suckling child who became one with a mother whose feeding was suffering, and that suffering saved the world."[218] Catherine's craving for Christ's blood, like her drinking of pus, was explicitly associated with a nursing Christ.[219] Eating and blood were prominent images in her interpretation of religious experience. In her writing, Catherine stressed the importance of the "drinking of pain" or bitterness as well as comfort, thereby underlining her own substitution of the filth of disease and the blood of Christ's agony for ordinary food. To hunger/suffer was to expiate the sins of the world. In hunger, according to Catherine, one joined with, "ate," Christ on the cross, and fused with his death throes that were also the bleeding/feeding of a nursing mother.

Thus, during the late Middle Ages, pious women clearly associated Christ's physicality with the female body. Fleshliness and sensuality (suffering) were linked with "woman." Catherine stressed repeatedly that Mary provided in her womb the stuff (i.e., the menstrual matter) from which was fashioned Christ's human body.[220] And she repeatedly called Christ's wound a breast.[221] Indeed, to Catherine, Christ was a nursing mother more often than a bridegroom.

Christ's humanity and fleshliness was perceived by many Western Catholics as an attribute of femaleness. This symbolic association of humanity with the female derived strength both from the association of humanity with physicality (and *woman* was the symbol of flesh) and from the associations of Christ's humanity with his mother: Christ's body was the occasion for human redemption, and Mary's body, the source of Christ's body, was the symbol of all human bodiliness.[222] Thus, to late medieval women like Catherine of Siena, Mary was the source and container of Christ's physicality: the flesh Christ put on was in some sense female, because it was his mother's. The roots of such theological interpretations lie partly in early medical theory.[223] Aristotelian physiological doctrine held that the mother provides the blood-stuff of the fetus, the father the form or animating principle; whereas a more Galenic interpretation held that the male and female substance together produce the infant (see Chapters 1 and 3). But whichever theory of conception a medieval theologian held, Christ (who had no human father) had to be seen as taking his flesh from Mary.[224] This sense that Christ, as blood and body, was formed from Mary's body led the German mystic Hildegard to argue that it was exactly *female* flesh that restored the world. Thus flesh was to her, in her visions and in the theological exegesis they stimulated, symbolized by woman: Christ's flesh was fashioned by and proceeded from the virgin womb—his mother's flesh.[225] The Flemish mystic Margaret of Oingt likewise wrote that Mary was the *tunica humanitatis*, the clothing of humanity, that Christ put on.[226] This emphasis on Christ as assuming Mary's flesh also appeared in fourteenth-century reflections on the eucharist.[227] A disturbing obsession with the bleeding host as a woman's placenta arose among female heretics in the context of a spirituality that laid graphic emphasis on the consecrated wafer as a product of, a fragment and exuding of, the female womb.

Such ideas of flesh, blood, and femaleness lie in the background of the theology of "God's motherhood," developed by Julian of Norwich in the late fourteenth century.[228] The use of *mothering* as a description for the nurturing and loving that the soul receives from God was not new with Julian, nor were her extended images of Jesus as lactating and birthing mother.[229] But according to Julian, God's motherhood, expressed in Christ, was not merely love and mercy, not merely redemption through the sacrifice on the cross; it was also a taking on of our physical humanity in the incarnation, a kind of creation of us, as a mother gives herself to the fetus she bears.[230] Thus late medieval theology and culture created an image of Christ as a birth-giving maternal figure.

God's motherhood was constructed around metaphors of "birthing" as much as his "lactating" (i.e., bleeding) wounds. This image of Christ as maternal—bleeding, feeding, nursing—had a long ancestry in twelfth- and thirteenth-century spirituality and must be understood against the background of contemporary physiological theory: "Medieval natural philosophers thought that that breast milk was blood. Thus blood was the quintessential food—and it was poured out as food or provided as the basic stuff of life only by female bodies. Therefore . . . the female body was an obvious image for a God who died to give birth to the world and bled to feed all souls" (Bynum 1987: 179). During the late Middle Ages, both men and women drank from the breast of Christ in vision and in image. Both men and women wove a complex sense of Christ's blood as the nourishment and intoxication of the soul. Both men and women therefore saw the body on the cross, which in dying fed the world, as in some sense female. Again, physiological theory reinforced image. To medieval natural philosophers, breast milk was transmuted blood, and a human mother—like the pelican that also symbolized Christ—fed her children from the fluid of life that coursed through her veins.[231] As early as the second century, Clement of Alexandria had spoken of Christ as mother, drawing out the analogy between a God who feeds humankind with his own blood in the eucharist and a human mother whose blood becomes food for her child.[232] In the twelfth century, nursing imagery often referred to milk and honey, but by the thirteenth and fourteenth centuries, the image of the nursing Jesus regularly stressed blood more than milk as the food of the soul.[233]

Mechtild of Magdeburg, for example, not only drew a parallel between blood and milk, she also spoke of blood as superior food and saw her own prayer and suffering for other souls as nursing them with blood.[234] When Catherine of Siena spoke of drinking blood from the breast of mother Jesus, she explicitly glossed blood as suffering, both Jesus' suffering, and her own.[235] Such an association of Christ's wounds with woman's body, and of woman with the food of the eucharist, is also found in late medieval art. One painting, reversing the usual image of the nursing Madonna, shows Mary drinking from Christ's side while holding him in her arms.[236] In another painting, a graphic image of Christ's flowing blood as food, the female figure Charity (herself often depicted with flowing breasts) receives the saving liquid in a chalice,[237] a remarkable iconographic parallelism of wounds and breasts. In some such depictions, it is not merely the breast as symbol of compassion or charity (and therefore of intercession) that is offered; it is the breast as food, parallel to the bleeding (i.e., nurturing) wound.

Since Christ's body was a body that nursed the hungry, both men and women assimilated the ordinary female body to it. Women mystics such as Mechtild of Magdeburg and Catherine of Siena used the metaphor of the nursing mother to describe their own suffering for others, sometimes clearly implying that their spilling of blood was a fusion with Christ's nurturing and inebriating wounds/breasts. Moreover, miraculous lactating, exuding, and feeding were characteristic female miracles in the later Middle Ages. The female body was seen as powerful in its holy or miraculous oozing, whether of breast milk or of blood and oil.[238] Male hagiographers saw women saints dripping holy fluids from breasts or fingertips. Stigmata appeared most frequently on women's bodies because stigmata (like the marks on the bodies of witches and the wounds in the body of Christ) were not merely wounds but also breasts. In this literal becoming of the crucified body, which a female mystic achieved by suffering or by eating the bleeding host (which fed humankind), women's wounds recapitulated the nurturing wounds/breasts of Christ.

Theologians underlined the fact that those who bled or exuded unusual fluids did not excrete or menstruate in ordinary ways. Closing herself off to ordinary food yet consuming God in the eucharist, the holy woman became God's body. And in eating a God whose body was meat and drink, women both transfigured and became more fully the flesh and the food that their bodies were. Women met God as flesh taken into, *eaten by*, flesh.[239] To eat God was to join with God: communion was consuming, that is, becoming a God that bled, suffered, and nursed. In union with the dying Christ, woman's eating, fasting, and feeding others were thus synonymous acts, a transfiguring and becoming of what the female symbolized: flesh, blood, nurture, suffering, and regeneration.

Gender and Consumption

The process of becoming God by eating God is, of course, a sort of cannibalism, and anthropological studies of cannibalism regularly stress it as a way of incorporating the power of what was eaten.[240] By consuming and digesting the spiritual forces believed to be physically constituted in human bodily substances, participants in cannibalistic feasts seek to enhance the power of the self, assimilating the other's vital essence into their own bodies. This equation of digestive and generative processes promotes the symbolic reconstitution of the world in a more general sense. By preventing decomposition of dead organic substance through the consumption of human bodies, acts of cannibalism and oral incorporation are always attempts at the denial of death, circumventions of the mortality of flesh.

Such efforts to enhance or reproduce life essence are particularly evident in cases of mortuary cannibalism, which is centered on the ritualized consumption of the dead.[241] The death rites (or funerary customs) of many non-Western band and village societies call for the consumption of portions of the remains of dead relatives: only the ashes, carbonized flesh or ground-up bones of the deceased are generally ingested.[242] Motivated by fears of decay and rot, the signs of total extinction, the consumption of bodies or parts of bodies negates the finality of death. Ingesting the transformed corpse of a kinsman reaffirms lineage continuity by promoting the transference of vital substance from one generation to the next.[243] The perpetuation of a group's vital essence is thus ensured. Cannibalism recycles and regenerates those forces that are believed to bind the living to their deceased ancestors. The eating of human bodies must therefore be interpreted as a ritual of social reproduction, a practice that conveys a sense of permanence and continuity to the members of a given community.

While cannibalistic customs and fantasies have conventionally been relegated to the margins of Europe, reflecting a colonial preoccupation with the "uncivilized" or "barbaric,"[244] corresponding dispositions are attested in the West. Christian theology focused its spiritual practices on the oral incorporation of a male deity: during the celebration of the eucharist, which dramatized the expressive affirmation of faith, worshipers consumed the deity's blood and body ritually.[245] Christianity taught that a god intervened in the history of humanity: through his incarnation in the body of a mortal man and his death on the cross, he bestowed upon the community of believers spiritual immortality. Identification, even fusion, with the god was subsequently made possible by the partaking of his flesh and blood. By ingesting the deity's corporeal substance, Christian worshipers were able to assimilate the god's spiritual and redemptive powers into their own mortal bodies. Biblical texts confirm the necessity for this alimentary embodiment of the divine: "I say unto you, unless you eat the flesh of the Son of man and drink his blood you have no life in you; he who eats my flesh and drinks my blood has eternal life, and I will raise him up at the last day. For my flesh is food indeed, and my blood is drink indeed. He who eats my flesh and drinks my blood abides in me, and I in him" (John 6: 53–56). One of the central rituals of Western Christianity was thus embedded in a cannibalistic fantasy. This was so whether one believed in the transubstantiated or in the symbolic presence of God.[246] Through the consumption of a male god, divine power could be appropriated and sedimented in the human body.

But these rituals of transference and embodiment were more than attempts to enhance the vitality or divinity of the self. Such exchanges were also enactments of power relationships, often conveyed through the idiom of gender. Peggy Reeves Sanday (1986) shows that in many cultures there is a connection between cannibalism and the use of the female body as symbol. Her analysis indicates that there may be an intrinsic connection between the emergence of specific bodily images for Christ in the later Middle Ages and the emphasis during the same period on the cannibalistic aspects of mass. Increasingly from the twelfth to the fifteenth century, worshipers saw "woman" as quintessential recipient, "man" as quintessential celebrant, maker, and controller of the body of God. More than occasionally they saw the celebrant as pregnant with the host. According to late medieval Christian dogma, a purifying male surrogate entered ("impregnated" or "inseminated") the body, bestowing consecration as well as sustenance. In Catholic scriptures of the late Middle Ages, celebrants (e.g., nuns, virgins, holy women) were described as pregnant with Christ.[247] Flemish and German female mystics used such images to express their fecundity, their ability to conceive God within. Moreover, medieval texts and medieval visions spoke of clerics as pregnant with Jesus.[248] In the mass, the priest became symbolically "woman": woman as food preparer, nurturer, and recipient of male substance (flesh, blood/semen).

Gender symbolism was encoded in body postures and the assignation of active and passive roles during the rite of communion. "During the celebration of the eucharist, the priest offered wine and unleavened bread at the altar, uttering the words of consecration: 'This is my body . . . . This is my blood.' The worshipers came forward and kneeled at the railing of the altar, facing the cross. Each of them was waiting to receive the *oblata* or host, a thin wafer, representing the corporeal essence of the deity. The priest approached with a gold platter, and the communicants, each in turn, raised their chins and tilted their heads backward. The priest made the sign of the cross, indicating the presence of Christ, and put the wafer into the communicants' mouths. They returned to their pews, kneeled down, made again the sign of the cross, covered their face with their hands and swallowed the deity's body."[249] Kneeling is a feminizing gesture, "a symbol of humility, inferiority, and subjugation" (Brandes 1980: 188). Open-mouthed, members of the congregation took in a male substance and through this act of oral consumption were cast in a subordinate, perhaps effeminate, role. Since religious authority was located in male figures, church services were traditionally performed by men: it was they who proffered the life-giving substance. "On the one hand, the priest was 'male' and the communicant 'female'; the priest was God and the recipient human. As is well known, Bonaventure argued that women could not be priests because the priesthood, the authority of God, had to be symbolized by a male" (Bynum 1987: 285). But in another sense, God's dying body was female, a birthing and lactating mother, and the priest was female too. He was Mary, for in his hands, as in her womb, Christ was incarnate; he was food preparer and distributor to recipients who ate. "The celebrant became food preparer, the generator of food, the pregnant mother of the incarnate God" (289). If male monopoly of religious leadership and descriptions of God as male mirrored social hierarchy, then these startling reversals at the heart of mass provided an alternative to and critique of the asymmetry between the sexes in the ordinary world.

The embodiment of generative male power was confirmed by visual symbols. Devotional images from the thirteenth and fourteenth centuries depict God's mortal body with an erect phallus. These signs of virility and reproductive ability after his sacrifice on the cross signified Christ's victory over death.[250] More explicit was the common practice of baking communion wafers, representing the body of God, in the shape of human testicles, which was not halted by the English church until 1263.[251] "The consecrated wafer, which the pious communicant received from the hands of the priest, on Easter Sunday, was made up into a form highly indecent and improper" (Warner 1791: 136). The ritual consumption of God's generative and nurturing body was focused on his blood and genitalia.

In the eucharist, the theme of cannibalism was thus conveyed through several interrelated images: on the one hand, the eroticism of the consumptive act; on the other, the inverted motif of female procreativity, which equated the dead male body with productive power. As in the cult of the sacred blood or sacred heart, late medieval doctrine frequently saw God's body itself lactating, giving birth, and clothing our humanness with his immaculate flesh. Christianity taught that it was men who, in death, gave their body and blood to constitute and nurture their followers.[252] Worshipers were made and sustained as they fed on the sacrificial male body, consuming his virile/nurturing substance.

Such notions of physicality and consumption provided organizing images for the social construction of gender. The symbolism of giving and eating God's body as food was central to societal definitions of masculinity and femininity. Comparative ethnographic evidence suggests that cannibalistic practices, when linked to death or mortuary rituals, were often associated with women and femaleness. In Christian theology, as elsewhere, the consumers of human flesh were typically endowed with feminine qualities. The takers of male essence were perceived as feminine, while the givers of bodies and providers of sustenance were defined as masculine. In non-Western death rituals, men exchange their bodies, their physical substance, for the gift of spiritual immortality. Women are commonly implicated in this transformational process through acts of generative violence. For instance, according to the world view of the Gimi, a peoples of the Eastern Highlands of Papua New Guinea,[253] cannibalism is the initial stage in the regeneration of the dead. By transferring human essence to other living beings, the continuity of existence is maintained. Until the early 1960s, after which the practice was abandoned, cannibalism was defined as a female activity: men's corpses were eaten by women. Gimi women were said to dismember a man in his garden, carry the sections of his body inside the men's house, and remain secluded there for days while they further divided up, ate, and digested his flesh.[254] Female cannibals, by ingesting male bodies, participated in the production of immortality for men. Women's consumption of human flesh was conceived as a ritual attempt to promote the rebirth of men. A man's passage through the regenerative female body engendered his transformation into a spirit being. Women ate the dead bodies of men in order to release their individual spirits, so that they could rejoin the ancestral spirits in the forest.[255] This release was carried out through a metaphorical model of sexual intercourse: by "going inside" female cannibals, a man's corpse functioned as a penis, whose virile substance was possessed and incorporated by women. The eating of a man's dead body permitted women to harness his vital or life-giving power, which (like the "eating of semen" during sexual intercourse) was understood as a necessary prelude to reproduction and as an essential prerequisite for the cycle of male regeneration.

These concepts were made plausible by a system of metaphors that equated oral incorporation and digestion with processes of female reproduction. As the male corpse was taken back inside the female body and devoured, it became the child, her ingested food, which awaited rebirth as a spirit.[256] Here, gender symbolism, by equating the act of sex with the act of eating, and the ingestion of a man's body with the ingestion of his semen, provided a tangible reality to cannibalistic fantasies of female oral impregnation, the child in the abdomen, and assertions of male rebirth through consumption.[257] Such a metaphorical model may be related to a simple physiological function: "For a woman, intercourse involves taking something into the body as one takes food (hence the myth of impregnation by mouth, the swallowing of the seed), whereas for a man it is the reverse" (O'Flaherty 1980: 264). This simple dialectic was encoded in cultural constructions of gender. Assertions of maleness often demand an outward projection and acting upon the world. Femaleness, in contrast, requires an ingestion of the world and a realization of internal regenerative abilities. In Papua New Guinea, as in Western Catholicism, acts of oral incorporation and consumption were typified as feminine behaviors. "Consumption, like production, [was] associated with the female gender by Hagen men. They [said] that women wanted to eat pork, while they themselves would rather give it away. The big-man, who represent[ed] male ideals, should not be a consumer but an investor of goods" (Strathern 1982: 115). Accordingly, men's pleasures and wants were focused on the establishment of selfhood by bestowing their wealth, and by divesting their bodies, into the world. In contrast, women's desires and pleasures were focused on a cycle of regeneration by incorporation, and by taking into their bodies what was outside of them.

In the New Guinea Highlands (as in Western Catholicism), the practice of consumption was inextricably linked to images of womanhood: the bodily pleasures of women were associated with visions of eating, using up, devouring, incorporating. Such notions of female consumption were thematically opposed to the expected patterns of male behavior and were therefore perceived as a potential threat: "Such 'female' values [could] invade those spheres controlled by men and disrupt them; men themselves [could] become 'unmanned'" (Strathern 1982: 115). When Hagen men participated in consumption, thereby acting like women, they were transformed, emasculated, thus experiencing a symbolic loss of manhood or maleness. Correspondingly, among the Gimi of Papua New Guinea, cannibalism was thought to fertilize women but to debilitate men. Whereas women were enhanced by eating human flesh, men were enfeebled, castrated, made unfit for battle. "Adult males who ate human flesh were referred to as 'nothing men,' as men of low status who, by eating the dead, made themselves weak like women. Eating human meat drained a man of his strength so that he was limply helpless before his enemies on the battlefield" (Gillison 1983: 33–34). The ingestion of human flesh, especially that of a man's corpse, enforced cultural assumptions about gender-specific behavior. It affirmed the sexual and reproductive roles of women but cast men into a state of effeminacy, stripping them of their manhood. As enactments of fantasies of female empowerment, and by dramatizing the feminizing consequences of consumption, cannibalistic rituals discouraged emphasis on masculinity or male participation.

This imagery of death and rebirth through the female body (possibly an archetypal male fantasy) provided a key scenario for rituals of cannibalism. In rites of mortuary cannibalism, where the principal agents were women, such notions could not be contested without calling into question the cultural premises that organize the relationship between procreativity and womanhood. The fantasy of male rebirth required greater symbolic elaboration when it was enacted in contexts where the principal agents were men and the male body was the only available vehicle of regeneration. In such cases, blood and bloodshed assumed enormous symbolic significance. Based on a model of female parturition, bleeding male bodies were presumed to nurture and give birth.[258] In non-Western rituals, the show of blood proclaimed men's physical potency and the generative independence of women. But blood took on a similar metaphorical function in late medieval Europe. According to Christian doctrine, it was the blood of Jesus that restored the world. Regeneration through the male body, and through male blood, was a crucial theological premise. Moreover, after the thirteenth century, the drinking of Christ's blood was denied to women, and its ingestion became an exclusive prerogative of the clergy. Priests, who controlled the reception and consumption of blood, were distinguished as the maternal body/womb through which the incarnate God was reborn.

In symbolic terms, and through the production and consumption of blood, ritual functionaries proclaimed themselves entirely independent of women.[259] In late medieval Catholicism, as in other male cults, the implementation of cannibalistic fantasies as well as the transformational and regenerative power of blood turned clergymen into birth givers. By enforcing strict rules of gender segregation, which restricted women's participation, and by enhancing the mysteries of the rites, priests were able to engage in blood consumption without having to acknowledge its feminizing consequences.

Although men performed the drama of eating and ingesting human flesh/blood, they tried to distance themselves from the connotations of such consumptive acts by displacing cannibalistic tendencies onto others. This is evident in ritual attempts to impute consumptive malevolence to women while emphasizing the protective or nurturing roles of men.[260] Cannibalistic monsters were portrayed in the form of dangerous women that had to be controlled or destroyed. The narrative plots and action sequences of such fictions were always identical. Initial trust was reposed in women. The women betrayed this trust and wantonly attacked those living under their auspices. They revealed themselves as cannibals who devoured human flesh, usually that of their own kin, their sons, or other young boys. In the end, the cannibal women/monsters were killed and their victims avenged.

The cannibal women, after having consumed their victims' bodies, either retained them in their bellies or regurgitated the devoured youths, vomiting up their half- digested remains. Among the Walbiri in Australia, such tales were performed by enacting a mythological plot: adolescent boys became men by being swallowed alive by two cannibal women, who — "crouching like hideous demons, with flies swarming into their gaping, bloodstained mouths" — later vomited up the ingested youths.[261] Since women might choose not to give up or release what they had ingested, their cannibalistic impulses were perceived as fearsome and threatening. The accompanying images of violence, death, and dismemberment revealed men's terror of the incorporating female body — of being consumed by women without the possibility of rebirth. This symbolic connection between fears of female consumption and emasculation (i.e., death) has been discussed at length by psychoanalytic theorists: the devouring woman, the vagina dentata, and the threat of castration are male fantasies of sexuality cast in terms of female oral aggression.[262] The mythic or ritual instances of swallowing and incorporation typify these male fantasies.

Consumption, as indicated by the comparative ethnographic evidence, was deemed especially dangerous when motivated by women's greed, hatred, or self-interest. In such instances, male bodies were annihilated and eaten as food, a practice that inhibited and negated the necessary regeneration of life. New Guinea Highlanders (the Gimi) thus presumed that without male supervision, the female tended permanently to retain and in that way destroy (i.e., reabsorb) what she nourished inside her.[263] Outside the context of male ritual operations, without control of its destructive propensity, cannibalism was perceived as a negative and antisocial force: cannibal women were regarded as monsters or witches. "The witch [was] pictured as a cannibal, who kill[ed] by eating the internal parts of the victim's body and/or practice[d] necrophagy as a means of obtaining human meat as such. [The witch] takes, consumes and kills: [she] does not behave reciprocally" (Strathern 1982: 112–13). Acts of self-enhancement and self-gratification transformed women's consumption patterns into a most dangerous feat. Under these circumstances, cannibalism represented a thematic opposition to the prevailing social order.[264] Women were expected to incorporate death by taking a man's corpse inside their generative bodies and to re-create life by regurgitating its corporeal or spiritual essence. Necrophagic cannibalism encoded precisely the reverse message: it repudiated the patterns of reciprocity and exchange upon which normal gender relations were premised. Since men were dependent upon women's bodies to complete the cycle of male regeneration, processes of female consumption and reproduction were closely guarded and controlled.

During the late Middle Ages, these same concerns organized public attitudes about the behavior of female saints. Women mystics fed on the body of Christ; they drank his blood in private visions. Not surprisingly, the bodily functions of medieval holy women were anxiously scrutinized. In many women's lives, eucharistic devotion, abstinence, and self-starvation were major themes. The stories of female saints were woven around the central motif of bodies: the closure and drying up of the flesh and the unusual exuding of blood. Holy women were often said neither to eat nor to excrete. Women, whose bodies bled in unusual ways, were often miraculous fasters, and theologians underlined the fact that those who bled or exuded unusual fluids did not excrete or menstruate in ordinary ways. Female saints thus exhibited behaviors that were directed toward shutting off menstruation, excretion, and other ordinary physical functions. In late medieval religiosity, such transfigurations were ways of fusing with a Christ whose suffering would save the world. Much was made of the fact that women suffered, hungered, and bled in the service of others. Women's bodily changes and miraculous effusions of blood were attempts at shaping themselves to Christ, at becoming or being the suffering body on the cross. Women mystics averted the stigma of the cannibal witch by repressing within themselves ordinary bodily functions: eating, menstruating, and excreting. They bled and consumed only to "nurture"—suffering in the service of others.

Anti-Semitism: Accusations of Ritual Murder

Images of the antisocial cannibal, the human monster who kills and eats to annihilate, not to regenerate, are attested in Christian blood libel accusations against heretics, witches, and Jews. Beginning in the eleventh century, European Jews were persecuted for the presumed murder and consumption of Christ and for the annual enactment of this deed on the body of a young male child.[265] Here, as in the case of the mythical cannibal monster/woman, such depictions were used to justify acts of societal vengeance against minorities—legitimating the killing and expulsion of Jews from medieval Christian communities.

The typical story line was that one or more Jews had murdered an innocent Christian infant or child, supposedly to obtain blood required for ritual consumption purposes, for example, to mix blood with unleavened bread to make matzo. The legend came into circulation in the twelfth century. It was told, in oral and written tradition, as historical truth.[266] The narrative plot revolved around acts of blood sacrifice and cannibalism and the eventual punishment for such crimes. The "killings" occurred most frequently on Christian religious holidays or on other ecclesiastical occasions when Jews were presumed to be in need of blood for their occult ceremonies.[267] The allegations led to lengthy trials, often involving torture to extract confessions, and the inevitable executions: "In 1171 at Blois, after due trial, thirty-eight Jews were burned at the stake; in 1191, at Bray-sur-Seine, the number of victims reached one hundred."[268]

One of the first blood libel trials took place in Norwich (England), where anti-Judaic sentiments inspired the following narrative. At the beginning of Lent, in 1144, William, a twelve-year-old boy, supposedly known to Jewish fur traders as a skillful apprentice, had disappeared in the town of Norwich. A monk named Theobald (himself a Jewish convert) swore that the boy had been lured into the home of a Jewish elder, who killed him in observance of the Passover ritual.[269] But when the boy's body was found, it showed no evidence of murder. This fact prevented a massacre of the Jews at the last moment. Nevertheless, the cult of William, the martyr of Norwich, had begun: the boy was sainted and enshrined in his home church. Later chroniclers failed to delete the gory fiction of the boy's crucifixion, giving prominence to the motif of ritual murder and the Jews' hunger for blood. Driven to reenact Christ's death and bloodshed, so the legend proclaims, "the Jews lacerated [the boy's] head with thorns, crucified him and pierced his side".[270] A Latin work, written about 1173, documents the ritual killing of the boy in gruesome detail:

[Judging] "from the marks of the wounds . . . the [boy's] left hand and foot were pierced with two nails . . . [And] from the presence of nail-marks in both hands and feet, the murderers were Jews." After additional "many and great tortures, they inflicted a frightful wound in his left side, reaching even to his inmost heart, and . . . they extinguished his mortal life . . . And since many streams of blood were running down from all parts of his body, then, to stop the blood and to wash and close the wounds, they poured boiling water over him."[271]

According to this narrative, the tortured body of the dead boy was found without any wounds because the Jews had "cunningly" closed the gashes with hot water.

Identical charges were brought against the Jews of Gloucester (England) in 1168: "A boy was secretly taken away by Jews" and then "tortured with immense tortures" in front of the assembled Jews.[272] Ritual murder accusations were levied against the Jews of Blois (France) in 1171: a servant claimed "that he saw a Jew throw a little Christian child, whom the Jews had killed, into the river"; on the instigation of a local cleric, thirty-one Jews were burned alive.[273] Blood libel charges were pronounced against the Jews of Bury St. Edmunds in 1181, Bristol in 1183, Winchester in 1192 and 1225, and Norwich in 1235.[274] The harassment of Jews in England intensified in 1255, following the disappearance of Hugh of Lincoln, the son of a poor washerwoman.[275] At the time, a large number of Jews had gathered in town to attend a marriage between prominent people. The day after the wedding, the body of a boy (who had been missing for several weeks) was discovered in a cesspool, allegedly bearing the marks of crucifixion.[276] A dramatic explanation of his death immediately suggested itself. Accused of having tortured, scourged, and crucified the boy, nearly a hundred Jews were arrested. Nineteen were hanged without a trial. The boy's remains were enshrined in the local church, and the final expulsion of the Jews of England was ordered by the king in 1290.

The anti-Judaic plot of the blood libel legend persisted throughout late medieval England. According to the oldest versions of the tale, dating back to the thirteenth century, a devout young boy was kidnapped, tortured, and murdered by Jews. The boy's body was thrown into a cesspool or a well. The crime, according to legend, was often revealed by miraculous means:[277]

The corpse was carried to the house of the Jews where its wounds began to bleed again. This persuaded the citizenry of the guilt of the Jews.[278]

The Jews were interrogated . . . and since, when they approached the dead body, the boy's wounds began to bleed again, something that, experience has taught, occurs whenever a murderer touches the victim, this [blood effusion] was taken as factual evidence that the Jews were to blame.[279]

A boy was found dead in a well . . . [T]he parents had "observed by definite surmises and clear proofs, especially by incisions in the bowels and veins, that he had been killed by Jews." In addition to this proof occurred "the renewed flowing of wounds when he was carried in front of the Jews' houses." . . . The Jews [were] accused because "the wounds bled afresh" as soon as the corpse was carried into town.[280]

The blood motif shaped the iconographic conventions of late medieval murder legends in fundamental ways, linking infanticide, sanguinity, and anti-Semitism. Perhaps most significantly, the prominence of blood imagery helped to promote the popular phantasm of the flesh-eating Jew. For example, when the death of Hugh of Lincoln in 1255 (told in gruesome detail by late medieval writers) became the subject of a famous British ballad, the connection between blood hunger and Jews emerged as a crucial theme.[281] In the narrative, a Jewish temptress induces a young Christian boy to enter her garden, where she brutally murders him, taking special care to catch his blood in a basin or cup.[282] In many variants of the ballad, the description of the killing has at least a suggestion of ritual to it, as indicated by a scene from an eighteenth-century Scottish text, which sounds somewhat like an altar sacrifice:

> She's laid him on a dressin-board
> Whare she did often dine;
> She stack a penknife to his heart.
> And dressed him like a swine.[283]

The cannibalistic implications of the killing were brought into association with blood extraction and wounding, merging images of "the dead child, the blood collected in jars, and the ritual of death" (Hsia 1988: 204). Many texts described a basin or container held to catch the boy's blood as he died, presumably to be used later in a ritual.[284] Detailing the alleged murder, fourteenth-century writers elaborated on the eucharistic/cannibalistic aspects of the event, and related how "the child was first fattened for ten days with white bread and milk, and then how almost all the Jews in England were invited to the crucifixion." [285] Here, the blood-drained body of the mutilated boy became a stand-in for the martyred Christ, who had offered his body for consumption. In the later Middle Ages, blood libel accusations (i.e., presumptions of a Jewish need for blood) relied on a conflation of ritual murder with eucharistic sacrifice and a concern with the salvific power of blood. The alleged motive of ritual murder represented nothing less than an inversion of the Christian themes of sacrifice and triumph,[286] with the Jews depicted as wanting to sacrifice Christian martyrs in order to gain resurrection and salvation by power of their blood.

The obvious parallels between the eucharist and the blood murder legend were pointed out by earlier writers: "The Jews . . . were pictured as doing in reality what the Christian worshiper was doing in fantasy, i.e., killing a child and drinking its blood" (Maccoby 1982: 159, 155). Orally incorporating the flesh and blood of their god, commonly perceived as the Christ *child* or *infant* Jesus,[287] a manifestation of one of his suffering personae, implied an act of cannibalism. Making the host (i.e., the incarnate God) bleed or wounding a child were parallel projective fantasies, symbolic of the motif of crucifixion. An important element of the crucifixion theme was the injury inflicted upon the eucharist, the charity of Christ, that is, the transubstantiated wafer, and the bleeding of this martyred or crucified oblata/matzo by the Jews.[288] In these anti-Judaic imaginings, the wounding of the body of Christ was fundamental: blood was redemptive and curative because of his death on the cross. The notion that Jews rubbed the blood drawn from a murdered child (the infant Jesus) into the dough of the matzo/host was clearly suggestive of the eucharist: the consumption of the body or blood of the murdered Christ/child.

The persecution of Jews in Europe began during a time, in the late eleventh century, when Christian crusaders reinvigorated the belief that God's suffering and death on the cross was to be blamed on Hebrew (not Roman) soldiers. Crucifixion and bloodshed, and later the ritual of the eucharist (with its motifs of blood and cannibalism), provided the root metaphors for anti-Judaic persecution. In the German Rhineland, in the eleventh century, Catholic theologians advocated that the blood of Jesus had to be avenged on the bodies of Jews.[289] Reports regarding the number of Jewish victims from 1096 who had been brutalized or committed suicide ranged from four thousand to twelve thousand. A renewal of anti-Semitic violence can be documented in urban centers along the Rhineland after 1187.[290] The brutalization of Jews intensified during the early thirteenth century, when the doctrine of transubstantiation was established. In 1235, the Jews of Lauda and Tauberbischofsheim were persecuted following accusations of blood libel and the murder of a Christian boy. During the next year, in 1236, Jews were accused of performing blood rituals in Fulda. Similar accusations of Jewish blood-hunger resulted in mob violence along the Rhine a few years later.[291] For example, in 1267 the Jews of Pforzheim were blamed when a child was killed and its blood collected on folded pieces of linen.[292] In Weissenburg, in 1270, Jews were accused of suspending a Christian child by the feet and opening every artery in its body in order to obtain all its blood. Jews were accused of kidnapping a child in Munich in 1285. A year later, in 1286 in Oberwesel, a boy known as "the good Werner" was allegedly tortured to death by Jews for three days. In 1287, the boy Rudolph was tortured and his head cut off in Bern, and likewise in Krems (on the Danube) the Jews supposedly killed a boy "in order to get his blood."

The events depicted, with their reference to the extraction and use of blood, were a perpetuation in simple form of the view that Jews had killed Christ (for which act they were held responsible by the Roman Catholic church until 1965). The alleged ritual murder of later Christians (i.e., the representatives of Jesus) served as a constant reminder of God's death on the cross. In all cases, the alleged murderers with great eagerness extracted the blood of their victims: "In 1235 Jews had, on holy Christmas Day, cruelly killed the five sons of a miller . . . [and] collected their blood in bags smeared with wax . . . [In another town, in 1270] Jews inflicted many wounds on the child and carefully collected the blood on a folded piece of linen placed under [the corpse]."[293] "In 1569 the body of a twelve-year-old boy was discovered near the road . . .

needle marks were visible on one side of the neck and the veins had been cut open, but little blood could be found near the body" which resulted in accusations of a Judaic blood sacrifice.[294] The notion of the magical potency of Christian blood emerged as a prominent motif in the subsequent trials. Emphasis on the ritual use of blood seeped into these stories only in the thirteenth century. It was first mentioned in 1235, when it was suggested that Jews needed Christian blood for their religious rites and cultic practices. The bleeding or bloodletting (with its emphasis on the ritual extraction of blood) was to become much more significant in some stories, "for instance if the victim [was] put into a head-down position like a slaughtered animal in a butcher shop, as in the case in Weissenburg, in 1270" (Rappaport 1975: 103). Such narrative plots reenacted the crucifixion of Jesus (signified by the bleeding Christ on the cross) and the rite of the eucharist with the unblemished body as food (the murdered boy/child), that is, the lamb of Jesus.

By the end of the thirteenth century, such accusations of blood-ritual murder were popularized in Franconia and Bavaria and throughout Austria. In the course of the violence perpetrated against Jews, nearly one hundred fifty communities were destroyed, and close to one hundred thousand Jews were killed.[295] By 1336, so-called Jew bashers (*Judenschläger*) carried out their violent intentions under the protection of several noblemen: these proclaimed to have received divine inspiration to "inflict the suffering and wounds that Jesus endured on the Jews' bodies and to avenge His death with their blood."[296] The bashers, organized in gangs, persecuted Jews in Alsatia, the Rhineland, and Swabia. But the greatest devastation occurred around 1348, when the blood accusations resulted in mass violence against Jews. For instance, in February 1349, several thousand Jews were burned on the grounds of the cemetery in Strasbourg. Nearly six thousand Jews died in Mainz, Cologne, and Basel through street violence, arson, and suicide.[297] This pattern of violent anti-Semitism was fused with frequent attempts at Jewish expulsion (e.g., in Speyer, 1435; Mainz, 1420, 1438, and 1462; Jütlich-Berg, 1461; Neuss, 1462; Rheingau, 1470). Late medieval Jewish settlements along the Rhine Valley, and in Germany more generally, were almost completely devastated by the aftermath of the blood/murder accusations.

It should be noted that there were opposing voices: a number of papal bulls on the subject of ritual murder (in 1247, 1259, 1272, 1422, and 1540), as well as Cardinal Ganganelli's famous investigative report of 1759, sought to diminish anti-Judaic sentiments by denouncing the blood libel legend.[298] The earliest official papal pronouncement from 1247, which was addressed to the archbishops and bishops of Germany and France, explicitly forbade faithful Christians to participate in the propagation of blood accusations: "But since Fulda and in several other places many Jews were killed on the ground of such a suspicion, we, by the authority of these presents, strictly forbid that this should be repeated in future." [299] Although several popes did honestly seek to repudiate and deny the blood libel legend, it is also true that the semi-official Vatican periodical, the *Civilita Cattolica*, from 1881 to 1914 promoted and systematically "documented" the legend, and this was the case as well with other nominally Catholic periodicals (e.g., *La Croix*, in the late nineteenth century). In some instances, Catholic priests and local clergy cleverly used the ritual murder accusation as a weapon against Jews. [300] Official attempts to suppress the popular belief that Jews used human blood in the preparation of their unleavened bread (and for this reason were guilty of the slaughter of Christian children) proved unsuccessful. As a result, Jews were unjustly deprived, not only of their possessions, but in many cases also of their lives.

During the late Middle Ages, blood libel had become a historical reality. Ritual murder discourse had lodged itself into the historical consciousness of Catholic (and later Lutheran) Germany. By the seventeenth century, poems, hagiographies, printings, and other iconographic representations portrayed the murder of the innocent child at Jewish hands. [301] The blood libel legend had become the basis of local festivals and commemorative rites and was remembered and memorialized in church decorations. [302] Religious engravings were fashioned to depict the boy martyrs: images of corporeal sensuality, pious suffering, and redemptive flesh—the sensuous iconographies of baroque Catholicism. [303] Legends proclaiming the Jewish ritual murder of Christian children or the desecration of holy wafers were celebrated in various European towns in such artistic forms as tapestries or stained glass church windows. [304] These artistic renderings of the legend provided daily reminders of the existence and, by extension, the truth or historicity of the story of Jewish blood-hunger. Likewise the revival of pilgrimages, which grew in the seventeenth century and reached a zenith in the eighteenth, also drew strength from the legend of the blood libel. Here, the use of relics (blood, bones, weapons, etc.), together with iconographic and written records, helped to sustain the belief in the historical reality of Jewish ritual murder. In one case, "the purported instrument of torture, a long curved dagger, was placed in a reliquary for display . . . and in 1800, the broadsheet commemorating [the supposed ritual murder], with woodcuts and verses describing the [event], and sold to pilgrims of earlier generations, was [once again] reprinted." [305] When in seventeenth-century Rinn (or Judenstein), a town near Innsbruck, the bones of a martyred boy were reburied in the parish church, his remains were treated as relics by local pilgrims. Soon the blood libel legend became a local cult worthy of wider Catholic recognition. The cult persisted into the late twentieth century, with the sanction of the ecclesiastical hierarchy.[306]

The climate of ritual murder suspicion was sustained by public iconographies that effectively drove anti-Judaic sentiments into historical consciousness. The blood accusation, the purported act of murder, and the eucharistic triumph were often celebrated through visual representations, paintings, and texts that could be seen and displayed in public places: the church, market, or roadside. For example, a tapestry in the village church of Loddon (England) depicted three Jews murdering a child; one had pierced the child's side with a knife and was holding a basin to catch the blood.[307] A similar scene had been re-created in the village church of Judenstein (near Innsbruck, Austria), where three figures, made of wood or wax, with knives in hand, menacingly surrounded a stone upon which they had placed the infant victim.[308] This exhibit had become a place of pilgrimage, where children—led by their parents—could see for themselves the reconstruction of the assassination by three Jews of a young boy.[309] Another example of such an artistic rendering, installed on the Frankfurt city gate, showed a naked child tortured to death by Jews.[310] Attempts to renovate the painting in the late seventeenth century gave rise to the printing of a scurillous broadsheet, with picture and text commemorating the purported murder. The top portion of the illustration reproduced the gruesome wall painting, which showed the boy Simon lying on a board, pierced by awls and covered with blood. Below, the rabbis and their families were depicted as the devil's servants, deriving their nourishment from the excrement and milk of a sow.[311] Demonization, Jewish bloodlust, and pollution through improper or incongruous (perverse) consumption were the central themes.

For many Germans, even after the eighteenth and nineteenth centuries, ritual murder was a historical reality. Documented in old chronicles, judicial records, and past writings, it lived on as the stuff of legend. Anti-Semitic circles professed to regard ritual murder as a fundamental Jewish practice. In the twentieth century, Nazi propagandists, even before their accession to power, issued periodic warnings to the general population to take special care of their children in view of Jewish ritual requirements.[312] The striking revival or perpetuation of the blood libel legend in the twentieth century was very much nurtured by Nazi Germany. "The legend was obviously made to order for anti-Semitic propaganda efforts. Leaflets circulated in Berlin and Dresden in 1933 telling of ritual murder accusations and calling for the prosecution of Jews" (Dundes 1991: 348). The political campaign of hate continued throughout the 1940s. The preoccupation with holy blood, initially fostered by the Catholic clergy, was finally adopted in Alfred Rosenberg's idea of a "blood mythos" and Hitler's concern over the purity of Aryan (German) blood. Nazi propagandists preached of blood and soil, and Heinrich Himmler founded a "blood order" for the Jew bashers of the fascist state.[313] Moreover, Nazi images of Jews drawing blood (a life source) from a body were similar not only to those of the Jew as vampire or sponge, a variation on the theme of the Jewish usurer soaked full with Christian money (blood), but also to the categorization of the Jew as a parasite who fattened himself upon the body of the nation, reducing its will and finally overpowering it. In the modern era, the motif of the bloodsucking Jew was gradually redefined in terms of a medical pathology, a biological threat that had to be expunged from the national body politic. Fears of blood loss and contagion (derived from a terror of Jewish blood-hunger) were crucial for the emergence of a Nazi aesthetic of race.

Part III
Blood in the
Modern Era

Chapter 5
Mapping the Modern Body
Blood, Medicine, and Magic

How did a secular aesthetic of blood come about? And what became of the religious iconographies of blood, women, and Jews amid the "progressive enlightenment" of modern science? Did the ordering and marking of social identities by blood emerge out of the late medieval preoccupation with sin, suffering, and contagion? Or was it based on an altogether different conceptual development? Indeed, the historical conditions that shaped the modern European aesthetics of race did not emerge until the second half of the eighteenth century, and it was some time before such notions became part of a common framework of perception.

According to Michel Foucault (1973), it was only with the sociogenesis of European modernity that blood, body, and race were created as biological entities. With the birth of the clinic, a new body perception became commonplace. The material body was seized by a dissecting gaze that embraced not only the entire organism, not only its surfaces, but also its recesses, orifices, and hidden crevices.[1] It penetrated inquisitively into bodies, relating living organs to gutted and eviscerated cadavers, to a visual image of a dead body. The penetrating gaze of the doctor was like a postmortem dissection: the sick patient was now treated in a way that once had been conceivable only with dead bodies. Foucault (1975) repeatedly points out that the impact of this new clinical discourse turned the body, and with it the patient who possessed it, into a discrete object. The modern medical examiner fabricated a biological body, which could be read and treated only through the grid of an "anatomical atlas." The material reality of the patient's body was a product of these clinical descriptions (and not vice versa); for what took hold was the belief that these medical descriptions truly grasped and reproduced a "natural" body. Assigned to the realms of nature and biology, the body was thus expelled from history.

As a result, contemporary histories of the human body examined cultural variations of the body's manifestations and attributes: the history of sleep and food, of sexuality and disease, of age and death. But the vehicle of all this activity, the body itself, was always thought of as a physiologically stable entity. As Barbara Duden so eloquently put it: "To us the body is essentially an anatomico-physiological collection of organs. Its inner processes, its secretions, fluids, and excretions, its sexual patterning and 'vital events'—birth and death, menstruation and menopause, nursing and ejaculation, procreation and pregnancy—are always thought of as physiological processes. This mental demarcation of a socially 'raw' corporeality has created barriers between historians and the body" (1991: vii–viii). What people of a past age and culture thought about the inside of the body—the stomach, blood, and excrement—was virtually unknown and rarely looked at. But, as I explored in Chapter 4, the very notion of the body as a kind of text, although written for divine purposes, existed already as a construct in late medieval Christianity. After death, holy women's bodies were "opened up" to be searched for anatomical evidence of their sainthood, and some women's bodily interiors were minutely dissected and examined for the visible presence of Christ's stigmata in heart, stomach, or blood.[2] Late medieval theorists imagined and described an osmotic or "magical" body and were fascinated by the ways in which the female body could serve as a vehicle for supernatural forces that worked unpredictable, and incredible, effects on female organs and functions.

After all, the body of woman was itself a source of power. Women's bodies housed the forces and substances that could produce good as well as evil: blood, the periodic flow, the afterbirth, the amniotic fluid, and finally the "mother" womb (*Gebärmutter*), which, like an oven, could bring forth or take life.[3] This power and task of infusing life and destroying it was embodied in woman. But in the wake of the European Counter Reformation, beginning in the seventeenth century, we observe an attempt to shift the source of power from the female body and the utterances of women to the institution of the church and its written word.[4] Priests demanded for the church the power to bestow the life that really mattered to ensure salvation from eternal death.[5] Thus the magical renderings of female bodies, including the "power over thunderstorms, which old women had long been able to command . . . by baring their buttocks, and the power of a virgin to influence weather by opening her bleeding vulva toward heaven were no longer simply accepted as strange and mysterious powers" (Duden 1991: 8). Regarded as threats to the institutional power of religion, such sanguine abilities were denigrated and negated. According to Robert Muchembled, what took place was a "persistent devaluation of the magic of the body," which was the medium of popular culture (1983: 151). From the seventeenth century on, the new bureaucratic power of the church worked to destroy this cosmic anchoring of popular culture: official dogma began to describe the female body and its ambiguous power as a demonic threat, and to explain its very nature as "natural" weakness.

During this same period (between the sixteenth and the eighteenth centuries), when the power of the modern state was being established, the anatomical makeup of bodies gained additional strategic importance. A new system of legal justice imprinted its gaze upon the bodies of its subjects. The public butchering and disemboweling of the executed or condemned person transformed the "opening" of the body into a strategy of political power.[6] The eviscerated body of the witch, heretic, or Jew allowed the acts of justice to become visible to all, "for the people crowd[ed] to the executions as onlookers."[7] These public executions were often stretched out over several days: a few hours each day, on a stage, the body was "opened" in full view of the public.[8] What took place was the dissecting of a living body, in which the act of justice was rendered visible first by dislocating the body on the scaffold, then by burning its skin, and finally by penetrating inside the body and drawing out the intestines. It would seem (from the perspective of the modern state) that the infliction of pain was secondary to the solemn act of taking control by means of the anatomy of the condemned.[9] The symbolism of punishment was conveyed by "opening" or exposing the innermost flesh. Indeed, anatomy was at this time still a public ritual that linked the penal process to an exhibition of the structure of the human body.

Gradually, in the course of the eighteenth century, the method of dissection changed: the judicial exposure of the inside of a human being gave way to a procedure in which doctors acquired professional knowledge in a closed dissection chamber.[10] This shift in dissecting practices did not, however, release the body from the hold of the state. To the contrary, the political meanings behind the anatomizing, the "dissecting," inflicted on bodies persisted and were reflected in a deep-rooted and tenacious aversion felt by ordinary people at losing their bodies to the court anatomists: peasants near Jena as well as London began to protect their corpses in order to escape this further intrusion of the state's power after death.[11] Compounded by religious ideas about resurrection, these feelings of horror at being physically fragmented and dismembered were expressed in a series of revolts against municipal authorities.

A comparison of these acts of undisguised violence (witch persecutions, the scaffold, and anatomy) suggests not only the strategic significance of the body but also the symbolic value of its integrity. According to Duden (1991) during the two centuries when the modern state rose to power, great importance attached to two interrelated developments: in scientific work and in corporal punishment, the inside of the body was "opened up" and examined: "In this way, the connections, deeply rooted in popular culture, between this (invisible) interior and the macrocosm were eradicated. [Around 1700], the act of dissection, which exposed things, and the reduction of the body merged into one process. The 'state' was able to gain power from this opening and isolating of the body because the 'biological' body and the 'social' body were connected, had a correlation in the culture's consciousness; whatever was done to the former was never done only to a 'private body'" (10). A violent process began in the seventeenth century, in which the body as the embodiment of localized social vitality was symbolically broken: demonized, atomized, and displayed, the body was deprived of its meaningful opacity.

The sociogenesis of European modernity was thus clearly implicated in an ever increasing objectification of blood and skin. Cultural historians, as I have briefly noted, insisted that what took place was a political devaluation of the magic of the body. In Duden's words, "before the body could be constituted as the object of descriptive observation, it first had to be devalued as a vehicle of symbolic meaning" (1991: 4). Yet paradoxically, it was precisely this symbolic valuation of flesh and blood that persisted in European popular culture. Despite the emergence of a biological model of the body in late eighteenth-century medicine, at least some fragments of body parts retained their magical value: the skin, fat, tissues, bones, organs, and blood continued to exert an intense magical attraction in the imagination and ritual practices of common people.

Thus in the historical archives of modern jurisprudence we find many recorded cases that describe how ordinary people insisted on the dissection and gutting of human bodies for healing purposes. For example, we learn that in 1822, "(based upon a case authenticated by documents), there lived in Napels an old doctor; he had [begotten], by several women, children, whom he inhumanly slaughtered amid special preparations and solemnities; he cut open their breasts, took out their hearts, and prepared from the heart's blood precious drops that afforded resistance to any disease."[12] There appeared in 1890, "before the court at Hagen, in Westphalia, a servant, seventy years of age, on the serious charge of robbery of dead bodies, and desecration of graves. The accused . . . dug up with a spade . . . a child's grave . . . and next day, after opening the coffin with a screw-driver, cut out of the thigh of the corpse a piece of flesh, which he laid on a wound he had had many years on his body . . . He even imagined, at least he said so in [the] hearing of the case, that the remedy had done good."[13] In the late nineteenth century, in the province of Prussia, "[t]hose who had fallen ill through a vampire's bite were healed by having mixed with their drink some of the blood (i.e., the thickish product of decomposition so described by the populace) of [the vampire's] head when cut off . . . Only a few months ago (March 1877), at Heidenmühl, in the Schlochau district, the body of a recently-deceased child . . . was mutilated in its grave, and a small bit of the corpse-flesh was given to a sick child as a cure [for vampire's bite]."[14]

According to nineteenth-century German and Prussian popular belief, inextinguishable lamps could be made of human fat; corpse fat was fashioned into candle wax: "If a thief gets the fat of a pregnant woman, [and] makes a candle of it, and lights it, he can steal where he likes without anxiety . . . [Thus] on New Year's Eve, 1864, a fearful murder was perpetrated at Ellerwald on Elizabeth Zernickl . . . A piece of flesh, nine inches long, and the same in breadth, had been cut out of her belly . . . [And] on the evening of February 16, 1865, . . . a working man, Gottfried Dallian of Neukirch, in the Niederung, was caught, and there was found on him a strange candle, consisting of a tolerably firm mass of fat, poured round a wick, and contained in a leaden container."[15] The motive for the deed was the delusion that a candle or small lamp prepared from the fat of a murdered person would not be extinguished by any draft, and the flame could only be put out with milk.

Blood, body parts, and excrement were used for medicinal purposes in Pomerania and West Prussia until the end of the nineteenth century. When a person had fallen ill and there was an urgent conjecture of witchcraft, the presumed perpetrator (typically a young woman) was seized and beaten till her blood flowed. In order to reverse the course of the disease, the extracted blood was given to the sick man to swallow or he was washed with it. The blood letting continued until the witch promised to withdraw the spell. A few of these cases came to the attention of the courts and the public:

[In 1867, in Styria] The son of a peasant was suffering from a leg injury. Instead of calling in a doctor, the father went to a "wise-woman" . . . She declared the boy was bewitched . . . and gave him the advice to use force, and in the following way. He must bind the witch fast hand and foot, then tear out a tuft of the hair of her head; dip this in the blood coming from a deep transverse wound in the sole of the right foot, and mix it with her excrement, and use the result as a fumigation cure for the leg. No sooner said than . . . done . . . At the trial . . . the woman, who had been crippled by the cut-wound [and] the accused, who was convicted, stood all the more upon the justice of the act because the leg had begun to heal.[16]

[In 1868] a peasant in Jaschhütte [Prussia] had broken his leg. He did not seek any professional help . . . Neighbours who visited him persuaded him he was bewitched by a woman in the village. The witch, a young relative . . . [was] made to enter the house of the possessed man, and asked by those present to give him some of her blood to drink . . . [She was] forced by blows of the fist from two of those present to let the salving blood be drawn from her nose. The attempt was a failure. One of the two men went to the courtyard, dirtied his hands with manure, whilst at the same time he made three crosses with it on them. Fresh blows of the fist on the nose with the blessed hands had the desired effect. The witch was now obliged to lay herself on the bed of the possessed man, and to let the blood trickle into his open mouth. [The curse] then indeed, seemed to give way, for soon after the patient was able to utter the words: "Nu wart me beeter" (I am better now!). The still-flowing blood was then collected in a cup for possible relapses.[17]

These examples illustrating the magical manipulation of blood, fat, and flesh clearly suggest that the making of the modern body was not the result of developments in science and medicine alone. In the course of the nineteenth century, the body gradually emerged as a multilayered entity, with each layer constituted as the text of a different episteme, a different field of knowledge, a different age, and each woven out of a distinct tropological fabric spun from earlier historical material. The metaphorical stratigraphy of body and blood, as I suggest in this chapter, reveals disturbing temporal densities: the "new" corporeal aesthetic was mediated by a tenacious stream of images and motifs that persisted over centuries. At times, these mythographic patterns seemed to blend and merge, but occasionally, and remarkably, they resurfaced in their original form.

Blood Magic

In late medieval and modern European folklore, immense power was ascribed to blood, especially human blood. Understood as the source and substance of life (a vital principle), blood was imbued with an assortment of mystical properties: healing virtues, destructive propensities, and magical potency.[18] In contrast to the modern insistence on herbal or mineral essences in pharmaceutical products, European folk medicine favored the use of organic materials and substances: blood, marrow, and bone. The hearts of certain birds and the flesh, blood, and fat of particular animals were purported to have curative powers.[19] According to these cultural premises, "the blood of birds and fox heals wounds; crow's blood bewitches; blood from a cockscomb or brain of a hare is medicinal";[20] "ox-blood can act as a violent poison; weasel-blood [or the] warm blood of a shrewmouse heals strumous patients; dry pigeon blood, mixed with snuff, reduces nose-bleeding."[21] Furthermore, "bat's blood [applied to eyebrow or lids] improves vision; goat's blood [smeared on a man's testicles] is good for impotence: [here] the magical relation is obvious" (Bächtold-Stäubli 1929: 1437). Given such notions, certain types of blood were endowed with powerful properties against evil. A late medieval panacea proclaimed that "the blood of a hyaena, black dog, or woman's menstrual flow, if applied to a door frame [or threshold], wards off witches." [22]

The use of human blood purportedly intensified the efficacy of certain magical practices, a belief that promoted a cycle of transgression, murder, and brutal punishment. Thus in 1784, in Hamburg, two women were put to death on the wheel because they had murdered a Jew for his blood, using the blood in their potions against the devil and in other attempts at magical enchantment. [23] However, according to Mosaic laws, medieval Christians (and Jews themselves) had to refrain from tasting blood because it contained the spirit of living beings; hence, animal or human blood was a polluting element. [24] But in the medieval German epic, as in Old Norse myths, blood was ingested to renew strength because it was widely believed that blood contained the power of the soul. [25] Thus blood was used in love potions to spellbind lovers in the Middle Ages. [26] This practice persisted into the modern period in the folk customs of Baden, Hesse, Bohemia, and Oldenburg. For instance,

In the Oberpfalz [Upper Palatinate], sweat [and] a few drops of menstrual blood are mixed into the drink of a person, whose liking it is desired to win . . . In 1885, in the circuit of Colmar . . . a barrister had to work on a divorce case, in which, among other things, it came out that the wife, in order to keep the affection of her husband, a farmer, had put a few drops of sanguis menstruus [menstrual blood] in his coffee.—In 1888, an unmarried woman B., . . . from Schleswig, gave her sweetheart some drops of her sanguis menstruus in his coffee. "He shall not run away from me," she shouted triumphantly; he was to be unfaithful nevertheless. [27]

As the embodiment of life, blood was also desired by the dead, giving rise to the legend of vampires: their hunger for blood is well attested in German and European folklore. [28] But blood was more than a substance of life: it became a symbol of the living being, the vital self. Thus, with blood one could sign a contract with the devil, an old Saxon belief that found its way into the Faust legend in the sixteenth century, when the unscrupulous magician signed over his soul with his own blood. [29] Fortified by the power of the devil, Faust, the magician, could even triumph over the crafty Jews: [30] by cutting off his own leg as collateral to a Jewish moneylender, in the end he won back not only his soul but more than his share of wealth.

Furthermore, blood was used as a protective agent: when painted on doorposts, it could keep away witches and demons. [31] Blood was also used for many cures in folk medicine: a Swabian pharmaceutical prescribed the application of warm blood for the alleviation of pain; an old German apothecary's recipe called for the blood of a young man as an essential ingredient in the preparation of *oleum rectificatum,* a medicinal ointment, which purportedly provided the basis for *balsamus antipodagricus,* an analgesic salve for the treatment of gout, and *spiritus antiepilepticus,* an elixir to cure convulsions.[32] Moreover, according to the records of the medieval and early modern rabbinic Responsa, the blood of a he-goat was recommended as a general medicine.[33] Further, "[e]ven during the last quarter of the [eighteenth] century, it was customary in some parts of Germany on St. James Day (July 25) to throw from a church tower or even from the guildhall, amid strains of music, a he-goat adorned with gilded horns and ribbons, and, as it lay below, to draw off its blood, which when dried was esteemed as a powerful remedy [against] many illnesses" (Strack 1909: 85). Likewise, among European Jews, the blood of sacrifice was used for writing the tetragrammaton on talismans as protection against pestilence.[34] In Christian Bavaria, to relieve cramps at childbirth, a father would let the laboring mother taste the blood from his finger.[35] Three drops of blood from the wound in the father's finger prevented convulsions in children; three drops of blood from the first joint of a man's ring finger alleviated attacks of distemper in small children.[36] And fresh blood, used with the consecrated host, presented a potent remedy against illness for late medieval Christians.[37]

Toward the end of the twelfth century, when the church promoted the doctrine of transubstantiation—whereby bread and wine, when consecrated by a priest during mass, were transformed into the body and blood of Christ while retaining their outward appearance—devotion to the mass and to the eucharist rapidly gained popularity among laity.[38] As a representation of Christ's sacrifice, his crucified body was depicted in gruesome detail in sermons, stained glass windows, sculptures and paintings.[39] Perceived as a reenactment of the humanation of Christ, the celebration of mass and eucharist were often reduced to the single moment of seeing the host.[40] Periodically, preachers and bishops condemned the disorder that marked the performance of mass: the elevation of the host tended to degenerate into a moment of commotion as people scrambled toward the altar to behold the Eucharist, hoping to reap benefits from beholding the sacred.

Not surprisingly, popular eucharistic piety nourished a vast paraphernalia of practices and ideas that existed alongside the official rituals of the late medieval church. Magical notions of blood played a prominent role in this unofficial eucharistic devotion, despite repeated condemnations by theologians. One of the most common uses of the eucharist was its application in love magic: according to popular belief, if a woman kissed a man with a host in her mouth, he would always be true to her; prostitutes applied the eucharist as a sexual device to seduce men;

the host, ground into powder, served as an essential ingredient in love potions.[41] Other powers were attributed to the blood sacrament at the altar: it protected one against dangers to life and limb; it helped one to achieve wealth and fortune; it saved one from drowning; it induced fertility in humans as well as in beasts and insects; and, finally, its presence kept the devil at bay.[42] When put to evil use, the blood of Christ in the host could cause destruction of life or property. It seems to have been applied frequently in attempted abortions: in his sermons, the Franciscan preacher Berthold of Regensburg, who died in 1272, warned women not to abuse the eucharist in unwanted pregnancies.[43] In stories dating from the fifteenth century, the eucharist was also reputedly used by witches in the preparation of magical potions, whose ingredients included bone powder and the blood of children.[44] According to these medieval legends, compiled by generations of monks, friars, and bishops, Christ himself often punished the culprits who had desecrated his sacrifice by turning his body, in the form of the stolen host, into bloody human flesh.

The German discourse about blood magic was typically anti-Judaic. The use of blood was central to Jewish ritual, according to Johannes Eck, a sixteenth-century Catholic theologian.[45] The nature of such blood magic was demonic: Jews needed Christian blood to make matzo, to anoint their rabbis, to cure eye ailments, to remove body odors, and to reduce menstrual bleeding; Jewish babies were born with two tiny fingers attached to the skin of their forehead (the very image of the devil himself), and without Christian blood it was difficult to remove these fingers without harm to the child; above all, Jews needed Christian blood to wash away the blood stain inflicted on them by God because they had crucified Jesus. "It is no wonder," Johannes Eck concluded, "that the Jews now buy the blood of innocent children, just as their fathers had bought the innocent blood of Jesus from Judas with thirty pennies."[46] In such anti-Semitic writings, Jews plotted to use the milk of Christian mothers to poison the blood of Christians, practiced blood medicine with the intent to kill, and were presumed to believe that Christian blood would wash away the stains of sin. Eck's assertions reflected the fundamentally magical mental structure of learned theologians of sixteenth-century Germany. Medieval medical lore posited that milk and blood were composed of the same substance.[47] In the world presented by Eck's text, magical (homeopathic) thinking was at work: opposites attracted one another, and a sympathetic substance forced the other out. Thus Jews could use milk to poison blood, and they needed Christian blood to cleanse their own bloodstains from the murder of Jesus.[48] Attributions of blood magic, and the notion that Jews as sorcerers practiced ritual murder, were entirely constructed by clergy and were particularly prominent in the German-speaking lands of central Europe.[49]

Blood as Medicine

In the late Middle Ages and into modern times, folk belief asserted that blood could be used as a curative, a powerful remedy, particularly when combined with magic. With sympathetic healing, a common practice in central Europe, the illness or pain was believed to travel (through the medium of blood) to an external substance or object that would take on the disease. The "sympathetic" substitute could then be manipulated and treated to cure the patient. In cases of epilepsy, fever, dropsy, freckles, toothache and gout, the ailing individual was instructed to find a suitable object, preferably before dawn. According to the case descriptions in old pharmaceutical manuals or in German folklore collections,[50] the patient often selected a plant, typically a young pine or oak tree. Then he had to scrape off a small piece of the tree's bark and use it to extract a few drops of blood from the aching body part. After soaking the bark in blood, the piece of wood was returned to the tree. Thereby the disease, through the medium of blood, had been extracted from the ailing body and was transferred to the tree.[51] Body, blood, and tree were thus magically connected. Concrete examples suggest that the ailment could be vanquished by the disposal of blood:

[Nuremberg]: He who is attacked by epilepsy should have his blood let. This blood should then be poured into a hole, which is made in a tree. Thereupon one must close the hole with the bored-out wood . . . In Nuremberg, they scratch the [affliction] till it bleeds, and plug some wool, soaked in blood, into the tree.

[Lower Franconia]: The invalid goes before sunrise to a small tree, scratches his left-little finger, smears the blood on the tree, and speaks: Go away, fever; go away into the tree, etc.

[Against freckles, Lower Franconia]: Go Friday morning before sunrise into the wood, bore a hole in a tree, put some blood from the nettle-rash into the shavings that have been bored out, put them back into the hole, and shut it tightly.[52]

According to German folk belief, as suggested here, a person's health could be restored by the careful removal or extraction of blood: the disease was dispelled by the loss and transfer of the infected substance. However, in some cases, under different circumstances, medicinal healing mandated the drinking of blood or required its external application in form of an ointment or salve. Examples of the diverse uses of human blood in German and central European folk medicine have been recorded by a number of sources. The celebrated physician Theophrastus Paracelsus of Hohenheim, who died in 1541, mentioned as remedy for leprosy "a dose of human blood," and he emphasized that the external "application of menstrual blood [would] change the course of the disease."[53] A Zurich professor and municipal physician, Johannes von Muralt, prescribed in his *Hippocrates Helveticus* (1692) the use of human blood for hereditary scab. Hildegard of Bingen, a German holy woman and late medieval theologian who died in 1179 documented the experiences of popular therapeutics in her *Libri subti litatum diversarum natur. creatur.* This work is probably the oldest compilation of monastic medicine in Europe. Another well-known source on blood remedies of the late seventeenth century is the *Curieuse Hauss-Apothec,* published in Frankfurt around 1700. The text recommends the use of blood as a generic heal-all, the *elixir vitae:* "The wondrous virtue of human blood is this. If one distills into an alembic the blood of a young, healthy person about thirty odd years old, it makes all poor complexions again blooming, is good for all weakness [frailties] of the brain, memory, and spirits, banishes all poison from the heart, cures all manner of lung complaints, purifies the blood beyond all other medicaments, and is good for diarrhea and lumbago, and increases the blood and semen, etc."[54]

From these and other texts, we learn that the magical potency of blood was strongest, assuming its most concentrated form, in the flow of the menarche. Hildegard of Bingen's work praised the use of baths in menstrual exudings for leprosy, and it recommended the application of a virgin's warm uterine blood to gouty limbs for the alleviation of violent pain: "The pains of podagra are relieved by the menstrual blood of a virgin, when it is smeared warm upon the [hurtful] place . . . Linen rags, steeped in menstrual blood, are poultices against gout — well known from of old. A shirt, stained with this blood, would protect against blow and stab and quench any outbreak of fire when thrown into the flames." Above all, "the first of a virgin's menses, preserved on the shift or a piece of linen is held in high esteem, and steeped in vinegar or rose-water, laid on diseased glands, small-pox, [and] apostemes, in accordance to the extent of the damage, and applied repeatedly, is prized as an excellent remedy."[55] The eighteenth-century apothecary book concurred with these observations about the medicinal potency of menstrual blood: "Take a piece of a virgin's shift, who has for the first time had the monthly flow [menses]. Wrap it in a new trousers' belt, which a pure [unblemished] virgin has made, and bind it on the naked skin beneath [under] the right arm, so wilt thou feel the effect."[56] Menstrual blood was also a good remedy for curing a woman's monthly problems. According to Frankish folk practice, a woman was compelled to drink water mixed with blood (from a first menstruation) to restore her own menarche; or she was advised to consume the bloody water in which another girl's menstrual shift had been previously washed; but even contact with a woman's menarche by wearing a shift moistened with fresh menstrual blood was expected to have the same dramatic physiological effect: the onset of her menstrual flow.[57]

The flow of the menarche, the blood of a still-born child, a bleeding placenta or a bloody umbilical cord, and the blood from a fresh corpse or an executed person (i.e., the blood of violence, murder, and death) were seen as powerful agents in the early modern struggle with illness and disease.[58] A treatment with such blood was to alleviate pain and dispel all ailments, including epilepsy, tumors, eruptions, outgrowths, diseased glands and swellings, leprosy, red birthmarks, infections, warts, gout, toothaches, brown moles, and apostemes.[59]

[According to Frankish folk belief in the nineteenth century] [b]irthmarks, red moles, and freckles vanish if they are smeared with warm menstrual blood, the placental exudings or the blood of an umbilical cord . . . from a woman bearing her first child. Moles are cured by being covered with the blood of a fresh umbilical cord, by being rubbed with a fresh afterbirth. [In Ennsthal, people say that] [t]he red moles [i.e., *Feuermal*] should be covered with a linen cloth moistened with fresh menstrual blood. [In Oberland, near Graz, folk belief holds that] [t]he brown moles, especially in the case of women, might be dispelled by soaking them with warm menstrual blood. [In Germany], [t]the smearing of warts with fresh menstrual blood is universally practiced.[60]

The blood from human beings who died a violent death, especially executed persons, was held to be even more efficacious than menstrual blood. In Swabia and Bavaria, "the blood of executed criminals, drunk warm, [was recommended] for epilepsy; somebody, to get rid of this complaint, [must drink] the still warm blood of an executed person."[61] In Wildeshausen, this same remedy was said to "drive away" physical afflictions: "Blood of an executed person, when drunk, helps against epilepsy and fever. One must, if possible, drink it fresh."[62] According to popular assertions in Siebenbürgen, the blood of the hanged is helpful in cases of epilepsy and convulsions.[63] The Danish writer Hans Christian Andersen described in his autobiography such an event, which he claimed to have witnessed at Skelskör in 1823: "I saw a poor sick man, whom his superstitious parents made drink a cup of the blood of the executed person that he might be healed of epilepsy; after which they ran with him in wild career till he sank to the ground."[64] The historical chronicle of the free city of Schneeberg makes mention of a similar practice in its description of a man's public execution on 15 December 1823, in Zwickau. The report concludes: "And with our own eyes we saw how a pot full of blood of the executed man was drunk dry by various persons, and how these persons, mostly children, were driven with blows from whips to run at utmost speed over the field." [65]

The use of human blood in pharmaceutical products, and as a popular remedy, persisted through the eighteenth and nineteenth centuries. The historical museum in Tetschner City retained the following document: a letter, dated July 1729, in which a J. M. Rühtenick of Leitmeritz requests permission to collect the blood issuing from the public execution of a convict. [66] The seal on the letterhead reveals that the writer was a priest, acting on behalf of a Jesuit pharmacy:

High and Mighty Noble
Especially Honorable Judge!
Having learned that the execution shall proceed at this time, I hereby request permission to catch the blood of the delinquent, since I need the same for very useful medicines in our pharmacy.

In Germany during the eighteenth century, it was the executioner's rightful privilege to sell (or give away) the blood of his delinquents after they had been put to death. [67] For instance, when the murderer Carsten H. Hinz was executed on 16 April 1844, the epileptic son of a farmer (P. Ketels of Gunsbüttel) drank, by permission of the Oldenburg executioner, some of the criminal's blood. [68] By granting such petitions, "the executioner and other town officials rendered lawful and promoted crass superstition" (Distel 1888: 160). The practice of drinking blood for medicinal purposes was transformed into a clinical or institutional commonplace in nineteenth-century Germany: "A woman [living in an] almshouse suffered from falling sickness [epilepsy], and received permission to go on the day [of the] execution to Trogen [in Appenzell] and try the gruesome remedy. Three draughts [of blood] must be swallowed whilst the names of the three Highest are invoked." [69] As attested by various legal documents, the German administration, including judges, attorneys, and town officials (perhaps for a commission), routinely approved formal requests for the collection of human blood:

On 6th June, 1755, K. G. Zeibig, who, when drunk, had murdered a man, was beheaded on the Rabenstein at Dresden [Saxony] . . . Before the execution, two senior apprentices of the guild of tailors from Dresden begged the prime minister, the imperial count Heinrich von Brühl, on behalf of their fellow guild member, Joh. Ge. Wiedemann, who suffered severely from epilepsy, that the same be allowed to drink the blood of the murderer for his restoration to health. An entry in the register announces that Brühl assented to the request, and also that Wiedemann, after drinking the blood of the individual beheaded "ran off." [70]

In German-speaking lands, these practices persisted well into the late nineteenth century. Thus a memorandum by a Mr. Woytasch, the attorney general of Marienwerder, dated August 1892, recounts in gruesome detail the witnessing of such an event:

I was a pupil of the famous Professor Herrmann at [the University of] Göttingen. At his suggestion, in early January 1859, I attended the public execution of [a murderess,] a female poisoner in Göttingen. It was done with a sword. When the head was severed from the body, and when the fountain of blood sprang up one and a half feet high, the populace broke through the square formed by [the armed guards] the Hannover *Schützen*, rushed upon the scaffold, and possessed itself of the blood of the dead woman, collecting it and dipping white sheets into [the puddles of blood]. It was positively a gruesome experience. To my horrified question [about the event] I received the reply that the blood was applied for the cure of epilepsy.[71]

Such documents and written artifacts (e.g., an entry in a town registry, a memorandum by a district attorney, a priest's letter requesting blood for a Jesuit pharmacy) are especially intriguing in light of the categorical prohibitions that the medieval Catholic church had placed on the commonplace eating and drinking of blood. These prohibitions and the accompanying theological doctrines and interpretations are well attested in the early medieval penance books and penitentials, which were written between the sixth and the ninth centuries.[72] Developed out of the monastic tradition of the confession of faults, these religious works (commonly referred to as "penitentials") were intended as spiritual guides for priests by providing descriptions of various sins and specifying correspondingly appropriate penances. These works contain many of the religious sanctions and ecclesiastical judgments concerning the consumption of blood for ritual or magical purposes:

If someone should eat the blood of animals unknowingly, or the blood and meat of strangled, deceased or sacrificial animals, or pigs having eaten blood, he shall do penance for four days over bread and water; but if he knew it, he shall live two years without meat and wine.[73]

The woman, who drinks the blood of her husband for curative purposes, or who gives blood to her husband as a medical remedy, must do penance for forty days.[74]

Whoever makes another person drink blood, semen, or urine for love or other reasons, they shall do penance for three years.[75]

The catalogue of offenses and the tariffs for sins were gradually extended to include the consumption of one's own blood.[76] In these medieval handbooks for priests, the magical manipulation of body and blood was clearly defined as an offense that was included in the list of prohibitions: as a sign of "barbarism" and heathen idolatry, the ritual consumption of blood was forbidden outside the celebration of mass, the eucharist, and the taking of communion.[77] The penitential restrictions were repeated well into the twelfth century, when Otto von Bamberg, for instance, took it upon himself to instruct the newly converted Pomeranians in proper devotional conduct. Yet while providing a core of canons dealing with matters of blood, and while repeatedly taking up "the question of women who mix their menstrual blood in food or drink and give it to their husbands to consume and the question of a woman who drinks her husband's semen,"[78] we know little about how the manuals were used in practice. But I suspect that as reference works and guides, these official pronouncements on the "sins of blood" were central to the compilation and transmission of a comprehensive code of a sanguine aesthetic in the Middle Ages. Regional transgressions, local violations, and traditional medicinal practices thus emerged as formative challenges in the development of a unified blood ethos.

Pure Blood—Clean Skin

Despite all efforts by the church, the clergy, and members of the religious orders to inhibit the popular uses of blood, the magical appropriations of the red flow remained an integral part of German folk culture. The concept that an immersion in blood could heal various ailments and result in an increase in strength and vitality was a common motif in traditional (postmedieval) German tales.[79] In these narratives, the ritual power of blood was enhanced whenever witches, sorcerers, monsters, giants, or wild men obtained such blood from virgins.[80] The blood of the innocent victim, including especially maiden women and young children, had the power to cure leprosy, congenital scabies, and other skin diseases.[81] A legend from the Swiss Aargau, at Lindenberg, "relates how a libertine, having become leprous, wanted to bathe in the blood of twelve virgins, so as to be healed . . . he had already killed eleven."[82] An Alsatian tale recounts a similar horror: "A giant [was] leprous and want[ed] to bathe in children's blood in order to cure himself. His servant ha[d] already kidnapped eight children, slaughtered them, and gathered their blood in a bowl," when the horror was discovered.[83] Perhaps such practices were motivated by the belief that "pure" blood absorbed impurities and thereby cured the disease:

Health, which has been shaken to its core . . . can only be restored by the application and invigoration of the *pure*. Ordinary aid by means of herbs, juices, [and] stones, which only operates for particular things, is futile; a complete annihilation of the evil and a new *rejuvenated* life are requisite. Leprosy and blindness were regarded as such generally incurable diseases that could only be removed by a miracle . . . The pure blood of a virgin or of a child was, above all, thought to be the source of life which would abolish those diseases and engender a new flourishing life . . . The patient had to be bathed in it or be sprinkled with it; whereupon he was pure and fresh, like a maid or a child. (Grimm and Grimm 1815: 172)

Many German and central European legends revolve around such a theme: pure blood, taken from a sacrificial victim, could expel all evil. Typical are the various narratives about selfless love, sacrifice, and male friendship. These tales usually begin by staging a context: two men, old friends, stand by each other when one of them becomes leprous. "When the other learns that a cure is only possible by children's blood, he kills his own children, and brings their blood to his friend. The friend is cured, but God rewards the other's loyalty by raising the children to life again."[84] This narrative exists in several different versions.[85] Typical is the tale of Ludwig and Alexander, which conveys the persistent belief in the medicinal power of children's blood: After learning of a cure for leprosy (from a mysterious healer), Ludwig "betook himself into the chamber wherein his five children lay, and killed them all five together, and took a vessel and filled it with the children's blood. Whereupon he went to Alexander and washed him all over with it. Now when Alexander had been washed with the blood, he suddenly became fresh and quite whole."[86] Some versions of this legend are more explicit in conveying their anti-Semitic intentions: the medicinal advice, which results in the killing of an innocent child, presumably issues from a Jewish physician:

King Richard of England, suffering from leprosy, sent for a Jew renowned for his skill, as no other doctor could help him. This doctor did his best, but the illness grew quickly worse. At last he spoke: I know of "a powerful remedy, if your Majesty had heart enough to employ it . . . Know that you will recover your health completely, if you can make up your mind to bathe in the blood of a new-born child, since I can swear to your Majesty by my Law that nothing in the world works so vigorously against the corruption that has settled on your body as the fresh blood of a new-born child. But because this remedy is only external, it must be helped out by an additional recipe, which extirpates even the inward root of the malady. Namely, the child's heart must be added, which your Majesty must eat and consume quite warm and raw, just as it has been taken from the body.[87]

The cannibalistic (and eucharistic) implications of these tales made plausible the extraordinary therapeutic power of blood. The narrative plot centered on the slaughter of an innocent male infant (i.e., Jesus), who was killed with the assistance or through the advice of a mysterious Jewish physician. These narratives are thus thematically connected to the anti-Semitic legends of blood ritual murder. Moreover, the image of the dead child (whose blood provided redemption) was in Christian iconography fused with the image of the eucharist, the lamb/flesh/body of God, whose suffering and bloodletting restored and healed the world. The legend about leprosy and child murder intensified this imagery through the coupling of two closely related motifs: crucifixion and martyrdom. The infant's death (and, as reported in some narrative versions, a man's selfless love for another) produced a concoction of blood that healed, rejuvenated, and purged.

The theme of suffering (and divine redemption) was central to these stories. Although the motif of the dead child was sometimes replaced by that of a selfless maiden (probably evocative of the gender ambiguity of the wounded Christ), the plot and the presumed power of blood remained unchanged. This is suggested by a narrative version attributed to the Swabian poet Hartmann von Aue, which dates back to the twelfth century. The tale, titled *Der arme Heinrich* (The unfortunate Henry), goes as follows.[88] The Swabian knight Heinrich suffered from leprosy as punishment for his arrogance. He consulted every known physician and was finally told that there existed only one remedy for his affliction: he had to find a young virgin who would willingly die for him; then her blood could cure him. Since Heinrich had no hope of finding such a girl, he decided to become a hermit and pray for his soul. He took refuge in the forest and lived on a small farm, where a peasant and his twelve-year-old daughter began to care for him. After some time, the girl learned of the cure of blood and finally offered her own body as a sacrifice. Heinrich accepted and took her with him to the (Jewish) physician, who was to extract her blood and kill her. In the end, the knight changed his mind about the ordeal and came to accept his disease. The girl was thus saved. For this decision, Heinrich was miraculously cured.

The eucharistic symbolism of blood surfaced again in modern legends: in these later narratives, the plot was often driven by a female protagonist—a villainous (bloodthirsty) woman. The tale reports how her vanity and desire for beauty (not her illness or suffering) drove her to lure "young girls into her castle, [where] she had their blood extracted . . . for the beautifying of her skin, and in which she bathed herself."[89] In such tales, blood had a cleansing propensity: bathing in blood washed away blemish and stain and restored the skin's youth and beauty. This purifying power of blood was linked to victimhood and murder: the killing of innocent children.[90] But here the motif of the dead child (i.e., the infant Jesus) was transformed into images of birth or rebirth from the female body: the catalyst for transformation was typically the blood of a young maiden, or virgin. These Western images of female victimhood and cannibalistic trangression are relatively recent historical productions.[91] From the late medieval period into the seventeenth century, accusations of blood libel were told and imagined with Jewish and female perpetrators.

Such legends of ritual murder not only reveal the inherently feminizing potential of blood consumption but also express a modern ambivalence toward women and power. European cultural historians have marshaled a wealth of evidence suggesting that fear of women grew from the sixteenth century on, and that the female body took on an increasingly threatening form in the popular imagination.[92] In narrative genres, this perceived threat of women's bodies gave rise to the motif of the female monster who killed and extracted her victims' blood for pleasure as well as self-enhancement:

A Hungarian woman, Elizabeth, was excessively fond of making herself up to please her husband, and spent as much as the half of a day at her toilette. It happened that one day one of her chamber-maids made some mistake in her coiffure, and received for it such a violent box on the ears, that the blood spurted on her mistress's face. When the latter washed the drops of blood off her face, the skin on the place appeared to her to be much more beautiful, whiter and more delicate. She at once came to the inhuman decision to bathe her face, nay her whole body, in human blood, so as thereby to increase her beauty and attractions. With this horrible intention, she took counsel of two old women, who accorded her their entire sympathy, and promised to assist her in the ghastly project. A certain Fitzko, a pupil of Elizabeth, was also made a member of this bloodthirsty society. This madman usually killed the unfortunate victims, and the old women collected the blood, in which that monster of a woman was wont to bathe in a trough about four o'clock in the morning. She appeared to herself always more beautiful after the bath. She therefore continued her operations even after her husband's death in 1604, in order to win new worshippers and lovers.

The wretched girls who were lured into Elizabeth's house by the old women under the pretense of going into service, were taken into the cellar on various pretexts. Here they were seized and beaten until their bodies swelled. Not infrequently Elizabeth tortured them herself, and very often she changed her blood-dripping clothes and then began her cruelties anew. The swollen bodies of the poor girls were then cut open with a razor. It was not uncommon for this monster to have the girls burnt and then flayed; most of them were beaten to death.[93]

In such popular imaginings, blood therapy was embedded in a new semantic field: eroticism and violence were fused in the legendary excesses of female self-indulgence.[94]

Bloodletting as Therapy

The popular preoccupations with blood, violence, and healing were deeply connected to a cultural thematic that had its analogue in certain branches of medical science: healers and physicians advocated the use of blood therapy "because it accorded with what educated men and women believed about their own bodies" (Sennett 1994: 162). Blood, when wrenched from the fleshly interior, had redemptive powers: it acted as a magical agent that healed or purged the body of loathsome afflictions. But the blood that remained inside the body, beneath its skin, lacked such redemptive qualities: enclosed within the corporeal interior, blood became a stagnant and foul accumulation that could cause illness. A medical handbook for German farmers, published in 1700, warns of the dangers of inert (brackish) sanguinity: "To preserve the health of human bodies, on occasion we require that the same be purged of the unclean and superfluous blood. For where it becomes overabundant [plethoric], it begins to putrefy, corrupt, and rot, and therefrom arise all sorts of diseases. In consequence, it is crucial that one knows how, where, and when blood-letting should take place. Remember not to let too much [blood be drawn], and beware that the purging proceeds in accordance with the advice of the physician, and it is best done in spring or autumn." [95] Ill health was linked to an excess accumulation of body fluids—to surplus blood, a condition called *plethora*. Induced blood loss, that is, the deliberate extraction of blood, was therefore an accepted medical strategy that aimed to restore the proper balance of organs, blood, and moisture.

Thus, throughout medieval and modern Europe, a standard therapeutic measure for disease was bloodletting, a practice that consisted of the deliberate removal of small amounts of blood from the body. Bloodletting, which was performed until the middle of the nineteenth century, served as a treatment for a wide range of ailments: falling sickness, convulsions, hemorrhoids, indigestion, palpitations of the heart, paralysis, plague, rheumatism, small pox, softening of the brain, suppression of urine, and other assorted disorders.[96] But bloodletting could also promote a general sense of well-being. A manuscript from the seventeenth century, written in verse form, recommends bloodletting as a healthful remedy for patients:[97]

> By bleeding, to the marrow commeth heat,
> It maketh cleane your braine, relieves your eye,
> It mends your appetite, restoreth sleepe,
> Correcting humours that do waking keepe:
> All inward parts and senses also clearing,
> It mends the voyce, touch, smell & taste, & hearing.

Bloodletting, as a medical therapy, redressed the disease-causing imbalance of internal fluids, humors, and sanguine substances that made up the constituent elements of the body.[98] The bodily interior, left to its own devices, could produce at least a temporary excess of blood—

accumulation, stagnation, rot—and the morbid lesions that constituted the disease. Medical intervention in this physiological process was perceived as necessary and therapeutic. Thus by means of "plethora" (and the treatment of an anomalous surplus of blood), physiology was connected with pathology.

European physicians developed elaborate methods for bleeding their patients: phlebotomy, cupping, venesection, cutting, laceration, and leeching. Manuscripts from the late Middle Ages prescribed ethical codes for physicians: doctors were advised to be courteous to their patients and to make small incisions when withdrawing blood, "so that from sinewes you all hurt do keepe."[99] Medieval recipes for bloodletting describe horns that were applied to the skin: the patient's blood was extracted by sucking out the air through the horn's upper opening, which was then sealed with a finger or with wax; these horns were gradually replaced by wide-necked vessels of metal or glass.[100] According to a sixteenth-century physician's manual, this method of bloodletting was medically less effective because it could only draw blood from the body's fleshy surface, leaving untouched the interior—the domain of the vital organs: "Bloodletting from the veins [*Aderlassen*] draws or pulls the blood up from the depth of the inner body, namely from the heart, the lung, etc. . . . . But cupping [*Schrepfen or Ventosen*] merely draws out the blood from the very body surface, where it resides [*steckt*] in the body's outer perimeter—in flesh and skin."[101] In modern times, such treatments were generically included under the so-called antiphlogistic regimen, which aimed to purge the body of accumulating fluids through the use of clysters (enemas), blistering salves, dietary restrictions, cooling lotions, and especially bloodletting in one form or another. By the early nineteenth century, this therapeutic strategy was recommended by English physicians for about two-thirds of all identifiable diseases.[102] The prevalence of this regimen can be estimated from the fact that for leeching, only one of the standard techniques for extracting blood, British physicians imported from France more than six million leeches each year.[103]

Physicians saw the body's morbid accumulation of blood as a pathological condition that threatened a person's state of health. Nevertheless, medical practitioners cautioned against the use of overly aggressive and extensive bloodletting. Thus a handbook for German farmers, published in 1700, attempted to impress upon its readers awareness of the dangers of generic bleeding: "But this one thing I will warn you about, and this you understand certainly: the heart-vein should never be bled. From my master I learned as an ethical duty that this vessel must never be injured. It often causes great damage . . . And when the bloodletting occurs . . . better give less blood than too much." [104] In order to prevent damage through excessive bleeding, the practice of bloodletting was typically localized. Physicians extracted blood from proscribed body parts to thereby affect a concrete ailment. A medieval physician's manual offers the following instructions: "There is a blood vessel [*Ader*] on the index finger; it is called *salvatellam* by anatomists. The same must cut on the right hand in case of a congested [blood-staunched] liver and bled on the left hand to alleviate constipation [blood-stagnation] of the spleen.' [105]

Specific veins were thought to be responsible for "feeding" or nourishing a complex of symptoms. A late medieval health code thus suggests:

A vein called *salvatell*
helps liver and spleen,
renders voice light,
it purifies around the chest and heart,
And thereby drives away pain. [106]

Once an illness manifested itself on the body surface through physical symptoms, physicians sought to purge the afflicted area of foul blood substances. [107]

Bloodletting manuals contain detailed descriptions about the spatial proximity of blood, veins, and disease. [108] A German handbook from the eighteenth century meticulously affixed various diseases and pains onto the body: a corporeal topography was charted and mapped, which could be consulted in an almost mechanical fashion:

Blood drawn from the *head* works for deafness and bleeding of the brain. Blood drawn from the *forehead* alleviates headaches, brain pain, and leprosy. Blood taken from the *temples* quenches headaches, bleeding, and boils on the eyes. Blood drawn from the *nose* heals scabs on head or eyes. Blood taken from *behind the ear* cures aches, improves memory, cleanses throat and face, and is good for breathing and the heart. Blood extracted from the *side of the mouth* heals facial boils and scabs on the head. Blood drawn from *under the tongue* works against toothaches, pain in the side, and a bleeding throat. Blood drawn from the *neck* shrinks boils on back and throat. Blood drawn from the *arm* is good for liver and spleen, a tight chest, headaches, stomach, and heart. Blood taken from the *elbow* strengthens heart and lungs, and reduces cramps and colic. Bloodloss from the *thumb* helps against headaches. Blood from the *smallest finger* works well for ailments of lung and spleen. Blood taken from the body's *right side* counters pestilence and anemia. Bleeding from the *buttocks* is advised for boils and small pox. Blood extracted from *knee, foot,* or *navel* is useful for gravel, gall-stones, bleeding in childbed, and pain in the hips. Blood drawn from the *big toe* reduces pains, boils, and menstrual bleeding. Blood extracted from the *small toe* helps against measles, epilepsy, pox, gravel, and dropsy. [109]

Every vein or vessel purportedly supplied specific body parts with sanguine fluid, thereby nourishing a localized symptom. Since brackish or spoiled blood fed the disease, its extraction (i.e., the draining of foul fluid) dried up or "starved" the sickness.

The art of bloodletting was performed under a variety of scientific and customary rituals. Medieval physicians developed elaborate methods for bleeding their patients, relying on astrological charts and religious sanctions to obtain the most favorable results. Blood extraction was considered most effective in April, May, and September.[110] Each month supposedly had characteristics that favored or promoted the bleeding of specific veins. For example, a blood vessel on the left arm, known as *Leberader,* or "liver vein," was bled in January; blood was drawn from hand or thumb in February; blood was extracted from any body part but the thumb in March; and the *Medianader,* or "median (center) vein," on the index finger was bled in April.[111] Since each blood vessel was thought to "feed" a concrete set of disease symptoms, different ailments were more effectively "starved" or diminished during certain times of the year.

According to these seventeenth- and eighteenth-century handbooks, the best season for bleeding was spring. The practice of extracting blood was less likely to be performed in winter and was considered especially dangerous during the summer. A bleeding manual from 1700 informs us that "the time of spring is warm and moist by nature, like the air: during this season, the blood grows, which is also warm . . . It is the best time of the year to take medications and be bled . . . [Summer] is the other time of the year, hot and dry; there grows the cholera, called the black or burned blood, which is analogous to fire, which is also hot and dry. The cholerics should abstain from bathing, bleeding, and all sorts of medication."[112] During the remaining seasons, bloodletting was possible, although it was not especially encouraged: "The third season [fall] is dry and cold, and there grows a wetness, which is called melancholy, and it is like the earth . . . One may take medicine and draw off blood . . . The fourth season [winter] is cold and wet, and there grows a wetness in human bodies called phlegm. One may take medicines and let out the blood."[113] No blood was ever supposed to be extracted in midwinter or midsummer, that is, the coldest and hottest times of the year.

The techniques of bloodletting were not only administered in direct response to illness; blood therapy and bleeding were also used as a preventive measure. Physicians tended to guard against disease by periodically drawing blood from their patients. Women were sometimes bled but much less frequently than men because, as physicians themselves acknowledged, female bodies achieved a beneficial cleansing through menstrual bleeding. Men could attain such a purging only through hemorrhoidal discharges or through artificial bleeding.[114] Indeed, physicians regarded bloodletting as an analogue to the female menstrual process. This view was promoted by the *Cyclopedia of Practical Medicine,* a scholarly publication from the early decades of the nineteenth century: "A tendency to plethora [i.e., flux, blood accumulation] in the head will be best counteracted by occasional revulsive bleeding from the lower extremities: as, for instance, the abstraction of a few ounces of blood from the feet . . . We have found this plan particularly useful in cases of suppressed or irregular menstruation, and by having recourse to it at the approach of the menstrual period, or on the first appearance of any of the symptoms threatening an attack of convulsions, we may often succeed in warding it off."[115]

Although European physicians usually did not make incisions in the male genital organs, "there were other parts of the [male] anatomy that were morphologically more similar to the female reproductive system" (Carter 1982: 226). Incisions were commonly made in the interior of the thigh, and leeches were applied to veins at the anus. Nineteenth-century physicians clearly regarded hemorrhoidal bleeding or men's blood loss through the "piles" as a beneficial equivalent to the menstrual discharge, and physicians thought of bloodletting as an artificial parallel to both.[116] Induced bleeding thus worked to counter the ill effects experienced from "the suppression of habitual discharges, such as hemorrhoidal and menstrual flux."[117] Examples from a nineteenth-century British medical encyclopedia further illustrate these connections:

[Should a suppression of the hemorrhoidal discharge be the cause of a disease], aloetic purgatives, and leeches applied *circa anum,* are the means to be employed. If the suspended menstrual discharge seems to be the cause . . . we try to assist the abortive efforts of nature at the ordinary period of the menstrual discharge, by determining [blood] to the uterus by means of aloetic purgatives, [and] by leeches applied to the interior of the thighs.[118]

[A physician] describes the case of a woman, thirty years of age, previously strong and healthy, in whom the menstrual discharge was in general remarkably copious. Having suffered from a fright immediately before the menstrual period, the charge did not take place, and she was seized with languor, loss of appetite, and dropsical swelling to such a degree that the integuments on the feet burst and discharged serum in great quantity. The menstrual discharge having taken place at the next period, all these complaints were removed . . . Similar symptoms have been occasionally observed in connexion with suppression of hemorrhoidal discharge after it has become habitual . . . Bloodletting is the first remedy demanded, and in almost every case this may and should be general.[119]

Various psychological attempts at interpretation suggest that woman's power, as perceived by men, was associated with her periodic loss of blood through menstruation.[120] What better symbolic expression could there be of a man's superior endowment than his ability to withstand the extensive losses of blood that "nature" extracted from woman? Thus, in being bled, his manhood was reaffirmed.[121] However, bloodletting redefined men's relationship not only to women but also to members of the lower social orders, none of whom ordinarily submitted to the ritual.[122] The sexual asymmetry was projected onto the social order, since bloodletting patients were drawn mostly from the nobility, clerics, and the wealthy.

Monks of the Middle Ages had to be bled from time to time under ecclesiastical law, and monasteries as well as churches had special rooms set aside for this purpose.[123] For members of the religious orders, the shedding of blood brought expiation and justification. Bleeding took on a similar role in the secular realm. There, the violation of social norms and the sins of overindulgence were mediated through blood atonement.

According to the emergent medical models, the bodies of the overindulgent, that is, those that ate or drank too much, who enjoyed beds too soft or too many warm baths, who were indolent, who had too much warmth, luxury and sex, produced at least temporarily an excessive accumulation of blood.[124] In such cases, bleeding was used to return the body to its normal state. A German physician's manual from the turn of the seventeenth century very explicitly pointed to bloodletting as a remedy for the consequences suffered from an excess of food and drink: "The enlightened Philippus Melanchthon used to say often and many times to his audience: We Germans eat and drink ourselves into poverty and sickness and into hell. Now if one has filled the body to the gills with a mixture of strange foods, and the next morning suffers from headaches, difficulty in breathing and pressure on the chest and other such things occur, then one should be bled quickly [*zur Ader lassen*]." [125]

Excess was a sign of wealth; overindulgence was not a problem for the poor. Because it was a class-specific practice, consumption and overindulgence created a social disequilibrium. By bleeding his patients and extracting their blood, the physician "mediated a kind of blood atonement for the excesses of his people" (Carter 1982: 227). The medical practitioner assumed the social role of a priest-physician who, by extracting blood, restored the symmetry of the social world: the blood of the privileged had to flow in imitation of Christ.

Sanguine States

These ideas about the inner world of fluids and organs derived from the medical and scientific assumptions of an earlier era, which were incorporated into medieval thinking with but little challenge.[126] Ancient ideas of body heat, sperm, menstrual blood, and the morphology of bodies passed into the medieval world with the authority of received wisdom; these beliefs were modified, often unwittingly, by the symbolics of blood in a Christian society that applied them a thousand years later.

Although the body and its interior had been the focus of systematic inquiry in ancient times, a principal means by which this medical knowledge passed into the medieval era was the publication of *Ars medica* by the Greek physician Galen, an edition that first appeared in Salerno before 1200 and was then adopted in Paris and other European centers of learning by the late thirteenth century. In this text, Galen defines medicine as "knowledge of what is healthy, morbid, and natural," a knowledge that depends on understanding how body heats and fluids interact in the principal organs of the body, the brain, heart, liver, and testes.[127] Body heat, Galen thought, ascended gradually along a sliding scale; body fluids, however, were of four types, or "humors": blood, phlegm, yellow bile, and black bile. The combination of heat and fluid produced in turn four psychological states, or "temperaments": Galen called them sanguine, phlegmatic, choleric, and melancholic. The manifestation of a temperament depended on how hot, cold, dry, or wet a person's body was at a given moment, and on which fluids were flowing hot and full and which trickled through the body slow and cold.[128] In Galen's view, emotionally charged behavior such as aggression or compassion derived from the temperaments that were created by an interchange of heat and fluids in the body. Thus Galen described the choleric temperament of a person, whose heart was warm and dry, in the following way: "The pulse is hard, big, rapid, and frequent, and breathing is deep, rapid, and frequent . . . Of all people, these have the hairiest chest . . . they are ready for action, courageous, quick, wild, savage, rash, and impudent. They have a tyrannical character, for they are quick-tempered and hard to appease."[129] This totalizing ethos was the very essence of Galen's model; it appealed to medieval readers under the sway of scientific humanism because it tied the body to the soul. The person sorrowing for others was in a melancholic state; compassion made the bile run hot in the heart. This was the physiology of a body experiencing the "imitation of Christ."[130]

Based on Galen's work and amplified by the observations of Arab and Italian researchers, the medical school at Salerno developed a regimen of health, which was gradually adopted by medieval physicians throughout central Europe. The treatment of illness was founded on the proposition that the human body contained the same four elements as those that made up the cosmos: in the body air was transmuted into blood (*sanguinity*); fire into yellow or green bile (*choler*); water into phlegm (*phlegmaticism*); and earth into black bile (*melancholy*).[131] The Salerno dietary code was filled with references to food that produced "bad" blood or "good" blood, and to the psychological states of "hot-bloodedness" and "cold-bloodedness."[132] This basic concept retained its popular appeal in German medical practice for several hundred years. The concept of humoral pathology prevailed until the early nineteenth century, and even appeared in the philosophical works of Immanuel Kant. In his *Anthropologie*, published in 1800, Kant suggested that mental states, or temperaments, were determined by the quality of body fluids and the elements of heat and cold that were involved in the processing of these humors. He derived the terminology for his classification of temperaments from a typology of blood. In four successive sections of his work, we find detailed descriptions of the sanguine state of the "light blooded person" (*des Leichtblütigen*) the melancholy of the "heavy blooded" person (*des Schwerblütigen*), the choleric temperament of the "hot blooded" individual (*des Heissblütigen*), and the phlegmatic character of the "cold blooded" man (*des Kaltblütigen*).[133] Such writings promoted the cultural persistence and revival of older beliefs about the properties of blood, resulting in a complete blurring of the boundaries between mental and physical afflictions. In these sanguine visions, the body emerged as a permeable organism: interior states were expressed externally through illness or mental disposition, which in turn were shaped by the external world, which impressed itself onto the composition of blood, fluids, and organs.

Indeed, the society of the early modern period did not yet conceive of a corporeality that was isolated or "disembedded" from the total network of social relations.[134] This becomes evident in attempts by European cities to prepare themselves for the approaching plague.[135] Under the pressure of this threat, the "scourge of God," varied activities unfolded in which the seventeenth-century gaze saw the presence of a "body" internally undivided and externally unbounded. The transitions from daily afflictions — evil and corrupting fevers, suppurating boils, watery stools — to the plague were as unspecific and vague as the boundaries between the corruption within the body and the decay of the entire cosmos.[136] The plague was perceived as a disease not only of the physical body but also of nature and the social body.

The physical body, on which the signs of poisoning were observed, was an "open organism," exposed to "evil" influences. The putrid vapors penetrated through the openings to the inside: through the pores (the pores of a hot-blooded person being more open than those of a melancholic person), through the mouth and nose, and then pushed on to the center, the heart. A constant exchange took place between the inside and the outside, "a relation of osmotic exchanges with the elements" (Duden 1991: 71). Efforts to cure the disease concentrated on calming the disturbed exchange between inside and outside with unguents, fumigation, massages, herbal pouches, and precious stones placed near the heart, while making sure not to clog the sensitive mechanisms of "reciprocal exchange and filtration between the inside and outside" (77). In this cosmos, the skin did not close off the body, the inside, against the outside world. In like manner, the body itself was also never closed off; it was composed of material that did not differ from the world surrounding it.[137]

The Permeable Body

How was such a permeable body experienced and constituted in everyday life? How did people in early modern Germany think about the inside of the body, the hidden world of stomach, blood, and excrement? In her exceptional history of the female body, Barbara Duden (1991) describes how a doctor and his woman patients in the German town of Eisenach around 1730 envisioned the inside of the female body, and how their ideas of blood, illness, and healing shaped their world. Duden's analysis draws on the voluminous works on *Weiberkrankheiten* compiled by Doctor Johannes Pelagius Storch, who in his old age excerpted his patients' case histories from a twenty-year span and compiled them into a multivolume handbook of instruction for younger colleagues. The volumes appeared over a six-year span, from 1747 to 1752. "In each of the more than 1800 cases Storch recorded, in a few brief lines or over many pages, the ailments of a woman and his own thoughts about her condition. Since he diligently padded his case studies with learned references and comparisons, the women's complaints are buried among quite fantastic details. Bits and pieces of medical theories that would have been circulating at the University of Halle are combined with elements from popular culture; self-evident bodily perceptions appear alongside things . . . utterly improbable . . . about . . . blood, labor pains, heart constrictions, or head cold" (Duden 1991: v–vi). Johannes Storch never physically examined his female patients, rarely performed autopsies, and therefore relied on the women's own descriptions of blood and pain in his medical analysis. Storch's perception of the inner body, as well as the women's narratives, are invaluable to our understanding of the cultural aesthetic of blood. In the remainder of this chapter, my aim is to convey this sense of social corporeality, a metaphorics of interiority and blood, as it was experienced by the men and women of eighteenth-century Germany. As we shall see, the notions of blood and the interior body dramatically shaped later social attitudes about contagion, health, and racial differences.

In early eighteenth-century Eisenach, the inside of the body was a realm of surprising changeability. The inside could be grasped only as a liquid interior, the place of a constant "flowing" that could be experienced but was invisible. Thus the external flows, the body's emanations and discharges, were aids to understanding the inside. The doctor and his female patients interpreted them as signs of inner movements. "Milk" could emerge from various openings and could resemble other secretions. The German doctor Johann Storch "cites several examples from the literature: milk was repelled from the breasts 'but issued forth from the mouth with the spittle'; a young girl had plasters placed on her swollen breasts, whereupon 'the menses broke out, which in color, smell, and taste resembled milk.' The discharge from the 'genital members' could be viewed as milk. We are also told about an incision for bleeding from which 'pure milk' had been drawn, and of the discharge of milk instead of urine."[138] What showed itself on the body's surface could be observed and examined, and it spoke of an inner process through smell, color, and taste, and through its likeness with analogous matter. Bodily discharges were interpreted on the basis of a belief in a continuous inner transformation.

The young wife of a tanner, who had developed an "oozing sore" on one of her legs while still unmarried, was pregnant. During the pregnancy this oozing on her legs disappeared. After the birth she ran a fever in childbed and developed an inflammation in her breast. When "the latter subsided, she said she got a red and itchy rash" and a "stopped-up-belly." Storch gave her prescriptions against these ailments, whereupon she had a "copious opening." She discharged "sedes" [feces] in good quantity, whereupon the rash "dried up." From this evacuation she got well.[139]

The doctor tried to explain to himself the course of the illness: the feces, the feverish rash, and the inflamed breast were external and internal forms of some "humoral matter, which prior to the pregnancy had issued at the thigh." From the multiplicity of complaints he had deduced an inner causal principle: it was *one* form of matter which in the body turned both inward, from the outer leg to the breast (inflammation), and outward, expressing itself as the rash. Eventually it was expelled as excrement. It was obviously bad and impure matter, which could move about in the body and had to be gotten rid of. All bodily matter, though ultimately the same, was involved in constant transformations. The inside was obviously a place of metamorphosis: "In this world, the fluid inside the body could apparently assume different forms, yet remain always the same substance. The inside was a porous place, a place of metamorphosis: fluids changed in the body, they transformed their materiality, form, color, consistency, and place of exit, and yet apparently they remained essentially alike" (Duden 1991: 109).

A pain, an external flow, was not simply "there," it was a sign of something. A headache could signal "agitated blood," an intensified inner movement, a maelstrom, which had turned upward from down below; the upsurge had an effect: the turning of the monthly blood to the head.[140] The ability to recognize the "characteristics of diseases" was the secret of medical learnedness, for the signs of sickness are those "clues whereby one can unravel and lay bare an obscure matter, or . . . they are visible manifestations that reveal a hidden and unknown matter."[141] The women had their own traditional means of understanding the signs; a myriad of phenomena could point to pregnancy, imminent death, the onset of the menses, or an impending consumption.

It is here, in the prognostic interpretation of personal signs and in understanding what the "signs of the women" meant, that the doctor and the women diverged most strongly. Their categories of meaning could be far apart. For the doctor, the body had the ability, even in a malady, to aim at something good: healing. A sign that was bad in itself could thus indicate a good as well as a bad prognosis: vomiting, spitting of blood, could be seen as nature's means of ridding herself of the filth of the upper body parts. The women spoke less of the body's healing power. The doctor sought to fathom the cause, the nature, the orientation of the inner body, in order to support it. Hence, he would "lure" the blood, show it the proper paths from the outside. The women, on the other hand, interpreted the same signs as a call to force open the stopped-up body from the inside. They wanted to "expel" the blood, to thoroughly "cleanse" the inside.[142] The signs of the body spoke to the women of an obstinate and stubborn interior threatened by stoppage. To the doctor they revealed an untimely or erroneous effort of the interior to rid itself of a burden. Johann Storch, the physician from Eisenach, thus frequently used the word *Reliquien* (remains, relics) for clotted blood, the blood remaining behind, inside. "Reliquien . . . among physicians . . . [were] the crudities, phlegm, and bad moisture that collect[ed] in a person's stomach."[143] But with Storch the "reliquien" remained in the womb: menstrual residues, stagnant blood, obstructed female matter.

The Menstrual Body

Blood in every form was central to all eighteenth-century reflections about illness. The rhythm of discharge, the periodic nature of bleeding, constituted womanhood—it was a necessary bodily phenomenon that gave women their special gender characteristic.[144] The menstrual flow, the "monthly affair," was regarded by some physicians as the necessary prerequisite for the "marriageable years" of a woman.[145] But this position required some qualification:

Except that this is attended with many doubts, since, first of all, there exist not a few stories that children also had menses, and second, there are also many who never saw the menses, and yet once they were married became happy and fertile mothers. The well-being of a woman in her marriageable years includes that she be well developed, have swollen breasts, and the menses; but it is not always part of her being. (Storch 1747b: 25, introduction) [146]

The medical literature recorded an abundance of stories in which even very young girls bled: a nine-year-old girl from Danzig, "who gets the menses, though irregularly";[147] a Tübingen bookkeeper's daughter, who began with the red flow in her eighth year.[148] Examples from all ages follow in the physician's manual. In 1732, Storch delivered a noblewoman of a "strong girl," "which . . . on the fourth day after the birth discharged several spoonfuls of blood per pudenda."[149] Monthly bleeding was not an exclusive mark of grown women.

Moreover, in eighteenth-century Eisenach, menstruation was not considered a prerequisite of womanhood, a "mark of their *esse,* their being-a-woman."[150] Johann Storch tells of Eisenach women who as adults never had the expected "menses," but instead bled from other parts of the body. In some women he observed a regular emission of "white flux," which could discharge below even in small girls or could collect as milk in the breast.[151] This white flow was also periodic.[152] The physician claimed that some women never had their courses while they were married until they were pregnant, in which case they had their monthlies regularly.[153] Other women experienced different habitual excretions. A "delicate and well-shaped" woman, who always observed only a few drops of the monthly blood on herself, reported "a large recurring blotch on the foot, which grew painfully at the usual time of her menses."[154] Then there were women who reported a periodic bloody sputum, diarrhea in the rhythm of the monthlies, a periodic flare-up of consumption, sweating in the monthly rhythm, a periodic "sadness and heaviness of the limbs," and piles, or hemorrhoids, that kept a four-week rhythm.[155] Other eighteenth-century physicians similarly reported the orderly or cyclical appearance of female afflictions: "[T]he itching rash observes a certain timing; the girls are afflicted by scabies at the same time as their cleansing should flow."[156] The movement of time inside the female body, a periodic internal, spontaneous surging, along with some cyclical excretion, seemed more constant than the sanguine consistency of the issued matter.[157]

The experience of temporary but regular cycles was not limited to women in their youth. Women who discharged blood in their old age were nothing unusual in the experience of local practitioners. A seventy-year-old widow complained in 1723 about pain in her hip, which she had contracted because the bloody "terms," which she had experienced "unwaveringly" until that time, had not appeared for two periods. After bloodletting, the menses returned. The woman came back only five years later, in 1728, to complain of a nosebleed that was troubling her.[158] The regular menstrual flow in old women was not common in Eisenach, but neither was it very rare.[159] A periodic, spontaneous excretion was understood as habitual to women. Yet the spontaneous issue of blood was not exclusive to women: it was also observed in men.[160] Evidently the discharged substance, blood itself, was not regarded as gender specific.

Unlike women, men did not have an inward disposition to bleed periodically from one location. Instead, they discharged blood flows from various body parts—some almost regularly, some sporadically: from nose, from piles, a wound, as bloody sputum.[161] The "bleeding piles" (e.g. hemorrhoids) especially were seen as analogous to women's "monthlies" by eighteenth-century German physicians.[162] "This discharge seems to be somewhat equal to the monthly cleansing of women"; the flow sometimes kept an orderly rhythm, "like among women."[163] In young plethoric men and in men with sedentary occupations, it served to discharge the superfluous humors. If the piles of a full-blooded man became "obstructed," said Johann Storch, then he instantly had ailments like those of a woman suffering from a "stoppage of the monthlies" (1747b:316). The "flow of the piles" was as sensitive as the "monthlies." It could be stopped up by a fright, by intervention in the wrong place, or by distempers, so that it never returned. When that happened, a man would get ill and possibly even die. As Storch reports, "a few years ago I heard that a forty-two-year-old corpulent merchant was having fluxum haemorrhoidum and let himself be persuaded by a boastful surgeon and medical quack to have a phlebotomy. The hemorrhoidal fluxus was immediately stopped up and the good merchant . . . died suddenly five days later" (1752: 34). Hemorrhoids and the menses were both seen as spontaneous evacuations of the body; they resembled each other and were interchangeable.[164] This similarity was not a marginal phenomenon; it was the subject of a great many learned treatises and disputations.[165] In his *Tractatus de Haemorrhoidibus*, published in 1722, Michael Alberti of Halle discussed the affinity or likeness of menses and piles, which he saw in their common task of relieving the body by discharging superfluous, troublesome, and impure matter.[166] The hemorrhoids were a healing if not a constitutive blood flow in adult men.

This similarity between men and women in the corporeal habit to relieve themselves through excretions also made possible the phenomenon of a "true" periodic menses in men.[167] In his great collection of the medical literature at the end of the eighteenth century, Wilhelm Gottfried Ploucquet (1809) cited the wealth of reported cases from the medical observations of the sixteenth and seventeenth centuries: with information on where they occurred and with detailed descriptions of the circumstances, the cases reported how men could experience regular menstruation. They bled from the fingertips (*per digitos*), from the left thumb at the full moon, through the varicose veins, and especially, in direct sympathy to menstruation, per penem, the male genital member.[168] Thus there was the case of a servant who, since his childhood, had "experienced regular bleeding in the thumb of his left hand. From the right side near the finger at the time of the full moon (it was rare indeed for this flux to appear the day before or after the full moon) and without any headache . . . the blood suddenly sprang forth from various rivulets."[169] Another case, recorded in the *Miscellanea* of the Natural Science Society, mentioned a peasant who diligently performed this monthly discharge from the time of his puberty to his seventy-sixth year and lived a healthy and cheerful life in the process.[170] Men issued forth blood and had corporal dispositions similar to those of women in terms of periodicity and body regions for their monthly bleeding. Thus, as Barbara Duden (1991: 118) points out repeatedly, it was only from the end of the seventeenth century that blood and milk were assigned to the functional sphere of physiological motherhood.[171] The new science of medicine did not acquire hold over the local understanding of the female body until much later. Biology was not yet the science of the body polarized by its sexual characteristics.

Women, with their disposition to spontaneous discharges, were less threatened by plethora (too much blood), than men. And yet they were weaker, colder; they collected more filth and humidity and therefore had to bleed regularly. In their "inferiority," as defined by Aristotle and Galen, they embodied the self-healing power of discharge from the inside. Bloodletting, which local physicians (like Johann Storch) prescribed, was supposed to be aligned, like proper menses, with the lunar phase, and it was interpreted explicitly in analogy to the menses. It was prescribed for men as much as for women; in fact, men needed it more. The inner blood had to flow, the internal fluids had to be drawn out: otherwise a serious disease would inevitably follow.

Body Openings

Seen from the outside, the body had a surface, the skin, and holes or orifices: eyes, ears, nose, mouth, breasts, navel, anus, urinary passage, vulva, and pores. In addition, the body had swellings and curves. The body openings were "exit points": "something [came] out of them, but what was voided change [could] also be excreted in some other place. The body openings [were] not clearly designated for a single substance."[172] We can see this when we examine several of the cases from Johann Storch's eighteenth-century medical practice in Eisenach: "The eyes run with tears, but there are girls who cry bloody tears; the nose runs, but there are girls who bleed from the nose. What comes out is the 'monthlies,' which are evacuated in this way. Spittle gathers in the mouth, but the menses can flow forth from a gap in the teeth or be vomited up in bloody sputum. Menstrual blood can also, though rarely be passed as bloody urine, or, more frequently, through the piles, especially in adult, full-blooded women."[173] The wife of a clergyman, who had her menstrual courses stopped by a fright, instead had bleeding piles;[174] and a "tall, choleric female cook, who was in the kitchen where she could eat well and also drink a glass of good wine," disclosed to her doctor that her "menstrual blood came by the stool."[175] The orifices had a different meaning during different phases of life: young girls bled above all from the upper part of the body, from the nose and the mouth. The bleedings could occur in the rhythm of the monthly period if the latter did not want to appear "below."[176] Among older women, hemorrhoids were more important. Unmarried women had fewer bleeding piles than did married women.

From the perspective of the doctor, the surgeon, and the women, wounds, lumps, and cuts were openings that could emit substances blocked from discharge through their proper passage. A tonsilar abscess was an issue: what came out there could be the menses or some other substance. The skin did not appear as a material seal shutting the inside off from the outside. Instead it seemed to be permeable from the inside: it had "sweat holes," which heat could open to allow the discharge of humidity, bloody matter, and impurities. A swelling, a boil on the skin, was a sign that some matter was pushing toward the periphery in search of an outlet. Wet scabs and ulcers evacuated "the reabsorbed foul matter in the skin."[177] The skin was a collection of real, minute orifices—the pores—and potential larger openings, especially where it was delicate, "seeing that a subtle skin can be easily . . . consumed or torn . . . by a caustic substance."[178] It was therapeutically perceived as a place where the body could be induced to open: "the porous periphery of the body, by means of which pungent, superfluous, or even noxious humors are expelled."[179]

Other phenomena on the skin were also considered as exits: varicose veins showed throbbing blood pushing toward the outside; "redness on the skin," facial burns, Saint Anthony's fire, were caused by impure matter breaking out; a rash issued from the inside; scabies seemed a salutary discharge; liver spots were impure stuff brought to the outside:[180]

all these cutaneous phenomena had a connection, a link with the inner blood flow, with the menses. They appeared above all when the menses was suppressed:

"A noble girl's birthmarks swelled when her menses were 'stopped up' owing to a fire; the spots diminished when the menses appeared in 'proper order.' "[181]

A maidservant from the country complained that for several years she has had her courses in small quantity, with an occasional stoppage. At the same time a spongy bump has appeared on her head. "When her menses eventually stopped completely, she reported that the bump grew bigger and spread."[182]

Natural body openings, epidermic ruptures, and skin discolorations were interchangeable. What happened at these places was similar: some superfluous or impure matter was ejected. The skin was fragile and it was a boundary, but it was not meant to demarcate the body against the outside world. According to Duden (1991: 123), it was above all a physical surface on which the inside revealed itself. The body's interior conveyed itself through the body openings, which functioned as points of exit for interior flows. In eighteenth-century Eisenach, the holes of the body, the continuous opening of all orifices, became a compulsive attempt to draw out the inner flow, the flux of menstrual blood, the impure monthly accumulation.

The Liquid Interior

In eighteenth-century Eisenach, the physical interior of bodies was flowing and indistinct, accessible only through the imagination. "The wide-awake consciousness found very few certain markers in this inner body, nothing solid, no scaffolding, no bones, no clearly demarcated organs. What it did find were metamorphosis, movements, urges, and stagnating resistance."[183] Since the fluids in the body could change into blood, milk, excrement, sweat, humidity, and scorbutic and impure matter, and could appear in so many places, how did physicians like Johann Storch conceive of these fluids? Was the body some kind of hollow space? What caused the inner flux of blood and its movements? As Duden (1991: 124) points out, blood circulation, the venous and arterial system, but also the traditional mix of humors, did not seem to come into play here. Storch sometimes adopted adjectives from humoral pathology for describing the bad blood, for example "black" blood (melancholic, thick blood) or yellowish white, phlegmatic blood; but he never explicitly referred to the doctrine of the humors. Humoral pathology was not a concept that systematically determined his choice of terms; "he merely dragged it along as an outmoded tradition."[184]

The Eisenach physician described the body as a place where the inner movement of blood responded, in a vague and unspecified way, to external stimulations. Scratches, small wounds, or bites attracted "moisture"—the blood—to the site of the irritation, luring it from the uterus to the head or limbs.[185] "A maidservant, twenty-three years of age, hit her head against the corner of a shop drawer and suffered a 'strong and painful contusion.' A few days later she swallowed purgantia [laxative] at the very time her menses were flowing. The menses became 'obstructed and regurgitated toward the head, which one could see from the swollen veins on her forehead and temples.' This threw the girl into 'confusion and melancholy thoughts.' Years later this melancholic attack recurred once more."[186]

In Johann Storch's thinking, the lump, the bruise on the head, attracted the blood upward, especially since the flow from the womb had become unsure and halting owing to the senna leaves the woman had ingested as a purgative. Moreover, this inner marking, or flux, remained virtually imprinted on the body.[187] "*Congestiones* press . . . from the obstructed evacuation of the menses for the most part toward the head, especially . . . so owing to former injury."[188] A stimulus lured the blood; it remained as an imprinting on the body. By means of a plaster, which irritated the skin to raise a blister and caused pain, nature could "be directed toward the ordinary excretion."[189] Through a stimulus (pain, purgatives, bloodletting), the direction of the flow, this newly embodied habit of blood, was diverted: pushed, lured, enticed, and driven upward or downward. The body remained merely an outer shell for this movement. "We are far from the inner body as described by the anatomists whom Storch cited: an interior where blood circulates, has the same quantity, moves in a circular flow, flows along predetermined pathways, and in which excess, stagnation, accumulation, and false paths are anatomically and physiologically impossible" (Duden 1991: 126). The eighteenth-century physician Johann Storch cannot reconcile these two ways of perceiving the inner body. In the case of a seriously ill woman, unable to turn in bed without help, he says: "for this reason all her blood sank to one side, and even before her death . . . she became blue and black on that side."[190] In the case of a pregnant woman, he remarks in general about the congestion of blood in her lower belly: "the return flow from the legs, which has to occur upward or rising, is burdensome for nature."[191] The blood seems to move in a vague space, and the paths along which it travels are like hollow vessels or a sponge.[192]

This image of the inner body—governed by notions of "urge" and "habit"—was entirely incompatible with the body system of the anatomists. The interior was seen as an unstructured osmotic space, and the errant wanderings within were given a vitalistic-physiological underpinning through the use of auxiliary categories from a mechanistic body model.[193] The medical categories of "urge," "enticement," "stagnation," "congestion," and "loosening" were perceived as interior phenomena governed by a tensive force: the *motus tonicus* (tensive movement). This impulse toward motion was nature's mechanism for bringing about excretions. The impulse toward expulsion and elimination moved the body on the inside, kept it together, and established a tensive linkage between body parts, muscles, and fibers. "Stagnant blood is contracted [by] spasmos" and pressed "from the outside inwards" and finally "ad uterum."[194] The greater the excess of blood, the harder the tensive force must work to move it, and the stronger the cramps. If abundant, thick, heavy, sticky, gross, and sluggish, then blood overburdened the movement's impulse and caused it to produce these cramps.[195] In Storch's words,

These spasms . . . do not always arise in the proximity of the lower body. Rather, nature also begins this impulse from afar in the very distant parts, and directs the tensive movement such that it contracts the muscles of the outermost limbs to press the blood standing or rising therein . . . toward the womb [*ad uterum*]: if then the veins and intervening spaces are too full of blood, the tensive movement [*motus tonicus*] cannot so easily and without obstruction move the same into circulation, and thus transforms itself into a spasm [*motus spasticus*] and causes such pains. Not infrequently nature even pushes the tensive movement to the point where, for the sake of this excretion, it turns into epilepsy.[196]

The many cramps that Storch had to tend to in his female patients were physiological exorcisms, internally driven, painful expulsions. The doctor's treatment supported this expulsion by extracting the "superfluous" blood. The surging was also calmed with internal medications (purgatives) and the matter was cast out.

This metaphorical physiology revealed itself with unique clarity at the end of one's life, when movement inside the body ceased. The doctor discussed in the following way the bleeding of a woman who had died: "A twenty-six-year-old, sanguine woman died in January 1730 in extreme poverty from infectious fever. For fear of contagion the relatives had not looked after her, though they had sent wine and beer. After her death the layer-out noticed 'that the monthly period had begun while she was dying and had flowed from her fairly strongly for several days even after her death.' The other women living in this room recalled the same incident had been observed with another inhabitant who had died in this house."[197]

How could a dead woman bleed, once her life, her impetus to motion, had gone? Storch suggested that "one can reasonably consider such expulsion of the blood in the act of dying *pro ultimo naturae conatu*, when frightened nature *in extremis* strives to thrust out." But how was it possible that after death the blood in the cold body not only "oozed out" but even broke out anew? "The very subtle, ethereal part in the blood is that from which the powers not only of the soul but also of the fibrarum motricium draw their sustenance, and this can remain concealed in the blood even when the person is already dead."[198] The soul, like the motive power of the fibers, drew its strength from a source: the blood. "Whatever was said metaphorically and physiologically about the blood's efforts toward expulsion spoke implicitly also of the soul, which was linked to the blood and mediated by it. In this instance, we can grasp not only an obvious but unspoken blending of physiological and religious layers of thinking . . . The language of the humors was the language of the soul" (Duden 1991: 129). And both separated at death in a manner inexplicable to Storch, "who could finally say beyond doubt how, when, and in what manner the soul [left] its body and dwelling, and whether the soul, for some time still united with the body, [might] not maintain hidden *motus vitales*."[199]

The Corrupt Body: Flux, Stagnation, Decay

Complaints about an "inner flux" were among the most frequent reasons why women turned to the doctor. The term "flux" (*Blutsturz*) described a host of things: pains felt inside from matter flowing in the body; fluids emitted—blood, the menses, pus; an oozing wound or open sore on the skin. The women of Eisenach, as documented by Duden (1991: 130–35), suffered from flux but were also fearful that the flow of blood might be driven back and become stuck inside. This stagnated flux caused pains: headaches, ringing in the ears, hardness of hearing, loss of sight, stone blindness, a "dull" or paralyzed tongue, gout and rheumatism, stomachaches, colic, suffocation of the womb, sharp pains in the legs.[200] The pains spoke of a laborious and viscous stream, a violent assault of blood on the woman's inner body.

The appearance of matter flowing out from the body was less of a concern. On the contrary, the outer flux—blood, pus, and white flow—ensured cleansing and unburdening. External fluxes included, in addition to the periodic discharges, the "oozing sores" that the body created for itself in order to discharge matter. In particular the thin segments of the skin, the swollen venous nodes, boils, and abscesses channeled these flows, these evacuations of "humoral matter" (white moisture, pus, and bloody matter); they were uncomfortable, itchy, even painful, but rarely a cause to consult the physician. The running flows did not constitute an illness, especially if they were periodic.

The opposite of an external ooze was something hard, an accumulation of solid matter. Here women spoke of a paradoxical inversion: the inner flow, if not drained off, engendered a hardening, a petrification; it became viscous and clogging. Flux on the outside was a healthy discharge; however, women became alarmed if an accustomed flow was "striking inward" and disappeared from the surface: "What fueled the fear was not the discomfort of an evacuation, but the perception of the inner space as a space of induration and stoppage" (Duden 1991: 132). An absent flow, an obstructed evacuation of the body, was interpreted as the cause of later ailments.

The wife of a shoemaker, forty years of age, "has had an oozing and sometimes foul-smelling sore under the breast for many years. Having dried up in February 1721, it moved to an untoward place, namely to the genitals, *ad muliebra.*" The pains, especially when passing urine, were so intense that the woman tried to soothe them with cold washes. This bottled up the flux, upsetting the stomach and the guts, causing great anxiety in the stomach and the lower body. During the next years whenever the flux, having returned to its old place, dried up, she immediately requested help, "for fear of dangerous ill effects." Storch gave her sudorifics and a mustard plaster. She placed the plaster under her breast, it dissolved the skin, and already within an hour "the flux could be lured out again, and the woman soon felt . . . relief." This woman died thirteen years later, and the cause of death was this: after she had fallen down the cellar stairs, the flux under the breast subsided and failed to return, whereupon all the matter got stuck in her head.[201]

In the doctor's eyes, as in the opinion of his female patients, the art of healing lay in supporting the external flow of impure, dirty, and pustular matter until the body had been sufficiently cleansed. Storch thus strove to prevent what, in medical terms, he called a "repelling" of the flux. To that end he used blister plasters, *vesicatoria,* and fontanels (literally "small fountains") to keep a wound open or to redirect the flow and to allow the continuous drainage of fluids.[202]

When the balance between the outside and the inside threatened to collapse, death began to cast its shadow over the sick person: with the onset of decay, "blood and matter clot in the womb."[203] If the deceased had not explicitly forbidden that her body be opened, Storch performed postmortem dissections on some women. And he now found in the opened corpse precisely what he had suspected: the site of the patient's fluxes and rotted blood.[204] "In the afternoon I had to dissect her," he writes of a woman who died suddenly and inexplicably. "In the navel hernia I found no bowels but only an accumulation of the peritoneum, which was all . . . rotten and gave off a black, foul-smelling water. I also found black matter like excrement."[205] The inside of the dead body showed traces of a process of decay, which the doctor expressed in terms of stagnation and foul matter. In his dissection reports, the organs interest him solely as the bearers of this decay within a kind of amorphous swamp. The images are very similar: a peritoneum is "rotten," a spleen is "large and blackish," a liver is "heavy" and "completely shot through by hard, cancerous excrescences and cavities"; a kidney is "scirrhous and yellow-white in color."[206] He described hollow spaces as stagnant pockets filled with foul-smelling moisture, as indurated petrifications or as spaces of putrid growths: the "womb is the size of an average pear . . . but in its cavity I found a hard, gristly ball the size of a nutmeg,"[207] or he discovered that it was "filled with ulcers the size of peas, beans, or nutmeg seeds," the "ovaries small, like nuts, and whitish-yellow in color."[208] These images speak of a perception in which the eye did not dissect but rather imputed the process of dying. As Duden (1991: 137–38) points out, the functional inferences that Storch drew always linked these three related processes: something was rotten, black, yellow-white, putrid—images of stagnation and *corruptio*; something was ulcerated, cancerlike, gelatinous—images of bad growth; something was callous, knotted, gristly—images of hardening, petrification. "All the metaphors point in the same direction. They speak of inner decay that had been set in motion by accumulation, stagnation, and hardening. The inside of the corpses confirmed the corruption that Storch suspected in the women during their lifetimes. Even in life there was already the threat of mortification inside the body."[209] According to Storch, the moist spaces of the body, the lung, the stomach, the womb, the intestines, were particularly inclined to accumulate something bad.

A noblewoman, with a hardened belly, was suffering from dropsy, "since a lot of water was locked up in the hollow stomach." Eventually she died from the inner stagnation of waste matter, "since the monthly period, in view of her age, was no longer issued and this excretion settled inside and caused fatal corruptions at the intestines." Since everything was "closed up" inside her, the menses was no longer discharged. All the bad matter, in particular the fluids of a copper-red rash that had been "struck in," had thus accumulated, corrupting, putrifying, and dissolving the intestines.[210]

A stagnating flow inside the body caused decay:

A young woman lay in childbed with pains in her "left groin." The lochia were stopped up, the pains in the side grew worse. A month later "black clots of blood" were discharged along with the menses. The woman "feared . . . that an abscess might be behind all this." For almost two months they waited and observed an aposteme forming in her left side, using compresses to promote its "maturing." Finally, the surgeon lanced the abscess. More than a pound of matter came out, and hours later "again more than one pound of mature pus without blood was drained."[211]

The procedure itself was called "drawing off," a term that was also used for treating bleeding patients. This abscess and the act of lancing it finished the illness; in this case, since the matter collected in the side near the periphery, the healers succeeded in preventing an inner "decay."

An abundance of fluids that could no longer be disposed off could collect inside and breed internal sores. If the regular monthly flow of blood "stopped," fear drove the women to seek prescriptions—"to keep a stubborn growth from forming in or on the womb," as one female patient told the doctor in 1738.[212] Excrescences, "cancerlike and wild growths," or hardenings, which spread and "devoured" the healthy tissue inside and grew larger, were caused by the same trouble the women complained about most and which stood in the center of everyone's attention: the stagnation of the monthly flow.[213] In the case of a soldier's wife, all of whose blood was flowing inward, "the superfluidity sat in the *cavitate uteri* and clotted":[214] menstrual blood stagnated, coagulated, curdled. Clotted blood (the "lumps" from the womb that were so often mentioned by the women in Eisenach) referred to hardened and sick blood: it was "burnt," sticky, viscous, stagnant, set, or thickened. The womb, from which blood flowed after collecting there for over a month, embodied this constant danger of stagnation by virtue of its shape as a collecting basin for blood. In the women's insides, says Duden (1991: 140), we see the flip side of their periodic flows. In the monthly discharge of their menses, women embodied the essence of medical treatment and the prototype of a healthful evacuation. But in their womb they embodied the other side, that of stagnation and hardening. In the middle of the body was the womb, a place of ever-present threat of stagnation. And stagnation eventually brought corruption, decay, and death.

Blood Mythologies and Medicine

The search for more precise anatomical knowledge, for regularity, order, laws, and causes—in contradistinction to the belief that the natural world was controlled by miracles and by forces of magic—was critical to a new understanding of the body in relation to processes of health and disease. Knowledge and explanation were sought not in the discovery of divine purposes but in the complex fluids, organs, and functions of the body itself. In the modern era, ever more radical explorations and interventions in the pursuit of knowledge began, inexorably leading the medical gaze into the interior of the body itself. Disease was associated with that which was taboo, contaminated, and filthy, particularly when it was supposed that disease posed a danger to the public health. Cleanliness was linked to political stability, and healthy behavior gradually folded into a capitalist definition of moral behavior.

Chapter 6

Between Blood and Soil
Body Politics in Nazi Germany

> Just as the Nazi goes back to the *peasants*, as the most organic caste, so for him the *personal physicians, racial doctors and hygienists* are his *social science* so to speak. They are also important to him in terms of state theory; hence not only the pathos of heredity and selective breeding, but above all the *national pathos of blood* . . .
>
> The nation thus becomes, in medical terms as well, a unity filled with blood, a purely organic river basin, from whose past humanity stems, into whose (most traditionally limited) "future" its children go. Thus "nationhood" drives time, indeed history out of history: it is space and organic fate, nothing else.
>
> Ernst Bloch, *Heritage of Our Times*, 1990

Blood and body metaphors emerged with particular force and nationalistic appeal during periods of German unification and fascism. The rhetoric of German fascists was permeated by organic images, and blood provided the metaphor through which National Socialists conveyed their political and racial doctrines. Blood thereby became a powerful symbolic tool in the promulgation of anti-Semitism.

Idealizing German Ancestry

National Socialism was founded on the doctrine that Germans were innately superior to others as a result of their descent from Nordic blood.[1] Idealized as a light-skinned, blond, and masculine body, the German was elevated by the inborn endowment of his blood. This assertion became the basic premise of Nazi ideology:

Der germanische Edeling leitet seine Herkunft von dem göttlichen Ahnenkern ab, dessen Blut (Keimmasse) von den Nachfahren in möglichster Reinheit weitergegeben werden musste. (Gütt 1936b: 4)

[The Germanic noble derives his heritage from the divine ancestral seed, whose blood (germinal substance) has to be passed on by the descendants in utmost purity.]

Similar statements appeared elsewhere:

Heute erwachte aber ein neuer Glaube, der Mythus des Blutes, der Glaube, mit dem Blute auch das göttliche Wesen des Menschen überhaupt zu verteidigen. (Rosenberg 1935: 114)

[But today arose a new faith, the myth of the blood, the belief that through the blood one generally also protects the divine essence of man.]

    Such an assertion of divine heritage involved a symbolic change of lineage. Members of the Nazi movement chose for themselves a new identity by renouncing their Judeo-Christian ancestry and by voting those who belonged to their lodge a different "bloodstream" from that of the Jews. Thereupon the former spiritual ancestors, the Hebrew prophets, became a "bad" father, that is, the persecutor.[2] Under Hitler's leadership, German society was unified by a sentimental attachment to Nordic blood and the revival of a cherished tribal past.[3] Drawing on ancient mythological constructs, genealogical tracing established a lineage to the Germanic community of warriors, central to which was the figure of Odin, the god of blood and war.

    Such an idealization of the ancestral bloodline led to an obsession with the culture of the past. Everywhere, attempts were made to consciously revive the ancient heritage. This involved a cultivation of Old Norse mythology as well as of Germanic symbols, customs, laws, and rituals.[4] Folklore as a whole was popularized because of its reflection of rural life, its intimate connection with the customs and heroic ethics of the German forefathers.[5] It was assumed that the exposure to national folklore would make Germans more aware of their ancestry and lead them to appreciate the simple way of life.

Blood and Soil

Such reasoning corresponded with Adolf Hitler's aversion to cosmopolitanism and what he considered the decadent lifestyle of the city. He proclaimed that urban residents had lost their German heritage since they were no longer bound to the land. The attitude was soon incorporated into Nazi ideology:

Gefahren drohen dem Volke, wenn es in die Städte abwandert. Es stirbt in einigen Generationen dahin, weil ihm die Bindung zum Boden fehlt. Der deutsche

Mensch aber muss bodenverwurzelt sein, wenn er am Leben bleiben will. (Rechenbach 1935:376).[6]

[Dangers threaten the nation when it migrates to the cities. It withers away in a few generations, because it lacks the vital connection with the earth. The German must be rooted in the soil, if he wants to remain alive.]

Nazi doctrines were permeated by images of "rootless" and "infertile" city dwellers, who remained separated from the "natural" soil by artificial layers of cement and asphalt.[7] Cities were unfavorably opposed to rural life and peasants, who were by contrast firmly "rooted" in the land. As a result, their bloodline had improved its quality through time, becoming "tough" and "resilient" by centuries of contact with the local earth.

The idealization of the German peasant effectively veiled Hitler's imperialist policies and redirected the symbolic focus toward concerns of blood:

Grundlage alles völkischen Seins ist die Verbundenheit des Blutes mit der heiligen Scholle unseres Vaterlandes. (Motz 1934: 7)

[The basis of all nationalist existence is the connection of blood with the sacred soil of our fatherland.]

The metaphorical image thus created gave rise to the formulaic Blut und Boden, or "blood and soil," which was elevated to a cultic symbol by Minister of Agriculture Walther Darré in 1930.[8] It stood for the fundamental assertion that "peasants were both food providers and an essential blood source for the nation" (*Der Bauernstand ist zugleich Nährstand und Blutsquelle des Volkes*).[9] The German nation continually received "a new influx of blood from the rural well of life" (*neuen Blutszustrom von dem bäuerlichen Lebensquell*).[10] These concepts of the food and blood producing peasant and the fertile soil were combined with notions of "blood sacrifice" in Hitler's rhetoric by 1939:

Vergesst nie, dass das heiligste Recht auf dieser Welt das Recht auf Erde ist, die man selbst bebauen will, und das heiligste Opfer das Blut, das man für diese Erde vergiesst.[11]

[Never forget that in this world the most sacred right is the right for a plot of land that one wants to cultivate by oneself, and the most sacred sacrifice is the blood which one sheds for this soil.]

Blood and soil were to provide the basis for the future of the German nation. In metaphorical terms, it became the foundation "from which a new tree shall firmly take root" (*aus dem einst ein neuer Baum die sichere Wurzel schlägt*).[12] Blood, tree, and soil became central metaphors of German nationhood.

Images of Contagion

Social theorizing proceeded in terms of these quasi religious, almost mystical concepts. Contemporary ideology had cultivated a vision of "blending" heredity, including the postulation of some metaphorical or perhaps even literal "mingling" of blood during sexual intercourse.[13] Since the "mixing" of different types of blood was said to result in blood "pollution," political controls were gradually extended to regulate the sphere of human reproduction. "Pure" blood was the teleological goal whereby the German nation would win its salvation. Such concepts are eminently apparent in Hitler's programmatic book *Mein Kampf*, which illuminates the essentials of the National Socialist world view.

The sexual symbolism that runs through Hitler's work can be easily characterized:[14] Germany in dispersion was the "dehorned Siegfried." The masses were "feminine." As such, they desired to be led by a dominating male. This male, as orator, wooed them—and, when he had won them, commanded them. The rival male, the villainous Jew, would on the contrary seduce them. If he succeeded, he poisoned their blood by intermingling with them. A few samples from Hitler's work serve to illustrate the point:

Der schwarzhaarige Judenjunge lauert stundenlang, satanische Freude in seinem Gesicht, auf das ahnungslose Mädchen, das er mit seinem Blute schändet und damit seinem, des Mädchens Volke, raubt . . . Sowie er selber planmässig Frauen und Mädchen verdirbt, so schreckt er auch nicht davor zurück selbst in grösserem Umfange die Blutschranken für andere einzureissen.[15]

[For hours, the black-haired Jewish boy, with satanical joy in his face, lies in wait for the unsuspecting girl, who he defiles with his blood and thereby steals her from her people . . . Just as he systematically corrupts women and girls, he does not hesitate to tear down the blood-barriers for others to an even greater extent.]

Much of the same imagery is repeated in other passages toward the end of the book:

Die Impotenz der Völker, ihr eigener Alterstod, liegt aber begründet in der Aufgabe ihrer Blutsreinheit und diese wahrt der Jude besser als irgend ein anderes Volk der Erde . . . Es bedarf aller Kraft, . . . um unser Volk noch einmal emporzureissen, aus der Umstrickung dieser internationalen Schlange, zu lösen und der Verpestung unseres Blutes im Inneren einhalt zu tun, . . . Wie will man unser eigenes Volk aus den Fesseln dieser giftigen Umarmung erlösen.[16]

[The impotence of nations, their own dissipation is, however, caused by the struggle with blood purity and the Jew preserves it better than any other race on earth . . . It requires all strength, . . . to resurrect our nation, to free it from the constricting snare of this international snake and to put a stop to the pollution of our blood inside, . . . How does one want to liberate our own folk from the fetters of this venomous embrace.]

By the method of associative mergers or metaphors, by using ideas as images, sexuality became tied up with death, rape, seduction, and immorality in Hitler's rhetoric. To him, intimate contact with others was a dangerous thing, a permanent and eternal source of infection. And when he was on the subject of "blood poisoning" by marriage, the associative connections of his ideas led naturally into attacks upon syphilis, prostitution, incest, and other similar misfortunes.

Anti-Semitic Imaginings: Jews as a Physical Threat

Hitler's rhetorical talent was to synthesize, and later to implement in a terrifyingly literal manner, a variety of racist notions already current. Thus for centuries, Jews had been accused of making use of Christian blood for ritual purposes.[17] German folk belief consisted of a whole repertoire of narratives, in which either a young virgin or a small boy was abducted and killed: later, the mutilated body, drained of blood, would be found. The murder was typically blamed on the local Jews. Such medieval legends were easily revived and exploited for Hitler's ideological purposes (Fig. 3). In popular newspapers (i.e., *Der Völkische Beobachter*), the motif of the blood-drinking and flesh-eating Jew was publicized and cast into nationalistic terms:

Der Jude mästet sich.
[The Jew feeds/fattens himself (on the German nation).][18]

Das Weltjudentum sucht seine blut-befleckte Fratze zu verhüllen.
[The world Jewry seeks to hide its blood-stained grotesque face.][19]

Jüdische Bluthunde.
[Jewish bloodhounds (victimizing unsuspecting Germans).][20]

Jüdische Bestien!
[Jewish beasts!][21]

Viehische Roheiten des jüdischen Untermenschentums.
[Bestial brutalities of the Jewish subhumans (directed against Germans).][22]

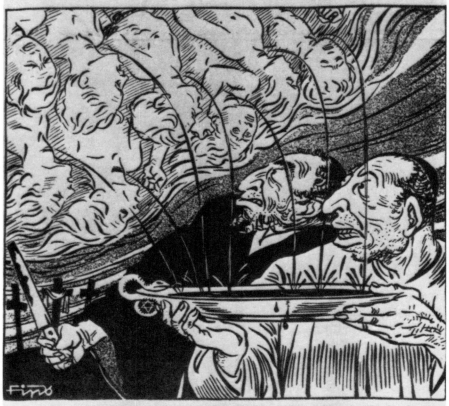

Figure 3. "Victims of the Jews! For centuries, the Jew, following a secret rite, spilled human blood. The devil still hangs on our neck; it is up to you to grab the devil's brood." The famous ritual murder number of *Der Stürmer* was withdrawn by Julius Streicher almost immediately as the Nazis did not want to spoil their "respectable" image at that time. From *Der Stürmer*, Sondernummer 1 (May 1934), front page.

The intentional creation of such animalistic images in published texts served to legitimate the force of German anti-Semitism. Similarly, Jews were equated metaphorically with "blood-sucking tyranny" (*blutsaugerische Tyrannei*) in Hitler's book, and their existence was causally connected to "the bloody extermination" (*die blutige Ausrottung*) of the German people and the "bleeding dry of our nation's body" (*das Ausbluten unseres Volkskörpers*).[23] Such metaphors were permeated by a fear of alien elements penetrating the societal body, resulting in the extinction of the German species. Such ideas became entangled in Hitler's death-linked imagery of wounded bodies, blood poisoning, rotting corpses, swamps, decay, open sores, venom, bacilli, vermin, snakes, parasites, maggots, leeches, and vampires. Among Hitler's obsessions was this concern with the verminous animality (the mere zoological quality) of his chosen enemies.[24] Although Jews were not the only objects of his racial hatred, they were undoubtedly the chief victims. Now viewed as an essentially subhuman, biological entity, they were portrayed as everywhere seeking the destruction of the German people. Among others, Alfred Rosenberg, Nazi Party ideologist, formulated this process in the following allegory:

Wenn der Sackkrebs sich durch den After des Taschenkrebses einbohrt, nach und nach in ihn hineinwächst, ihm die letzte Lebenskraft aufsaugt, so ist das der gleiche Vorgang, als wenn der Jude durch offene Volkswunden in die Gesellschaft eindringt, von ihrer Schöpferkraft zehrt bis zu ihrem Untergang.[25]

[When the hermit-crab pierces itself through the anus of the pocket-crab, and gradually grows into it, sucking from it the last vital force, then this is the same process by which the Jew penetrates into society through the open wounds of the nation, and draws from it all creative power until its final demise.]

The projection of such destructive tendencies upon Jews seemed to justify the use of any degree of violence, to any extent, to save the German nation. Defined by a language of death, with its associations of dirt, anality, animality, and corrupt sexuality, Jews had to be exorcized and placed into a locale suitable to their own nature.[26] Hitler's drive to exterminate them became a mania as German racism progressively turned from the depersonalization to the utter dehumanization of its victims.

Violence in Metaphor

Later, when Hitler became a successful orator, he insisted that revolutions were made solely by the power of the spoken word. National Socialists subsequently attributed a paramount role to the manipulating power of consciousness through language and the mode of action that it inspired. The Austrian cultural critic Karl Krauss had already analyzed the Nazis through their verbal rhetoric in 1933, when he attempted to show through satirical analysis that Hitler was in fact negating the metaphorical nature of language. The expressions that referred to parts of the body especially were interpreted not metaphorically but literally.[27]

The result was the brutality and inhumanity of language, which progressively intensified as time went on:

> Wenn diese Politiker der Gewalt noch davon sprechen, dass dem Gegner "das Messer an die Kehle zu setzen," "der Mund zu stopfen" sei, oder "die Faust zu zeigen," wenn sie überall "mit harter Faust durchgreifen" wollen oder mit "Aktionen auf eigene Faust" drohen: so bleibt nur erstaunlich, dass sie noch Redensarten gebrauchen, die sie nicht mehr machen . . . Vollends erfolgt die Absage an das Bildliche in dem Versprechen eines Staatspräsidenten:
> "Wir sagen nicht: Auge um Auge, Zahn um Zahn, nein, wer uns ein Auge ausschlägt, dem werden wir den Kopf abschlagen, und wer uns einen Zahn ausschlägt, dem werden wir den Kiefer einschlagen." Und diese Revindikation des Phraseninhalts geht durch alle Wendungen, in denen ein ursprünglich blutiger oder handgreiflicher Inhalt sich längst zum Sinn einer geistigen Offensive abgeklärt hat. Keine noch so raffinierte Spielart könne sich dem Prozess entziehen. (Krauss 1955: 122–3).

> [If these politicians of violence still talk about "putting the knife at the throat" of the enemy, "of gagging his mouth" and "showing him the fist," if they want "to come at him with a clenched fist" or if they threaten him "with actions of their own bat": then it is astonishing that they are still only using these expressions but not acting them out . . . The renunciation of the metaphorical is complete in the promise of a certain president:
> "We don't say: An eye for an eye, a tooth for a tooth, no, he who knocks out our eye will have his head cut off, and he who knocks out our tooth will have his jaw smashed." And this revindication of the content of such phrases permeates all expressions in which the originally bloody and corporeal content has long since been filtered into a mere metaphorical attack . . . No matter how crafty the metaphor, it couldn't possibly avoid this process.] [28]

Anti-Semitism continued to be present and, as part of the official Nazi doctrine, it was increased to the level of a grotesque hate campaign against every Jew. In one of the many anti-Semitic works, a part of which was entitled "Out with the Jews" (*Hinaus mit den Juden*), the author quoted numerous proverbs to back up the expulsion of Jews because they were "born criminals" (Hiemer 1942: 164–68). A few examples from this text show the increasing brutalization of a language that could no longer retain its metaphorical disguise:

> Schneid ihm die Hälse ab,
> dem verdammten Judenpack.

> [Cut the throats
> of the damned Jewish pack.]

> Jud spei Blut,
> Spei! in eine Ecken,
> Morgen sollst du verrecken.

[Spit blood, Jew,
Spit! into a corner with you,
Tomorrow you shall croak.]

The publication of these gruesome texts reinforced the Nazi drive to murder all Jews.

The Cultural Politics of Race

In a systematic effort, party ideologist Alfred Rosenberg had developed as early as 1933 a highly specialized and detailed mechanism of controls in order to carry out more effectively the cultural politics of the Third Reich. The major institution responsible for the anti-Semitic "guidance" of the German people was the *Reichskulturkammer* (Office of Imperial Culture) with its various branches created to censor art, literature, theater, the press, radio, music, and language. Officially, the Reichskulturkammer was under the leadership of propaganda minister Josef Goebbels in matters concerning the ideological training of German citizens.[29] Less obvious at first was perhaps the party's conscious revival of German anti-Semitic folklore, including particularly the image of the Jew as presented in legends, tales, and proverbs. Gradually, folklore and its various genres were turned into a blatant political tool.

This process has been of particular interest to historians of German folklore, some of whom have examined the interrelation of language and politics during the Nazi era.[30] Much of the existing scholarship consists of detailed surveys, collections, and dictionaries of Nazi terminology in use during the 1930s and 1940s. Some studies concentrated on the political manipulation of everyday language, analyzing either the use of single words and phrases or the style of political speeches, while others discussed the symbolic efficacy of language in specific folklore genres, such as tales or proverbs.[31] Nazi rhetoric seems to have been effective because of its *emotional appeal*, the frequent use of repetition, the use of "common" or "vulgar" language, and the incorporation of simple proverbial phrases into political slogans. For instance, it is not surprising that Hitler particularly liked the expression *jemanden in Fleisch und Blut übergehen*,[32] literally "to enter into one's flesh and blood," which meant "to become second nature to somebody," in light of his ideas of racial purity. Such expressions added familiarity and imagery to his lengthy and verbose speeches.[33] They also helped to increase the efficacy of Nazi persuasion.

The politicized use of proverbs turned language into an effective tool for the conscious construction of culture: "A number of publications concentrated on proving Nazi racial theories through proverbs, while others assembled dozens of anti-Semtitic proverbs to add to the racial hatred already rampant in Germany. The proverb texts were usually taken at their literal level without any contextual consideration, and they were amassed blindly to convince the reader by mere saturation. It was here that proverbs played directly into the propagandistic hands of the Nazis, since proverbs are usually used to spread insights and wisdom in an authoritative generalized fashion" (Mieder 1982: 448). Under National Socialism, a number of proverbs were used to instruct people in matters of heredity, choosing proper marriage partners, hygiene, and children. Some of these were published as a small collection in the Nazi folklore journal *Volk und Rasse* in 1936 under the title "Living racial hygiene in the German proverb" (*Lebendige Rassenhygiene im deutschen Sprichwort*):[34]

Heiraten ins Blut tut selten gut.
[To marry into the blood (close relatives) is seldom good.]

Nur die gleichen, sollen sich die Hände reichen.
[Only those who are alike should exchange their hands in marriage.]

Art lässt nicht von Art.
[Race sticks to race.]

Je näher ans Blut, je schlimmer die Brut.
[The closer to the blood, the worse the offspring.]

Es steckt im Blut, wärs in the Kleidern, könnte man's ausbürsten.
[It is in the blood; if it was in the clothes, one could brush it out.]

Some of the texts merely stressed the need for healthy marriage partners and warned of the consequences of incest. But in Nazi racial doctrines, even these proverbs took on new meanings, that is, purity in reproduction and the need for more German offspring. These isolated texts became dangerous slogans of confrontation and racial discrimination.

The preoccupation with the "sin against the blood" and racial purity in marriage culminated in this proverb: "Three things make the best couples: same blood, same passion, same age" (*Drei Dinge machen die besten Paare: gleich Blut, gleich Glut und gleiche Jahre*).[35] Proverbs on marriage were interpreted as "laws for the protection of the hereditary health of the German nation,"[36] as the racial interpretation of the following proverb shows: "First healthy blood, then a large estate and a pretty hat" (*Erst gesundes Blut, dann grosses Gut und schöner Hut*).[37] The political use of Nazi proverbs was intended to be educational. The goal was to instruct Germans in the need to increase "valuable Aryan blood" and to eliminate "bad" blood through the physical extermination of the Jews and other "worthless" life.

Toward a Community of Blood

Ideologically, society was conceived as a "new community," a unitary body based on the common substance of blood.[38] Such notions were based on Adolf Hitler's assertion about the invariability of blood: "Classes vanish, classes alter themselves, the destinies of men undergo changes, but something always remains: the nation as such, as the substance of flesh and blood."[39] The prevailing conception is best summarized by the following quotation:

Blut bedeutet uns, in unserer gesammten Betrachtung, nicht etwas nur Leibliches, sondern: Seele in artlicher Verbundenheit mit ihrem Ausdrucksfeld dem Leibe. (Clauss 1936: 147)

[To us (National Socialists) blood not only means something corporeal, but it is in a racial sense the soul, which has as its external field of expression the body.]

In order to fortify the central racist tenets, great effort was expanded on examining and measuring the subleties of human anatomy, thereby continuing the nineteenth-century anthropological preoccupation with the physical reality of the body. Almost any physical feature was usable in the elaboration of complex statistical relations between racial and cultural characteristics. Still, craniology, the comparative examination of the size and shape of skulls, coordinated with a range of imputed racial and social qualities, remained the most central concern of the German fascists. Debates on topics like the relative merits of certain types of profiles, of "broad heads" and "long heads," engaged the attention of many. Great effort was devoted to discovering the proper proportions of beauty, which could be measured and mathematically expressed in the geometry of a human face.[40] Such an elaboration of anatomical details and the subsequent classification of types were all repeated in the racist writings of the 1930s.

A New Aesthetics of Race

Nazi ideology suggested that physical beauty, as once possessed by the German ancestors, had retreated into the soul, into the blood,[41] and could be projected outward only through a reconstitution of the body. Political power thus took hold of the body, instituting programs toward the reformation of a healthy, athletic, and aesthetic body. Adolf Hitler himself even created a set of comparisons for his vision of the reconstituted German male youth that became proverbial in fascist Germany:

In unseren Augen, da muss der deutsche Junge der Zukunft schlank und rank sein, flink wie Windhunde, zäh wie Leder, und hart wie Kruppstahl.[42]

[In our eyes, the young German male of the future must be slender and tall, quick as a greyhound, tough as leather, and hard as Krupp steel.]

Thus invested with a novel form of power, the body became an object of numerous disciplinary practices. Action was thereby taken in an area in which the revolutionary structural change of society could be produced most efficiently: in the field of education. It was here that Nazi propaganda turned to the body as an important symbol of German racial superiority and military strength. Educational programs, exercise, and training were supposed to produce a body "hard as steel": upright, firm, strong, and rigid.[43] The goals of National Socialism could thus be displayed visibly as they assumed realization in the physical appearance of the masculine body. Hitler himself disclosed the ends to which he wanted his youth and their bodies to be educated: "I want a violent, haughty, dauntless, cruel youth . . . The free and glorious beast of prey must gleam again through their eyes. Strong and beautiful I want my youth. I shall have them trained in all bodily exercises. I want an athletic youth. This is the first and most important goal. Thus I shall eradicate the thousands of years of human domestication. Thus I shall have the pure, noble material of nature at hand. Thus I can create the new Man."[44]

While on the one hand attempts were made to reeducate and reform the outer manifestation of the individual body, the inner essence of the social body was reconstituted by taking control of human reproduction. Such a body politic had to be achieved through an integrated, carefully focused program.

Gleichlaufend mit der Erziehung des Körpers hat der Kampf gegen die Vergiftung der Seele einzusetzen.[45]

[Synchronous with the education of the body, there must begin the struggle against the poisoning of the soul (that is, blood).]

In a speech delivered at the annual Party Congress in 1937, Hitler made explicit that his political aim was the "rebirth of the [German] nation by the conscious breeding of the human body" (1937: 25). It was the reproductive body that thereby became the target of knowledge, power, and control. National Socialists began the conscious practice of population politics and racial hygiene, and they issued a corpus of laws promoting the "purity" of German blood.

Protecting the Blood

The protection of German blood came to be the primary political purpose and goal of the state. By exterminating all that was alien and by regulating marriage, the state could serve as an instrument whereby the Germans could accomplish the rebirth of their nation.[46] Hitler, in a speech delivered to local party leaders in the south of Germany in 1937, states:

Wir Nationalsozialisten haben für den Staat eine ganz bestimmte Definition gefunden . . . Sinn hat er nur dann, wenn seine letzte Aufgabe doch wieder die Erhaltung eines lebendigen Volkstums ist. Er muss sein nicht nur der Lebenserhalter eines Volkes, sondern damit vor allem der Wesens erhalter, der Bluterhalter eines Volkes. Sonst hat der Staat auf die Dauer keinen Sinn.[47]

[We National Socialists have found a very specific definition for the state . . . it has only a purpose if its final task is the preservation of the living folkdom. It must not only be the life preserver of a people, but thereby primarily the preserver of the inner essence, the maintainer of a nation's blood. Other than this, the state has no purpose in the long run.]

Recognizing this, a number of practices regulating marriage, descent, and birth were put into effect. By September 1935, National Socialism had created laws for the "protection of German blood and German heritage" (*Blutschutz- und Erbgesundheitsgesetz*), which on the one hand prohibited sexual union with "Jewish blood" and which, on the other hand, attempted to prevent the "German blood stock from dissipating its value to the Jewish lineage."[48] The political aim was the "growth of healthy blood" by preventing the "infiltration of alien blood."[49] Mandatory sterilization for purposes of "racial hygiene" (*Erbgesundheitspflege; Erbpflege*), proof of German descent (*Abstammungsnachweis; Ahnenpass*), and the certification of racial eligibility for marriage (*Ehetauglichkeitszeugnis*) by the Ministry of Heredity and Health had become a terrible reality.[50]

Such practices were coordinated with plans for breeding human beings like cattle. Hitler himself had already suggested in *Mein Kampf* that "the time has come for the German nation to become racially aware; besides the breeding of dogs, horses and cats, it should also have mercy with its own blood" (1939: 732). It was suggested that laws promoting the purity of blood were passed to regulate "proper breeding" through the state-approved selection of mates.[51] "It is the task of the German state to subject young men to a performance test before granting them the right of marriage and to educate them in mate-selection in accordance with the idea of the preservation of the Nordic blood" (Darré 1931: 144). Such educational practices were designed to promote the future of the German "community of blood" (*Blutsgemeinschaft*).[52] In order to accomplish this task, Nazi legislation also had to "secure the family as the germinating cell of the state" and to increase the reproductive capacity of "women and mothers, who are the source of German blood."[53] National Socialism thus attempted to place human reproduction under state control.

Orchestrating the Internal Flow

While the state was to protect the flow of German blood, the political party became in a metaphorical sense its "blood vessel," channeling, directing, and controlling the movement of blood inside the social body. Thus Hitler suggested in 1937:

Ich halte es weiter für notwendig, dass die Führer der Partei immer und immer wieder versuchen, die lebendigste Verbindung mit dem Volk herzustellen, . . . weil es notwendig ist, eine souveräne Kenntnis der Volksseele . . . zu besitzen. Und das ist auch das Wunderbare in unserer Organization, dass sie Dank ihrer Verzweigung bis in den letzten Fabrikshof hinein und jedes Hinterhaus, dass sie hierdurch, ich möchte sagen, ein Blutnetz hergestellt hat, bei dem aus tausend Adern fortgesetzt lebendiges Blut nach oben fliesst und damit auch Kenntnis nach oben fliesst und umgekehrt, Energie und Willenskraft und Entschluss-kraft.[54]

[Furthermore, I consider it necessary that the leaders of the party try again and again to establish the most vital connection with the folk, . . . because it is necessary to possess reliable knowledge about the soul of the folk. And that is the most wonderful thing in our organization, that, thanks to its multiple blood vessels, it penetrates into the last factory, and into every home, and that it thereby, shall I say, created a blood network (a blood system), in which living blood continuously flows upward through the thousands of arteries and veins, and thereby also flows knowledge, and energy, will power and determination.]

Here the penetration of political power into every sphere of life was conveyed metaphorically in terms of the blood circulatory system inside a single body. In turn, the governed populace was seen as an organic entity, projected as an image of the unitary body, the *Volkskörper*, which had become an object of knowledge, glorification, and violence.

Hitler attempted to organize society under the sole authority of the party so that it became manageable for his political purposes. Everyday life became permeated and regulated in such a way as to mobilize and equalize society under the rule of the party. There was hardly a way to extricate oneself from this effect:

If one was not a member of the party or one of its numerous organizations, from the SA down to the Association of National Socialist Women (*NS-Frauenschaft*), one probably was a member of the Association of Civil Servants (*Beamtenbund*) or the Association of Labor Unions (*Deutsche Arbeiterfront*), both dominated by the party. If one did not participate in the cultural activities of the National Socialist *Kulturgemeinde*, one perhaps spent leisure time or vacation in one of the countless programs of the recreational organization *Kraft durch Freude*, and on top of that one was permanently inundated by all sorts of activities, like the compulsory weekly Stew Day or the incessant collections of metal, paper or money. (Vondung 1979: 400)

Theories about National Socialism itself have tended to ignore the importance of these daily rituals, organizations, and cults, which eventually provided the essence of fascist politics in Germany.[55] Ideologically, society was conceived as a unitary body based on the common substance of blood. Corresponding to this belief was the ritual actualization of that concept in the National Socialist cult. Scores of holidays, festivals, and ceremonies were developed during the Third Reich, designed to commemorate Hitler's putsch of 1923 or his seizure of power in 1933, and to celebrate many other events in the course of the year. Such celebrations were designed to actualize the sociopolitical image of reality through ritual visualization.

After 1933, the most impressive self-celebration of the "new community" was the annual Party Congress at Nuremberg. As its main event, the nocturnal "hour of consecration" (*Weihestunde*) of the party functionaries, 240,000 people were massed together in the *Zepplin* Stadium, underneath Speer's "dome of light," surrounded by tens of thousands of illuminated red Swastika flags on the walls, and interspersed with 25,000 red and golden glittering standards which, all having been consecrated by Hitler's "blood banner" of 1923, symbolized total devotion as well as the unifying substance of the blood. (Vondung 1979: 400)[56]

Thus German politics during the Nazi era moved in an archaic world of blood mythology and symbolism. What was new was the concretization of these blood metaphors as an instrument of political control.

Chapter 7
Gendered Difference, Violent Imagination
Blood, Race, Nation

What, then, became of the "symbolics of blood" after 1945, follow-ing Hitler's defeat and the collapse of the Third Reich? How were the themes of health, progeny, and race inscribed in German memory after the war? And what happened to the mythical concern with protecting the purity of blood in postwar Germany? According to Michel Foucault (1978), the thematics of blood, specifically a sanguine aesthetic of race, had their origin in a premodern age, in which the genealogical prin-ciple (with its emphasis on birthright, descent, and kin) had maintained the ancient forms of rank and privilege. In the twentieth century, as Foucault observed, the blood myth was disinterred to serve the political interests of a modern state apparatus: "Nazism was doubtless the most cunning [in its deployment] of the [old] fantasies of blood [and] power. A eugenic ordering of society, . . . in the guise of an unrestricted state control, was accompanied by the oneiric exaltation of a superior blood; the latter implied both the systematic genocide of others and the risk of exposing oneself to a total sacrifice. It is an irony of history that [under Hitler] the blood myth was transformed into the greatest blood bath in recent memory" (149–50). But did the death of the Nazi state and the end of the regime of terror successfully eradicate these long-lived pre-occupations with blood, gender, and race? Was the traumatic shift in political systems able to dislodge the sanguine aesthetic from its firm hold on the German historical unconscious? While no longer endorsed as an official ideology after 1945, the blood mystique was often visibly inscribed on the historiographic surface of postwar Germany. Residing at the margins of awareness, fantasies of blood were rendered visible in fragments, each appearing by itself in a "scene," thereby providing the performative labor of social memory. For instance:

In 1983, during an air show at an American military base in the Rhine Palatinate, German peace protesters staged the occurrence of a nuclear Holocaust by simulating mass-death: dressed in black costumes to symbolize the victims' charred bodies and skeletal remains, the protesters arrayed themselves on the ground. When the military police finally intervened, the event turned into a form of dramatic poetry in which members of the German audience played out familiar roles, becoming participants in the physical brutalization of their political opponents. One spectator, a man with a small son, proclaimed that he wanted to "rip the heart" from one of the protester's bodies. Another shouted that the activists "should be run over with a tractor." A man to his left, who until then had been contentedly chewing on a hot dog, suddenly poured his cup of beer over a young woman lying on the ground, and began to shout "Blood! Blood! Blood!" while rhythmically stomping his foot up and down. A female spectator, while kicking and spitting at the protestors, screamed: "Beat them to death, beat them all to death!" As the peace protesters were loaded onto the waiting military trucks, another man proclaimed: "And now into the gas with them!"[1]

What are we to make of these violent imaginings? Zygmunt Bauman, in *Modernity and the Holocaust* (1989), argued that genocide in Germany must be understood as a central event of modern history and not as an exceptional episode. The production of mass death was facilitated by modern processes of rationalization. Exterminatory racism was tied to conceptions of social engineering, to the idea of creating an artificial order by changing the present one and by eliminating those elements that could not be altered as desired. Genocide was based on the technological and organizational achievements of an advanced industrial society. A political program of complete extermination became possible in modern times because of the collaboration of science, technology, and bureaucracy.

Such an interpretation of mass violence requires a critical reconsideration of modernity as a civilizing process—as a progressive rationalization of social life.[2] It requires rethinking genocide, not as an exceptional episode, a state of "anomie" and a breakdown of the social, a suspension of the normal order of things, a historical regression, or a return to primitive instincts and mythic origins,[3] but as an integral principle of modernity. Comprehensive programs of extermination are neither primitive nor instinctual.[4] They are the result of sustained conscious effort and of the substitution of organizational discipline for moral responsibility.[5]

This concept of modernity emphasizes the normalcy of the perpetrators. In the 1930s and 1940s, ordinary German citizens participated in the killings. "As is well known by now, the SS officers responsible for the smooth unfolding of operations were not particularly bestial or, for that matter, sadistic. (This is true of the overwhelming number of them, according to survivors.) They were normal human beings who, the rest of the time, played with their children, gardened, listened to music. They were, in short, civilized" (Todorov 1990: 31). The genesis of the Holocaust offers an example of the ways in which ordinary Germans—"otherwise normal individuals"—could become perpetrators by their passive acceptance of the "political and bureaucratic mechanisms that permitted the idea of mass extermination to be realized" (Mommsen 1991: 252–53). The technocratic nature of Nazi genocide attests to the "banality of evil" (Arendt 1964), that is, the sight of a highly mechanized and bureaucratized world where the extermination of entire groups of people, who were regarded as "contagion," could become a normal occurrence. From this perspective, race-based violence and public machinations of mass death cannot be understood as regressive historical processes:[6] they are manifestations of new forms of cultural violence and the centralizing/monopolizing tendencies of modern (state) power.

But such a modernist conception of genocide also implies the existence of a powerful political imaginary through which everyday understandings of national belonging, race, and body are defined. How do we analyze a cultural history of genocide? Seeing nationalism as a generalized condition of the modern political world, Liisa Malkki (1996) suggests that "the widely held commonsense assumptions linking people to place, and nation to territory, are not simply territorializing but deeply metaphysical" (437). This chapter is a schematic exploration of further aspects of this metaphysics. I examine the ways in which specific national identities are dissociated from the fixities of place and geographical implacement that are normally associated with the modern nation-state. The formation of German nationality is complicated by a corporeal imaginary: blood, bodies, genealogies. My intent is to show that the naturalizing of the links between people (i.e., the national community) and the state is routinely conceived in specifically organic metaphors. German images of "the national order of things" (Malkki 1995b) rest on metaphors of the human organism and the body. Among the potent metaphors for the national community is blood.[7] Nationality is imagined as "the flow of blood," a unity of substance.[8] Such metaphors are thought to "denote something to which one is naturally tied" (Anderson 1983: 131). Thinking about the German nation thus takes the form of origins, ancestries, and racial lines, which are "naturalizing" images: a genealogical form of thought.

Much recent work in anthropology and related fields has focused on the process through which such collective representations are constructed and maintained by states and national elites.[9] Here I focus on powerful metaphoric practices in everyday life, and I examine how media discourse and political language are deployed to understand and act upon the aberrant boundary conditions of blood and nationhood in postwar Germany. I examine the location of violence in German political culture, and I inquire how subaltern bodies, as racial constructs and potential sites of domination, are imagined in public discourse. My aim is to shed light on postwar Germany, where the feminized body of the outsider (foreigner, refugee, Other) has been reclaimed as a signifier of race and contagion; where violence defines a new corporeal topography, linked to the murderous elimination of refugees and immigrants; where exterminatory discourses have once again begun to colonize the national imaginary; where ordinary citizens with divergent political beliefs participate in the reproduction of cultural violence;[10] and where notions of racial alterity and gendered difference are publicly constructed through iconographic images of blood and liquidation.

I trace the (trans)formation of these conceptual models from the turn of the century through the post-unification era, thus illuminating the persistence of German ideas about racial purity and contamination. I propose that modern forms of violence are engendered through regimes of representation that are to some extent mimetic, a source of self-formation, both within the historical unconscious and the fabric of the social world.[11] I begin by drawing attention to the racist biomedical visions of blood that emerged under fascism. The representational violence of such blood imagery, which entered the popular imagination through political propaganda, emerged as a prelude to racial liquidation. Genealogies of blood were medicalized, conceived as sources of contamination that needed to be expunged through violent bloodletting. Documenting cultural continuities after 1945, I explore the implications of a racialist politics of blood for the German nation-building process in the postwar period. I analyze more closely the linkages of blood to gendered forms of violence, focusing on the central role of masculinity and militarism for a German nationalist imaginary. Images of women, blood, and contagion became fused in the fascist visions of the corporeality of German nationhood. I explore the metaphorical extensions of a "symbolics of blood" in postwar German culture, and I show how easily a misogynist militarism is reconfigured to (re)produce a violent body politic that legitimates the brutalization of immigrants and refugees. Throughout, I emphasize the interplay of race and gender against the background of medical models, documenting how fears of natural disasters (women, Jews, refugees) and medical pathologies like dirt and infection (i.e., bodily infestations) are continuously recycled to reinforce a racialist postmodern.

The Symbolics of Blood

The production of death and the erasure of Jewish bodies were central to the fascist politics of race. The aim of genocide was to maintain the "health" of the German body politic by enforcing a strict regimen of "racial hygiene."[12] German political fantasy employed a model of race in which the images of difference were not visibly written on the skin but had rather to be carefully constructed in order to identify the Other.[13] The axiom for this construction of ideas of difference derived from a typology of blood. Race, disease, and infection were imagined through blood metaphors. Blood became a marker of pathological alterity, a signifier that linked race and difference.[14] The attempt to expunge the racial subaltern (specifically, Jewishness) was thus imagined as a multilayered discourse of "liquidation": the consumption by fire *and* the reduction to blood. Images of blood were invoked both through the genealogical ordering of society, in which blood functioned as a verbal signifier of descent and citizenship,[15] and through the violence inflicted upon subaltern bodies, thereby effecting the transfiguration of the linguistic construct "race" into its physical signs: blood, pain, and contagion. Imagining racial differences through the blood motif became a prologue to extermination, effectively feeding the political rationalizations of death. As early as 1916, these images of blood and liquidation were popularized through lyrics that were later adopted into Nazi political songs:

> Blood, blood, blood must flow
> Thick as a rain of blows
> To hell with the freedom of the Jewish republic . . .
> In blood we must stand
> In blood we must walk
> Up to, up to our ankles . . .
> We are ready for the racial struggle
> With our blood we consecrate the banner . . .
> Keep from the Reich the foreign Jews
> Let Aryan blood not suffer destruction.[16]

In these songs, German fascists expressed both the mandate of National Socialism and the manner in which it was to be carried out. I suspect that these visions of blood (much the same as the visions of fire and burning bodies) existed as a core fantasy of fascist violence: a way of publicly imagining (and visually anticipating) the dissolution of bodily reality, the termination of identity and difference in a river of blood.

The German politics of blood and the discourse of liquidation were thus closely connected. Both sought to reduce the salient Other into an undifferentiated mass. Such attempts at liquidation tended to follow a fixed sequence: death was indexed first by fire, next a flood, then blood. For instance, in German war prophecies from 1914, events of mass death were predicted through the symbolic chronology: a fire year, a flood year, a blood year.[17] This same sequence of fire, flood, and blood reappeared in fascist writings in the 1930s.[18] In each case, the flow of blood was tantamount to a logical consequence: Blood was equated with race; Blood was expected to flow; The murdered were expected to bleed.

The construction of this idea of genocide, the very discourse of liquidation by blood, has analogues in the postwar German understanding of alterity, an understanding shaped by a deep-seated revulsion to racial difference and facilitated by a vocabulary of race that originated during the Nazi period. For instance, in Fall 1991, the prime minister of the state of Schleswig-Holstein, Björn Engholm, a liberal Social Democrat, referred to persons seeking political asylum in Germany as a threatening "counter race" (*Gegenrasse*) whose continued existence "had become a question of survival for Germany."[19] Around the same time, the mayor of Vilshofen, a member of the conservative Christian Democratic Party, announced his opposition to Germany's constitutional guarantee to protect political refugees: "Today we give the asylum-seekers bicycles, tomorrow our daughters."[20] German politicians are surprisingly candid in their articulation of these ideas about the dangerous Other. A councilman from the city of Dormagen thus explained his position on German refugee politics in 1991: "Some people talk . . . about integration, others about amalgamation. I speak about the adulteration and filthy mishmashing of blood" (*Blutverpanschung und -vermanschung*).[21] In November 1988, Bavaria's minister of the interior, the conservative Christian Democrat Edmund Stoiber, claimed that Germans were becoming "hybridized and racially infested" (*durchmischt und durchrasst*) by the influx of foreigners and those "not of the blood" (*blutsfremd*).[22] In painting a picture of a "mongrelized society," Stoiber, who is now Bavaria's head of state (*Ministerpräsident*), thus not only naturalized but also sanctioned xenophobic tendencies as necessary for German ethnic well-being.[23] Popular notions of "genetic identity" are here subsumed by fears of racial impurity. For Stoiber, the racial/blood purity of the German people is threatened by the mere presence of ethnically diverse groups. His assertions are deeply embedded in biological images of difference: blood and blood contamination. In German popular culture, according to Stuttgart's mayor Manfred Rommel (1989: 4), such notions of blood origins, that is, concerns about "where the blood comes from" (*woher das Blut kommt*), are at work in the determination of racial otherness.

This vocabulary of blood as an index of difference and genealogical placement is used not only by political conservatives. Derived from a West German understanding of the past, the language of race appears in the public discourse of liberal politicians and, sometimes, even the more radical left.[24] In January 1989 in Berlin, at a working dinner with representatives of the major political parties,[25] Gabi Vonnekold, the evening's Green/Alternative spokeswoman, declared that Germany's politics of repatriation (which actively encouraged the return-migration of ethnic Germans from Eastern Europe and elsewhere) were legitimately based on ideas of "blood right" (*Blutrecht*): ethnic Germans, she asserted, were granted citizenship because of their "blood ties" (*Blutsbande*) to the German nation.[26] Supporting similar statements made by the other politicians, Vonnekold argued that such verbal images had no racial connotations because they originated in the commonsense reality of kinship. She noted that it was this meaning of "blood relatedness" or "kinship by blood" (*Blutsverwandtschaft*) that had been adopted as law by the postwar West German state. Several weeks later, after a successful election campaign for the Berlin Senate, a militant faction of the Green/Alternative party (*Gruppe Grüne Panther*) distanced itself from Germany's policy of repatriation. The practice was denounced in a public forum, however, without making the concepts of blood right and citizenship through blood a critical issue.[27]

In the German political imagination, cultural differences tend to be constructed as differences of blood. For instance, a commentary by Herbert Gruhl, one of the conservative founders of the Green Party, is suggestive of the habitual infusion of ethnicity and nationality with biological overtones. In Gruhl's opinion, most refugees are biologically or organically incompatible with Germans. In a 1990 interview, in which he outlined his differences with the Greens, Gruhl stated:

If one thinks ecologically, one must acknowledge that there are organic peoples, languages, and cultural communities. The Greens, on the one hand, consider all human beings in the world to be interchangeable, like numbers. That is unacceptable. It simply is not true that everyone is the same. If someone comes from India, South America or the GDR [East Germany], it makes a big difference . . . It is after all most natural that one accepts those with whom one already shares a common historical fate and with whom one even has direct blood ties.[28]

Apparently exempt from critical inquiry in political debates, the judicial field of German nationality seems to have rendered "normal" a modern conception of race: the citizenship law of the Federal Republic determines national membership through the idiom of descent, as expressed by the Latin term *jus sanguinis*, "power/law of blood."[29] Enacted in 1913—and still in effect today—the German citizenship law permits, and even encourages, the nations's social/racial closure: individuals born within the territory of the German state cannot automatically acquire citizenship. German nationality is determined by an understanding of a community of descent, shaped by an "ethnocultural" or "ethnonational" perception of statehood.[30] Deeply embedded in Germany's imperial history, the blood principle of citizenship is defined by racial premises, which were established at the turn of the century to deny colonial subjects inheritance and voting rights.[31] Once inserted into the German legal system, the concept of the modern nation as a "reservoir of blood" was rendered unremarkable. But this iconography of nationhood, defined by a symbolics of blood, has retained its association with violence and racial contagion.

In the German imaginary, the invocation of blood, whether in the context of genealogy or racial liquidation, presupposes an act of violent transformation. This violence is aimed at producing a particular condition of the racial body: its dissolution, liquification, and reduction to blood. Such a transformation of the body (flesh to blood/solid to liquid) is probably intended as a form of cleansing. When in June 1992 a Dresden city councilman, Günter Rühlemann, announced that "he wanted to cause a bloodbath among foreigners," this plan seemed somehow to be connected to the expectation of a rebirth, the beginning of a new era without the threat of "blood contamination" (*Blutverschmutzung*).[32] Coordinating attitudes of violence with fears of pollution and dirt, the German discourse of death requires the transfiguration of racial Others into blood, an act of ritual purging.

In Germany's racialist mythography, the external production of blood takes place within a particular field of meaning. On the one hand, blood loss through violence is perceived as cleansing: a release, a sacrificial libation, which purges the body of ritual impurities. But blood effusion takes on sexual connotations whenever this image of the bleeding body is symbolically connected to the periodic emission of women's menstrual flow.[33] This analogic affinity of menstruation and blood spillage confirms the metaphorical linkage between "sexuality and those diverse forms of violence that invariably lead to bloodshed" (Girard 1979: 35). Masculinist ideology can thus reconfigure the flow of blood as a social threat, an attack on manhood and the national body politic. On the other hand, blood spilled by violence is read as a stigma, a red stain of contagion; it contaminates, inundates, and subsumes everything with which it comes in contact. This discourse of blood is formative within a particular regime of representation: "When violence is [unleashed], . . . blood appears everywhere—on the ground, underfoot, forming great pools. Its very fluidity gives form to the contagious nature of violence. Its presence proclaims murder and announces new upheavals to come. Blood stains everything it touches the color of violence and death" (34).

The flow of blood visibly exposes or unmasks everything that is undesirably different: women and women-associated Others (e.g., Jews, revolutionaries, homosexuals). Blood metaphors thus establish a "sanguine connection to sexuality, gender identity, and the biologization of the Jew" (Geller 1992: 254). Moreover, violent bloodshed creates an observable physical condition: liquidity, sexual contagion, and carnal femininity. The bleeding body (in much the same sense as the menstruating body) becomes a mark—a stigma—of femaleness: a (dangerous) liquid corporeality. The German discourse of *liquidation* (in both its genealogical and its violent form) is thus integrated into a pattern of domination that transforms the racial Other into woman.

Imagining Jewish Bodies

The feminization of the racial subaltern, particularly the Jewish body, emerged as a construct of the European cultural and religious imagination. Assumptions that Jewish males menstruate, for instance, can be traced to medieval notions of difference that continued at least into the late eighteenth century.[34] Likewise, the existence of the presumed link between blood, ritual periodicity (or cyclicity), and Jewish sexuality has been chronicled through centuries of European history, from medieval Christianity to twentieth century Germany.[35] Fears of sexual degeneracy and bleeding male bodies merged in the modern German mythographies of race: "Here it is necessary to point out that the stereotyped depiction of sexual 'degenerates' was transferred almost intact to the 'inferior races,' who inspired the same fears. These races, too, were said to display a lack of morality and a general absence of self-discipline. Blacks, and then Jews, were endowed with excessive sexuality, with a so-called female sensuousness that transformed love into lust. They lacked all manliness. Jews as a group were said to exhibit female traits, just as homosexuals were generally considered effeminate" (Mosse 1985: 36).

Furthermore, the development of modern scientific disciplines, with their allegedly objective epistemic discourses, provided these constructions of difference with a new form of legitimation. The emergent sciences offered a grammar of truth that treated the reproductive system and the female body as a language through which difference could be expressed as "a fact of nature."[36] This emphasis on reproduction led to representations of the "abnormal" that were increasingly biologized. Femaleness and difference were now defined by a medical model.[37] Through the ascription of disease and pathology, the female body became a repository of sexual identity and race.

The medical model, which defined Germany's nationalist agenda in the early twentieth century, was anchored in the complementary discourse of descent and reproduction; blood was the common icon. Encoded with qualities characteristic of the ideological construct "woman," blood became the iconic marker of pathological difference: a signifier of sexual disease and racial contagion.[38] These fantastic images found political expression in the 1930s, when the promotion of glorified hypermasculine values, and an emphasis on proficiency in physically aggressive activities like sports and warfare, were intertwined with a fear of pollution from "bad" blood. In the late 1930s, German fascism became obsessively concerned with controlling both women and reproduction.[39] Politically effective images of difference were drawn from fantastic fabrications about female carnality and visions of the destructive power of the vulva and its fluids. Society's energies were subsequently directed inward toward "containing" the penetration of the masculine (political) body by racial impurities. The eradication of racial difference, through the evisceration of the feminized Jews, thus emerged as a central template of violence in Nazi Germany.

Racializing Female Bodies

The violent obsession with the female body, and its reduction to blood, is documented in Klaus Theweleit's *Male Fantasies* (1987/89). Mapping the collective unconscious of the proto-fascist warrior, Theweleit examines these men's motivations for terror against women and the linkages between racial hatred and male power. Theweleit focuses on the fantasies of a particular group of men: members and officers of the *Freikorps*, the private, mercenary armies that fought the revolutionary German working class in the years immediately after World War I. These "white" troops (consisting of former imperial soldiers, anticommunist youth, and adventurers) regarded the socialist labor movement as the greatest threat to their image of the nation and German manhood. After suppressing the communist insurrection of 1919, under the leadership of the socialist chancellor Friedrich Ebert,[40] the Freikorps soldiers came to play a crucial role in the rise of Nazism. In several cases, they emerged as key functionaries in the Third Reich: "The Stahlhelm, the SA, and the SS all recruited many of their most prominent leaders from the alumni of the *Freikorps*."[41] Rudolf Höss, a former Freikorps officer and influential Nazi, was appointed commandant of Auschwitz.

The excavation of Freikorps literary remains, of novels, letters, and autobiographies, uncovered the terrifying visions of these proto-fascists, visions of hatred and fear in which women were reduced to a series of blood images: the red tide, the red flow, a sea of blood. Women, perceived as sources of contagion, were equated with dirt, pits of muck, effluvia. The nature of femaleness and womanhood, envisioned in terms of bodily emissions or secretions (blood, mucus, excrement) was experienced as menacing. The Freikorps soldiers hated women, specifically women's bodies and sexuality. Their hatred surfaced in an endless series of liquid images, in which women were associated with everything that threatened to flood or deluge the boundaries of manhood. It was a dread, ultimately, of dissolution, of being swallowed, annihilated.

Fascist soldiers always depicted women and female bodies through a lens of violence. A military operation against the primarily female participants of a labor protest is recounted with an emphasis on blood and dismemberment:

"They're probably spitting there again," thought Donat [a Freikorps soldier], knitting his brow. Suddenly, he saw a mouth before him. It wasn't really so much a mouth as a bottomless throat, ripped wide open, spurting blood like a fountain . . . They certainly were spitting. But the men of the brigade didn't take it lying down. Quick as lightning, they turned their carbines around and ground them into those spitting faces.[42]

The same discourse of violence, with the aim to obliterate the female Other, characterized another military expedition against women demonstrators:

A rain of spittle hits the soldiers . . . The spitting woman . . . stands before the barrel of his gun—his sight is pointing straight into her mouth, into the center of that slobbering hole, so wide open with hysteria that he can even see the gums. "Get away!" he screams again, as if he afraid of himself. It's really her. Now he recognizes her. "Fire!" . . . Everything turns suddenly to frenzied flight. Yet [the soldier] sees nothing of this. He sees only the woman who was standing there before him a moment ago. It threw her onto her back, as if she had been blown over by some gigantic wind. Is that thing at his feet really her? That person without a face? The head isn't really a head anymore, just a monstrous bloody throat.[43]

In these violent encounters, specific parts of the female body are attacked: "[A] woman is punched in the mouth; she is clubbed in the teeth with a rifle butt; a shot is fired into her open mouth. The mouth appears as a source of nauseating evil, a 'venomous hole' that spouts out a 'rain of spittle.'"[44] According to one soldier: "Women are the worst. Men fight with fists, but women also spit and swear—you can't just plant your fist into their ugly pusses."[45] The men's attacks destroy those parts of a woman's body that are perceived as a threat to manhood: her head, her mouth, her genitalia.

Mouths can symbolically represent the vagina and the effluvia pouring out of them can represent vaginal secretions.[46] It is possible that all the objects with which the soldiers' attacks were carried out represent the phallus: whips, boots, rifle butts, bullets. Following this framework, we might conclude that we are dealing with violent erotic advances: the murders or attacks were committed against women with whom the perpetrator was engaged in violent sexual intercourse, an act of rape.[47]

But it is the mutilated female body, rather than the soldiers' actions, that assumes primary symbolic significance. The men's violence aims to expose woman's horrifying sexual potential. Female bodies are penetrated, opened up, and exposed to the male gaze. All that remains is a bloody, bottomless throat, ripped wide open. "[T]he killings are conceived as corrective measures, which alter the false appearances of the women so that their 'true natures' can become visible" (Theweleit 1987: 196). The women's wounds magnify the men's source of terror, revealing what the soldiers knew all along: women are whores, vehicles of urges, emasculators. They are treated accordingly.

The men's desire to perceive women in the condition of bloody masses seems to be the driving force behind the killings. The assault itself is a means to this end. Consider the following example, in which Marja, a communist woman, falls into the hands of the German Freikorps soldiers and is beaten to death: "Moving along the stream, [the soldiers] are astonished to see it blocked by the bodies of Bolsheviks. The soldiers must have been given an order . . . to toss all of the wounded into the water . . . The last body they ride past seems to be that of a woman. But it's very hard to tell, since all that's left is a bloody mass, a lump of flesh that appears to have been completely lacerated with whips and is now lying within a circle of trampled, reddish slush."[48] The woman is reduced to a pulp: a shapeless, bloody mass, trampled flesh. This same imagery appears in other narrative descriptions of women's bodily remains: a blood-drenched mass; naked and cut to pieces; a pulp of blood and excrement. The soldiers' reduction of the murdered woman to a "reddish slush" meant that the victim had lost her outlines: her solid body, her identity. Her wounds were no longer discrete entities nor was the body to which these wounds belonged.

Fascist violence was preoccupied with this dissolution of the body and of the woman as bodily entity. The soldiers' attacks fit into a series of repeated attempts at exposing the *woman* in the body: through the infliction of wounds (i.e., bleeding vagina) and by the production of blood (i.e., the menstrual flow). In the violent imagination of the fascist soldiers, women's bodies had to be transfigured into a deluge of blood, causing total obliteration. The point seemed to be to make everything red, a color that (like blood) functioned as a dominant metaphor for the men's erotic desire and fear.

The Freikorps soldiers' fear of and revulsion toward women manifests itself in the incessant invocation of metaphors of an engulfing fluid or flood, the terrifying deluge. Fearing that which they both see and expose (the erotic female Other), the men want to be freed from all that could be identified with women's bodies: liquidity, emotional warmth, sensuality. Theweleit (1989) believes that this desire gave rise to a fascist body politic that tried to elude and repel feminization. The hardened male body with its stiff military pose became the armor men used to protect their inner selves. Repulsed by their own corporeality, the Frei-korps soldiers attempted to subdue and repress the woman within: it was she, or what she stood for, that constituted the most radical threat to the men's own integrity. "[T]he most urgent task of the man of steel [was] to pursue, to dam in and to subdue any force that threaten[ed] to transform him back into the horribly disorganized jumble of flesh, hair, skin, bones, intestines, and feelings that call[ed] itself human" (Theweleit 1989: 160). The soldiers' repudiation of their own bodies and of femininity became a psychic compulsion that equated masculinity with hardness, self-denial, and violent destruction.

The armored organization of the male self depended on the use of violence to maintain its integrity. In the act of killing, the corporal boundaries of the victims were transgressed while the inner cohesion of the male self remained intact: by penetrating and dismembering women's bodies, the men's own bodies became armored and whole; by liquifying female bodies, theirs become hard. The men's destructive im-pulse derived from their inability to feel or sustain any sense of bodily boundaries without inflicting violence. The symbolic construction of the dangerous female Other, and her eventual obliteration, served as a mechanism of self-cohesion. Threatened by imaginary "floods," "tor-rents," and "raging waters," the men stood firm against these onslaughts of surging womanhood. Hardened by military procedures, the male body was transformed into a machine, the man of steel. "Fear of the inner body with its inchoate 'mass' of viscera and entrails, its 'soft' geni-talia, its 'lower half,' is translated into the threat of the 'masses' in the social sense of classes or—especially in those chaotically mixed groups with women and children in the forefront—mass demonstrations. The mass is diametrically opposed to the need for a rigidly, hierarchically structured whole" (Rabinbach and Benjamin 1989: xix).

To the Freikorps soldiers, communists, like individual women, were an undifferentiated force that sought to engulf: "a sea of blood, a flood, a swamp, a tide, a threat that came in waves." [49] Consider the follow-ing examples: "The wave of Bolshevism surged onward, threatening . . . to swallow up the republics"; "The Reds inundated the land"; "the Red wave surged onward"; "the raging Polish torrent"; "The stream of insur-gents pours like the Great Deluge over . . . against . . . the Germans"; "the all-destroying flood . . . advancing toward the west." [50] The fascist soldier wanted to keep the red flood of revolution away from his body.

He wanted to hold himself together as an entity, a distinct body with fixed boundaries. He wanted "to stand with both feet and every root firmly anchored in the soil" (Theweleit 1987: 230). His fear that contact with women would make him cease to exist as a discrete entity was here reproduced as a fear of being inundated, flushed away, dissolved. The dread of women, which existed at the core of the fascist movement, was thereby linked to anticommunism as well as race hatred. "All that [was] rich and various [had to] be smoothed over (to become like the blank facades of architecture); all that [was] wet and luscious [had to] be dammed up and contained; all that [was] 'exotic' (dark, Jewish) [had to] be eliminated."[51] In the end, it was the men's battle against feminization that led to the use of violence, and ultimately murder.

As Barbara Ehrenreich emphasized in her foreword to *Male Fantasies* (1987), the boundaries that delineate the proto-fascist warrior cannot be precisely defined. The lines between fascist militarism, the soldiering male, Nazism, and male fantasy are intentionally blurred by the author. This blurring of historical distinctions raises some important questions. If these desires or fantasies are not limited to the men of the Freikorps, if they are the common property of bourgeois males, then what distinguishes these Freikorps men from other men? Is it that they are military men? "Military culture divides itself from non-military culture in its equation of civilian life with femininity, the existence of 'masses' or 'classes' with unpermitted pleasures of the body. The fascist warrior turns nation, race, and volk into instruments of the militarization of the self—the pain principle" (Rabinbach and Benjamin 1989: xviii).

Theweleit himself posits a continuum between ordinary male fantasy and its violent counterpart. His work suggests that the militarization of German society was accomplished by incorporating, and often intensifying, existing notions of misogynist masculinity. Fascist soldiers, who used terror against women as a strategy of war, were dependent on peacetime constructions of society and gender.[52] German fascism created a culture of terror by accentuating the everyday forms of violence against women, privileging those cultural images of masculinity and manhood that were driven by a desire for bloodshed: the brutalization of woman, her reduction to a bloody mass, was fundamental to the making of the German fascist. Using the soldiers' revulsion toward women as a starting point, Theweleit's work uncovered the "military's heavy reliance not just on men as soldiers, but on misogynist forms of masculinist soldiering" (Enloe 1995: 224). In fascist Germany, as in other modern nation-states, military violence, militarization, and everyday cultural practices shared resonances that mutually reinforce these masculinist visions of power.[53] Sexual violence and female mutilation were fundamental to fascist militarism because such physicality, the imagery of broken bodies, was also a cultural phenomenon. Blood (bleeding corpses, menstrual flows, a threatening fe/maelstrom) existed as a dominant metaphor for the German body politic.

The German militarization of violence, directed against a perceived feminine threat, was deeply connected to the social fabric of race. The soldiers' efforts were directed against women and other forms of contagion that could be imagined through the threat of (female) blood pollution. In recognition of such a linkage, some scholars have begun to trace the connections between military patterns of rape, on the one hand, and racial stratification on the other.[54] Such studies seek to expose how societal systems of racism need particular forms of sexualized violence in order to survive. Given this pattern, we should not be surprised to find evidence of a certain kind of fantasy material, a misogynist/racialist politics of representation, in contemporary Germany.

In German media culture, visions of female liquidity and foreign flows have merged into a common frame of reference: liquification/liquidation. But what are the specific implications of finding the threatening image of a "raging flood" applied to immigrants or refugees? How do we interpret the rhetorical invocation of public images of dissolution and subsumption by "streams of refugees" in a united Germany? My comparative tracing of fascist imaginings and postwar representations of racialized bodies shows how such powerful tropes are maintained in cultural systems to emerge in wartime militarization or in peacetime reactions against immigration, and how such schemata can motivate violent civil aggression against foreigners and women in present-day Germany.

The Threat of Foreign Bodies: Blood, Flood, Contagion

Soon after 1945, after the end of fascism in Germany, the spatial proximity and mingling of racialized bodies emerged again as an unresolvable dilemma. In the postwar period, during the era of economic reconstruction, German cultural politics continued to perpetuate racial prejudice, invariably keeping the Other at a distance, "under control"— a recipe for psychological terror. Relations between Germans and racial Others came to be socially organized and regulated, the object of laws.[55] Economically, foreign workers and immigrants were needed, even as politically the German state sought to eliminate them.[56] Feeding on images of otherness and difference, ultimately taking control of them, German capitalist culture nourished the symbolic constructions for its own ends. The postwar German state depended on racial otherness as an ideological and structural phenomenon, which it simultaneously sought to exploit and destroy.

Beginning in the late 1960s, German industry attempted to alleviate its temporary labor shortages by recruiting foreign workers. These migrant laborers (brought from southern Europe and its immediate periphery) were hired on short-term contracts. They were employed in the service sector or in production, there taking on the unskilled, manual, and often most dangerous jobs.[57] "Initially called *Fremdarbeiter*, foreign workers, in a carry-over from the forced laborers imported during the Third Reich, they were quickly rechristened *Gastarbeiter*, 'guestworkers.' All Germans believed that these guests, who were considered *Ausländer*, foreigners, would eventually return to [their home] countries" (Borneman 1992a: 206–7). Inserted into the capitalist economy, migrant workers were soon reduced to the function of surplus labor. After the onset of the energy crisis in 1973, and a deepening economic recession, West Germany closed its borders to foreign workers, initiated elaborate (and costly) programs of repatriation, and tightened its laws concerning refugee and immigration rights.[58] This period of state repression and racial tension persisted until the early 1980s.

Germany's closure of national boundaries was complicated by a legal system that defined political asylum as a basic human right. In commemoration of the terror and dislocations caused by the war, fascism, and the concentration camps, the West German state had made the protection of refugees an integral part of its judicial foundation. This foundation, the very basis of postwar German state authority, was deemed threatened, attacked "at its core,"[59] in the early 1980s, when German officials observed a sudden increase in refugees from Africa and Asia who, as victims of political persecution, were seeking asylum in Germany. Administration officials interpreted this influx of refugees as a direct result of attempts by foreigners to circumvent the state's increasingly restrictive immigration policies.

In discussing the influx of foreign peoples, German politicians began to conjure images of an invasive "flood" of bodies, a "rising tide" that threatened to inundate the country. "A hundred-thousand, perhaps more, foreigners are expected to enter the Federal Republic this year and appeal to the constitution which promises asylum for victims of political persecution . . . [T]his stream of foreigners pouring into Germany is regarded as a wrong. Politicians acknowledge this by talking about dams that should be raised against the 'flood of asylum seekers.'"[60] German politicians envisioned the threat of alien bodies as a liquid mass—inundating, flooding, surging. Their terror of and revulsion toward this liquid Other continued to find tangible expression in the compulsive use of metaphors that described political events as natural processes.

By the early 1980s, refugees were thus reconfigured as a menace, a "deluge" of unimaginable proportions: "The stream of asylum-seekers [is] pouring in," a "human flood";[61] a "rapidly rising stream of foreigners,"[62] which "pours into the Federal Republic";[63] the "river rose to nearly fifty thousand immigrants";[64] "West Germany [is] inundated by a wave of foreigners";[65] a "torrent," a "river";[66] a "deluge," "streaming into the country."[67] There is "wide-spread uneasiness about the foreign flood" in Germany;[68] "the flow of refugees";[69] the "rising tide," the "wave," the "in-pouring of foreigners";[70] "the stream of asylum seekers into the Federal Republic."[71] It is an "untamed stream";[72] a "dangerous surge of foreigners";[73] a "fearsome flood."[74]

These same images of Germany's inundation by asylum seekers reappeared in 1990 after unification: Germans began to "fantasize about an invasion by millions, the flood of refugees, that threatened to subsume them" (Kreft 1991: 28). These signifiers functioned to prefigure public images of refugees as a negative presence. In public speech, discussions about asylum seekers were "often coupled with nouns denoting some natural and/or uncontained disaster: flood [*Flut*], river [*Strom*], mass [*Masse*]" (Mattson 1995: 66). The natural energy of this torrential flow was encoded as "foreign"/"Other": untamed, dangerous, destructive. Its manifestations inspired terror as well as repugnance: mighty streams were pouring out over Germany, transforming it upon contact, leaving it substantially altered.[75] "Does the Federal Republic have the strength to cope with the so-called 'economic refugees' who are inundating the country? At the moment, these problems are still manageable. But how will it be in three, four years, if the river pouring into Germany remains constant or becomes even greater?"[76] The terror of the external invasion was combined with a fear of dissolution. Contact with the "flood" killed: it posed a threat to the nation's bodily integrity.

Within this roaring cauldron, the men's own bodies appeared — struggling to contain the terrifying deluge — but also a larger, external body: the metropolis. The city was conceived as a human body (perhaps even a female body) inundated, depleted, weakened.

The rising stream of foreigners into the Federal Republic is taking on precarious forms. Many cities are literally flooded by the refugees . . . The German council of mayors urged the Federal Minister of the Interior, Gerhard Baum, to correct the processing of refugees. If it proved impossible to dam the flood, then the bearers of public responsibility at all levels might no longer retain control of the events [*Herr des Geschehens bleiben*].[77]

Metropolitan centers like Stuttgart, Frankfurt or Berlin no longer have the strength to handle the surging flood of asylum seekers . . . The Eritreans have reduced the city of Leinfelden-Echterdingen to such a state of desperation that the Chief Mayor threatened to issue a temporary decree of emergency unless the government agreed to move the Eritreans out into other communities, beyond the inundated city: "If the state does not take charge of a larger proportion of the refugees, then emergency in-take camps must be constructed in order to retain control of the human flood" [*der Menschenflut Herr zu werden*].[78]

The flood metaphor is abstract enough to allow processes of extreme diversity to be subsumed under its image. Their common linkage is the politicians' fear of transgression, which threatens to destroy the cohesion of the nation, cities, and the German body. The symbolism of the foreign "flow" provokes (or agitates) particular racial and historical memories: it unleashes something that has been forbidden.

Germany's political men demand that "something be done" about the "mighty stream": they want to stop the flood, "dam up" and "contain" the flow, "stem the tide," "halt" or better yet, "reverse the flow" of immigrants.[79] Gerhard Baum, federal minister of the interior, "wants to dam up the tide of refugees with his emergency program."[80] Former chancellor Helmut Schmidt wants "to dam and contain the rising stream of foreigners by changing the constitutional right of political asylum."[81] "The stream of asylum seekers has risen to such enormous proportions that the administrative agencies and the courts no longer have the strength to cope with the flow."[82] Herbert Ehrenberg, minister of labor, intends "to stop the Turkish invasion," the "surge of foreigners"; and the German government promotes such efforts as a form of "self-defense" (*Notwehr*).[83]

The spatial proximity of refugees inspires growing fears of "over-foreignization" (*Überfremdung*).[84] The term, conjuring an undesirable transgression of race, refers to the estrangement of a people from their cultural or genetic heritage through the superimposition, a "grafting," of alien bodies. "The refugees were soon so numerous that onto every village dweller came one asylum seeker" (*so dass auf einen Dorfbewohner ein Asylsuchender kam*).[85] "Germany is 'over populated' and 'racially inundated' by foreigners" (*von Ausländern übervölkert*).[86] Such visions articulate a fear of "racial inundation" that appears to be resilient, persisting after 1990.[87] Frankfurt's city councilman Daniel Cohn-Bendit, a prominent member of the leftist Green Party, received hate-mail letters, which accused him of being an "enemy of the German people" because he did nothing to prevent "the foreign inundation" (*Überfremdung*).[88] By contrast, the conservative Steffen Heitmann, who had declared his candidacy for the German presidency in 1993, promised to "protect the nation from the racial superimposition by foreigners" (*Überfremdung*).[89] In southern Germany, the Christian Socialist Union party (CSU) renewed its commitment to transform the German fear of "over-foreignization" (*Überfremdung*) into a political platform.[90] The head of this same party, Theo Waigel, affirmed that the "threat of foreign inundation" (*Überfremdung*) would become a central campaign issue in the forthcoming election.[91]

These anguished visions of the foreign "flood" are governed by recurrent images of weakness, disorder, and loss of control. Germany's politicians articulate their fears of extinction through images of emasculation and impotence. Control of the foreign "invasion" is construed as an assertion and display of manhood: to "remain a man/master/ruler over the events" (*Herr des Geschehens bleiben*); "to become the man/lord of the human flood" (*der Menschenflut Herr werden*). The common German title *Herr* means both "man" and "master," in the sense of "lord," "ruler," "head." The plural form of this term is linked to expressions of racial superiority: German *Herrenrasse* means "master race." It refers (quite literally) to a "select breed of men." In the German imaginary, the subduction of the foreign flow, its containment and annihilation, is perceived not only as a rightful assertion of masculinity but also as an act of racial domination.

Defined as a threat against the German state, the containment of refugees requires "drastic measures": the construction of "camps for foreigners" (*Ausländerlager*),[92] "residency camps" (*Wohnlager*),[93] "emergency in-take camps" (*Notauffanglager*),[94] "the setup of mass camps" (*Massenlager*),[95] "concentration camps" (*Sammellager*)[96] and "federal internment camps" (*Bundessammellager*),[97] that is, the "placement [of refugees] in fenced barracks with armed guards."[98]

The language we encounter in these political visions curiously resembles that of the Freikorps soldiers: perceived reality is annihilated and reconstituted in order to preserve an ideational representation and to "see" reality in terms of an existing paradigm. The hated foreign Other is feminized by reduction to a series of liquid images: a "flood," a "tide," a "deluge," a "dangerous flow" of bodies. The images that vivify these fantasies of extinction are few and almost always the same ones. The racial subaltern is equated with the destructive potential of "woman" and is reduced to her bodily functions, a beast of consumption capable of producing much waste and devastation.

German statemakers communicate the "feminine" threat through the affective intensity with which they talk about the imminent catastrophe: the coming of the racial Other who seeks to inundate, engulf, swallow. Germany's political men, like their fascist counterparts, feel threatened by the "natural" manifestations of devouring "femininity": her flooding, surging, streaming. The refugees, according to media depictions, exhibit signs of unrepressed (and uncontrolled) consumption: the nation has been "ravaged" by a wave of foreigners that was "hungry" for it.

The source of this dangerous (all-consuming) torrent can thus be localized more specifically. It seems to flow from *inside* those foreign bodies: their yearnings, their wants, and their insatiable "hunger" for a better life. "There is the growing realization among politicians that the rising stream of refugees . . . is driven by the desire to improve their standard of living . . . to find in the Federal Republic of Germany the promised land: work, high salaries, security, generous financial support, and carefree leisure."[99] This image of the flood represents a maelstrom of terrifying desires: the emotional, the irrational, the uncontrollable, and the female.[100] Its significance lies in its ability to convincingly displace the exaggerated desire for consumption onto a fantastic (and nightmarish) manifestion.

Refugees, as depicted by the German media, possess a voracious appetite for wealth, money, and status, and an unquenchable craving for power and Western affluence. German imagemakers presume that the foreign "flood" is solely driven by economic interests: "to find work or to receive social welfare payments";[101] to "open the flood-gate to the land of economic miracles," to enter "the promised land";[102] to find an "economic paradise."[103] This process of inverse projection transforms the German nation into "the object of longing by millions of people."[104] Reconfigured by alien desire, the German nation is equated with the sensual and the feminine. Picturing the nation as "female" makes it seem so much more vulnerable to conquest: "[M]any of those, who set out from far-away lands, are economic refugees, enticed in their home-countries by the reputation of the Federal Republic as an island of the blessed, where one can easily gain a foothold."[105]

Shaped by these visions of foreign desire, the German nation is consistently described as "a utopia," a "paradise," a "garden of delights," an "island," a "treasure mountain," a "resort." The naturalism and eroticism of these cultural themes[106] provides the German imaginary with the elements of powerful stories about the origins and rationality of gender and race distinctions: refugees, equated with the category "woman," are perceived as devourers, pleasure seekers, freeloaders. Such a configuration of the racial Other as "consumer" is no less fantastic or violent than its literalization in the vagina dentata myth, for it is a conception that functions to erase the true labor, the true productivity of "woman" or her symbolic stand-in: in this case, the refugee, the foreign worker, the immigrant.[107] Yet this erasure forms the very possibility of exchange.

It is ironic that these conceptions of the racial Other were unwittingly encoded in the German constitution, or "basic law," which was drafted shortly after 1945. In these legal documents, victims of political persecution were described by a language saturated with consumer images. According to the juridical rhetoric, the right of asylum was granted unconditionally. Political refugees were entitled to protection: they "enjoyed" (*geniessen*) the right of asylum. The German term *geniessen* means "relish," "taste," "enjoy," "consume." It refers to the pleasure and sensual gratification that a person derives from acts of consumption. More specifically, it conveys a sense of the experience of "partaking" in cultural commodities, an experience that is centered in the body: the sensuous immersion of the inner "self" in things of pleasure (leisure, food, travel, sex). The choice of this term (which rarely appears elsewhere in the German constitution) [108] suggests that in the judicial and political imagination of the German founding fathers, the right of asylum was conjured as a commodity, a gift of leisure (and value).

Such a conception of political refugees (as unproductive, antisocial labor) facilitated the revival of the Aryan (Nazi) racial aesthetic: conventional notions of race and difference were patterned by a booming German postwar economy and linked to a nationalist aesthetic of consumer culture. Images of the materialist behavior and devouring promiscuity of foreign refugees came to be identified as perhaps the most radical threat to Germany's attempts at national reconstruction.

Out of the experience of war and defeat, Germans had generated a story of their own postwar victimization. The state reemploted these experiences into a romantic, future-oriented narrative. The appeal to tradition, virtue, and assimilation into a prosperous community of Germans became an antidote for this sense of victimization.[109] The state's master narrative was restoration. By the 1950s, the propagation of consumer images and the stimulation of consumer desire was encouraged as an integral part of the reformation of German national identity:[110] Western democratic freedom came to be identified with material prosperity and consumer choice.

The integration of German citizens into consumer culture was thus desired by postwar West German governments. The state's official narrative encouraged participation in the economic miracle of the 1950s by buying consumer goods as a reaffirmation of Germanness. "Prosperity forms the integument of West German identity, enabling them to erase their past, both in memory and physically, and to allay their fears of disorder and dirt" (Borneman 1992a: 236). Work and prosperity were the central organizing tropes of their life constructions: they saw virtue in work; pensions and free time were understood as rights earned in exchange for labor.

In Germany's postwar economy, conspicuous consumption became emblematic of a national "birthright": it was a symbol of nationhood and citizenship. Attempts by foreigners to partake in these privileges of a "closed" community were experienced as transgressive, as a threat to German personhood and statehood. The writings of political analyst Rudolf Wassermann are a compelling example of such discourse. In a critique of Germany's asylum politics, he equates refugees with economic opportunists: "The motivation is understandable. Legally, however, they are—and one must, for the sake of terminological clarity excuse the hard word—asylum con-men [*Asylbetrüger*]. They conjure up facts purportedly pertaining to their political persecution that do not correspond to the truth. And they do this in order to force the German state to grant them the status of political refugee, which is bound up with the right to settle in Germany and is tied to financial advantages" (1992: 12).

By conjuring images of refugees as "economic parasites" (*Wirtschafts-schädlinge*), Germany's political men foster an atmosphere that legitimates the use of racial violence. German public discourse imputes criminal intent to applicants for refugee status: fraudulence, illegality, corruption, and a fierce materialism are among the inherent traits ascribed to Third World or Eastern European peoples.[111] Foreigners are transformed into villains as politicians attempt to tear the masks from their faces and the disguises from their bodies, thus revealing their duplicity and deception. In doing so, they seek to justify the persecution of the "pretend-refugees" (*Scheinasylanten*), the "non-authentic asylum seekers" (*unechte Asylanten*) possessed by economic self-interest, the "economic refugees" (*Wirtschaftsflüchtlinge*) marked by their illicit appetites, unrelenting materialism, and grotesque bodies.[112]

Upon closer inspection, German politicians began to "see" the foreign flood as an indistinguishable tangle of bodies, a mass of brown flesh. Foreign corporeality was deemed a racial threat, which was connected to a repugnance toward disorder and dirt. Housed in public facilities, refugee bodies invaded the nation's interior spaces: schools, gyms, lecture halls, and hotels were now occupied, seized, and appropriated for alien purposes. The inundated (besieged) city eventually burst, rupturing its bounds of order. When its interior reached German men's bodies, the latter were destroyed. Their corporal boundaries were exploded, liquefied. Thus the more directly the men were exposed to the events, the more overwhelmed they were by fear: the fear of dirt, contamination, death.

In the German imagination, the proximity of racialized bodies was linked to processes of deterioration and filth: "[G]overnment officials discovered houses in the inner city, in which Pakistanis and Indians had been packed together, houses in a state of disrepair and decay."[113] "Where there had been 60 available openings . . . there now lived 160 foreigners."[114] Crammed into impossibly small spaces, those foreign bodies evoked images of dirt, improper hygiene, the grotesque: they were "anti bodies," endangering the clean and proper German bodies. Refugees, defined as "matter out of place,"[115] were conceived and experienced as sources of contagion. "Officials wade through unbearable hygienic conditions, spray-can in one hand and note-pad in the other. But, on occasion, people lie there packed together so tightly that the door does not even open and the official inspectors cannot advance at all into the rooms."[116] The inspectors were standing "in filth," disgusted. Direct physical contact with "dirt" (the contamination of the bodies' peripheral areas) rendered them "lifeless": they are felled, cut down, knocked unconscious (*Das haut uns schlicht um*).[117]

The consequences of Germany's "racial inundation" are closely connected to processes that occur within the human body. Dirt dwells in the depths, in the bowels of the body: there, nothing is solid; everything is sloppy mush. According to media depictions, the nation's interior had become a morass. And the morass became simply human filth, a pit of liquid manure teeming with bodies. This type of contamination "seeped" through the walls of judicial containment, seeking to subvert the German legal system: "Most of the applicants for refugee status spill into the black labor market."[118] According to German political commentators, the implementation of more restrictive immigration laws or even constitutional changes was unlikely to prevent desperate individuals from entering Germany, thereby exacerbating the nation's problem with illegality and the perception of refugees as criminals.[119] During political debates about German refugee laws, Konrad Weiss, an elected member of the leftist Union Greens (*BündnisGrüne*), formulated this possibility in his parliamentary address in 1993: "Human beings, who as asylum-petitioners are still tolerated today—at least for a while, will soon vegetate in the underground [the black labor market]—in a gray zone of illegal work and criminality that we will no longer be able to control. This pre-programs the rise of serious social conflicts compared to which today's situation will appear harmless" (1993:4).[120] Equated with illegality and unlawful practices, foreigners were presumed intent on disappearing, "diving below the surface of detection" (i.e., *versinken, untertauchen, wegtauchen, abtauchen*), seeking shelter underground in cellars and sewers, roaming in darkness and in dirt: slowly "seeping" (*versickern*) into the German body like a toxin that permeates the soil.[121]

The government's task was to get rid of any "dirt" that settled on the "body of the nation." The political order thus appeared to take on the same function as the fascist soldiers' body armor: it became a protective enclosure that "bottled up" the nation's seething interior. German politicians, like their fascist predecessors, took comfort in imagining themselves and their nation as an "armored enclosure" preserving a "pure interior." In the everyday experience of those men, the "wave" of refugees had managed to break and transgress their defensive barriers: the nation's interior fell prey to erosion, becoming "hollowed out" by the torrential foreign flood.[122] Weakened by the foreign onslaught, the integrity of the law and the strength of the state were perceived as threatened.[123] Defense was now located in a social body whose protective armor had been ruptured, its interior contaminated, flowing with filth and dangerous water. "Excrement poses a threat to the Center—to life, to the proper, the clean—not from within, but from its outermost margin. While there is no escape from excrementality, from mortality, from the corpse, . . . the (social and psychological) goal is to get rid of it quickly, to clean up after the mess" (Grosz 1994: 207). Violence, even murder, could be imagined as a viable form of defense against this threat.

Blood, Gender, Violence: Thinking the Nation

The nation-state is a political configuration of modernity,[124] which, as an "imagined community," a "conception of peoplehood,"[125] relies on traditional iconographic repertoires for the construction of its symbolic universe. Burdened with myths and metaphorical rigidities,[126] there probably exists no "privileged narrative," no "normal" way for a modern nation to be or to define itself.[127] Nevertheless, the German state clearly exemplifies the powerfully homogenizing version of the Western nation that seeks to constrain, oppress, and eviscerate difference.

Modern states tend to constitute their subjects in a gendered way: the sphere of the political project itself is defined as essentially male in its capacities and needs; the sphere of the nation, in its symbolic figuration, is constructed as female.[128] The modern state thus works in part through a process of politicizing gender roles: "[I]t politicizes or constructs the kinds of citizens women and men are supposed to be under the state's jurisdiction" (Moore 1988: 149–50). Predicated upon gender difference, the modern state inscribes this difference into the political process. "According to some writers, women are relegated to the margins of the polity even though their centrality to the nation is constantly being reaffirmed. It is reaffirmed consciously in nationalist rhetoric where the nation itself is represented as a woman to be protected or, less consciously, in an intense preoccupation with women's appropriate sexual conduct. The latter often constitutes the crucial distinction between the nation and its 'others'" (Kandiyoti 1994: 377). Control of women and their sexuality becomes central to the national project.[129] Implicated in gender relations, each state embodies a definable "gender regime."[130]

The trope of nation-as-woman draws on a particular image of female selfhood: she must be chaste, dutiful, daughterly, maternal.[131] The representational efficacy of such depictions of the nation as a female body, whose violation by foreigners requires its citizens to rush to her defense, "has served to bolster colonial conquest and racist violence throughout

Western history" (de Lauretis 1988: 16). In the German case, however, the violent imaginary is centered on the equation of the woman's body with the "grotesque," envisioning the "fluidity" of female corporeality as filth, death, and contagion. "[I]n the West, in our time, the female body has been constructed not only as a lack or absence but with more complexity, as a leaking, uncontrollable, seeping liquid; as formless flow; as viscosity, entrapping, secreting; as lacking . . . self-containment—a formlessness that engulfs all form, a disorder that threatens all order . . . women's corporeality is inscribed as a mode of seepage . . . liquidity" (Grosz 1994: 203).

This iconography emerges most clearly under German fascism. The corporeal metaphysics of the fascist soldier were encoded in two basic types of body. The first type was the soft and liquid female body: a quintessential negative Other, lurking inside the male body, a subversive source of contagion that had to be expunged or sealed off. The second was the hard, phallic body, devoid of all internal viscera, which found its apotheosis in the machine. This body-as-machine was the acknowledged ideal of the fascist warrior.

While the peculiar characteristics of these imagined bodies were forged and culturally encoded by the gendered world of fascist politics,[132] images of the unaesthetic racial Other reappeared in postwar Germany, albeit displaced onto a different field of relevance. Like the fascist soldier's fear of his inner body, with its inchoate mass of entrails, and his terror of women, Germany's political men transformed their revulsion with physicality into a repugnance toward "otherness," specifically the "feminized" racial Other. During the 1980s, almost forty years after the last World War and the end of fascism, we encounter the vision of the "armored (male) body" and the "inundating (female) flood" in the purely civilian context of German racial politics.

In contemporary Germany, we see the conflation of foreignness with femininity: refugee bodies are depicted as wet, devouring, filthy. Media images of "invading masses" are transformed into a public discourse about dark-skinned Others, a racial threat. The language of German politics contrasts the "femininity" of the foreign "mass" with the need for a rigid, hierarchically structured whole: assertions of manhood and state authority are translated into images of control, mastery, containment, law, strength. In these images, race is always a subtext.

Such allegories of gender and race are implicated in the murderous elimination of subaltern bodies in contemporary Germany. In the 1980s, racial violence defined a new corporeal topography: the purging of foreign bodies from German territory. Such a "cleansing" of the national landscape, the erasure of refugees and immigrants, emerged as an indispensable element in the recolonization of the physical interior of the modern state, and of German manhood.

The Contaminated Body: A Ruined Modernity

In this chapter I have attempted to show (through a critical analysis of German public culture) the highly ambivalent and stressed relation of the national order to the modern, and its eventual escape from modernity through the essentialisms of blood, race, and gender. My ethnographic material was drawn from a diversity of historical sources, not only to illustrate the diachrony of events, but also to highlight the fact that German history and cultural memory overlap and appear as repetition—a frozen continuum—in which certain templates and motifs are reencountered or return again and again, and where the new is mediated by a refurbished sameness via the essentializing metaphors of blood and body: a tropology of liquid corporeality. This mode of historicization, of memorializing the anatomy of German nationhood, exposes historical experience as a pathology, a traumatic syndrome.

In my analysis, our understanding of German historicity is mediated by the concept of the unconscious, of dream work, and of fantasy formation. Recognizing the material force of the historical unconscious, my emphasis has been on the formation, inheritance, and devolution of essentialist symbolic systems, of grids of perception. What are the building blocks of these essentialist constructs? My work seeks to contribute to an archaeology of essentialist metaphysics in the public sphere of modern Germany. Throughout, I have inquired how essentialism is made. How does it achieve such a deterministic and habitual hold on the experience, perception, and processing of reality?

My treatment of essentialism as a formative construct (a content-filled, yet murky, density) and my orientation toward the notion of a historical unconscious mean that the point of emergence of ethnographic data in this type of study does not conform to the highly localized/bounded profiling or extraction of data typical of conventional anthropological analysis. A major historical condition for the replication of essentialism (as I have demonstrated in this chapter) is a continued oscillation between free-floating fantasy formations (haunting various cracks and crevices of popular culture) and the frightening instantiations of fantasy formations in precise locales and specific performances. From what discrete sites of social experience, class affiliation, and gender identity does essentialist fantasy originate? We are no longer within the circumscribed space of childhood socialization, the nuclear family, the residential community. Popular culture and the mass media have deterritorialized fantasy, although instantiations of fantasy can be given a discrete coordinate or topography. In many cases, the fantasy formations, particularly those embedded in linguistic and visual icons (as I demonstrate) criss-cross divergent class and political positions: thus, the powerful thrust of excavating a common symbolic grammar of blood between the neo-fascist right and the leftish Greens; or the disturbing evidence for a common logic of liquidation between the Social Democratic left and the Christian Democratic right. Such essentialist ideological/fantasy formations gather force and momentum precisely due to their murky and indistinct parameters in cultural repertoires.[133] This fuzziness evades simplistic cause/effect style analysis. Rather, as my research suggests, it requires ethnographic exploration on a heterogeneity or montage of discursive and image-making sites: political demonstrations, the mass media, popular memory, linguistic substrata, and symbolic geographies, which all share a translocal, national scope.

The German instrumental imagination of current ideologies of violence works with mystified bits and pieces of materiality, rehabilitating old positivities in the search for social anchorage as well as personal and class efficacy. We are in the material culture of blood and the linked somatic and medicalized nationalism that has specific German (but also trans-European) coordinates. A root metaphor of the German state defines citizenship by blood (as opposed to soil—i.e., place of birth—in the case of France). Blood and soil, body and space, constitute the materialist theory of national interiority and foreign exteriority. There exists a fundamental contradiction between the liberal state's promotion of tolerance and diversity and the founding charter of familial blood membership, which underwrites stigmatizing imageries of otherhood. For the pathos of the nation-state, that is, the political community as an object of patriotic feeling, derives from the liberal revolution, with its infantilization and gendering of the subjects of the "fatherland."

In the twentieth century, however, the familial model of the organic nation was medicalized. By the early 1930s, fascist sociologists began to envision nations as "units of blood." A good deal of German social theory during the first part of this century was in effect a medical anthropology, a diagnostic science of the racial body. The nation was imagined as a genealogical reservoir for a "healthy" German body politic: "hence not only the pathos of heredity and selective breeding, but above all the national pathos of blood" (Bloch 1990: 90). The nation thus became, in medical terms as well, a "unity filled with blood," a "purely organic river basin," "from whose past humanity stems and into whose 'future' its children will depart. Thus 'nationhood' drives time, indeed history out of history: it is space and organic fate, nothing else" (90). Nationality came to be accepted as a medical fact by the fascist state and its supporting racial ideologies. Such a medicalized vision of nationhood resulted in the transposition of earlier forms of state culture into the political vernacular of everyday life (as is evident in contemporary Germany). My ethnographic data show that a retrograde archaism of national state culture is continuously repositioned in the present. Crucial to this reappearance is the fact that the current manifestations of the civil state, as I have noted, remain both neutral and even opposed to these ideologies of organic unity and spatial purification, but nevertheless abet them. This is dialectical necessity, since it is precisely such residual archaeological strata, older sediments, earlier ideological manifestations and cultural memories of the state, that are thrown up and expropriated to organize the political perceptions of the present. Thus blood imagery and organicism, as a devolved language of the nation-state, also inflects the discourse of the German left. There exists, as I have tried to show, a cultural complicity of the left in the organistic iconography of the right. The left unwittingly accepts the fascist polarity between defilement and sealed armorment, the national body. The historical project of this masculinist en/closure (as characterized by Theweleit) is focused on the containment, indeed, the eradication, of feminized flows and streams of foreign bodies. When thus attempting to decipher this logic of German national fantasy, as Allen Feldman has noted:

[W]e cannot escape the image of the archeological ruins of Nazi state culture emerging from a forest of public memory as a substructure of everyday life—like one of Max Ernst's brooding cityscapes. It is as if a flea market of former bureaucracies and ideologies opens up for ideological traffic, with its used dusted-off contents of gas chambers, military campaigns, racial hygiene, racist economic rationalities, war imagery, and formulaic linguistic codes. These antiques are excavated by the anxieties of everyday life, and are super-imposed on and redecorate contemporary German social space, endowing it with the aura of authenticated ruins—a ruined modernity. Struggles for political legitimacy mobilize an attic full of authenticating artifacts by both left and right.[134]

The ideological ruins of the Third Reich, of race and soil and the Other, are thus required by left and right for a massive remetaphorization of the political landscape—a performance that indicts the poverty of available "nonviolent" political depictions and of the failure of existing institutional optics, which can no longer visualize contemporary experience with any public satisfaction.

Epilogue
Symbolic Places
An Iconography of Gender, Blood, and Race

May 1990, Frankfurt am Main

The following are excerpts from a proposal by a German initiative to commemorate the Holocaust and the Jewish victims of National Socialism by building a memorial on the ruins of a former synagogue in Frankfurt.

"Until 1938, the largest synagogue in the city of Frankfurt was located at Friedberg park. The National Socialists destroyed it, removed the physical remains, and built a bunker there. We recognize the entanglement of Jewish and German history at this site. It is therefore a suitable location for remembrance, for coming to terms with this part of German history, for sorrow and commemoration. At this place, the suffering of the Jewish population and the consequences of war for the German civilian population are brought into proximity. The site therefore offers itself as a stage for preservation and historical representation . . .

"The intent to construct a memorial inside the bunker requires the remembrance of all those human beings who, at the risk of their own lives, helped those who were persecuted by the Nazi regime.

"Trees should therefore be planted all around the bunker; they should be dedicated to the remembrance of these human beings. The job of planting and maintaining the trees, in memory of the human beings who helped the anguished, would be a meaningful task for schools. In this context, the teachers, together with their students, should attempt to uncover biographical details about these benefactors of the past . . .

"Near the bunker, and in the immediate vicinity of the trees, the flow of a narrow stream should symbolize the vitality which the benefactors, through their brave engagement, passed on to future generations. This representation is also an attempt to counter those forces which desire to suppress the public remembrance of these human beings as well as of the victims.

"This watercourse should flow into the bunker and at the threshold turn to blood through the symbolic use of red dye. There are alternative proposals to present the stream either as black or as a torrent. Inside the bunker, the watercourse ends in a pond. On its shore, the multitude of human suffering is personified by four statues of a mother and her child, standing in varying postures and distances from the blood-red water. In the immediate vicinity of the bloody pond, two unclothed women, a Gypsy and a Jew, embrace their naked children with both hands, in a gesture of deep humiliation. A third mother represents the suffering of the Slavic peoples . . . The fourth mother symbolizes the contradictory role of the German woman. She maintains the greatest distance from the bloody pond and is completely clothed. The child, in contrast, embraced by only one maternal arm, is also naked. With the other arm, the mother executes the Hitler salute. The physiognomy of the women and their children is similar, not however their distance from the blood-filled pond . . .

"The closeness to or distance from the bloody pond symbolizes the differences in the extent of the sacrifice made in blood and the suffering and hardship endured. — On the other hand, blood is also a symbol of life, a vehicle of the soul. The symbolic content of the bloody pond is therefore multivalent.

"However, within the total field of meaning surrounding the memorial, the symbolism of the blood-filled pond will probably be interpreted almost exclusively in terms of violence and victimization. Thereby, more specifically, an intense emotional response can be achieved as well, similar to what is labeled 'red-shock' in psycho-diagnostics. Its linkage to aggressive drives (war, violence, etc.) would then offer the possibility of exposing the associated repression of guilt and letting it become a starting point for purification . . .

"Since the neolithic, the representation of mother and child is a commonly used and understood cultural symbol of life, love, and safety. The mother/child unity guarantees the continued existence of life. The template of the child appeals to instincts of protection and nurturance. That it must do because the child is dependent on adults. Hardly anyone can resist this instinct or turn away from the helplessness of a small child.

"The morally reprehensible and thereby culpable act (Hitler salute) of the fourth mother and the simultaneous embrace of her child shows the entanglement of this woman, who as it were gives up her identity and thereby inflicts harm on herself and her child, and at the same time suffers victimization.

"The four mothers, through their separate placements and positionings, refer in an unsurpassed manner to the unscrupulous way in which the former [Nazi] rulers dealt with the primordial values of human life. Their attack was so comprehensive that it put into question the continuity of their own nation. The disdain for human life did not exclude Germans who resisted the regime; it transcended the nation's indigenous threshold of pain. The German woman stands for the willingness of many Germans to participate. Her role as victim may not be overemphasized or downplayed. She raises her hand in enthusiasm and thereby overlooks how much this movement is directed against herself and her child . . .

"Independent of the above proposal, one might consider whether additional levels could be added to the existing bunker. This development would proceed provided that the newly constructed premises be transformed into urgently needed living accommodations for immigrant families from various ethnic groups that are resident in Frankfurt. In this newly available residential space on top of the bunker, the attempt would be made to put into practice the principles, whose tentative theoretical foundations are being tested inside the bunker."[1]

Notes

References to all primary and secondary sources, which provided ethnographic data used in this work, have been placed in the notes. Bibliographic references pertaining to any material not directly quoted are also in the notes. Sources for quoted commentary are cited in the text.

Preface

1. See Röhrich (1967: 49).

Chapter 1. Artifacts of Gender

1. See Martin (1989), Turner (1984), and Douglas (1973).
2. See Needham (1973), Hugh-Jones (1979), and Theweleit (1989).
3. See Lévi-Strauss (1966, 1969), Ortner (1974), Ardener (1975), and MacCormack and Strathern (1986). Marilyn Strathern (1980) has convincingly argued that what is considered "natural" cannot be assumed a priori nor be applied as a universal category. Yet while the construct "nature" itself might be called into question as a Western concept, it would appear that corresponding analogies and binaries exist in other societies—wild/domestic, raw/cooked, violent/tame, chaos/order, and so on.
4. See Bloch and Parry (1982), Brandes (1980), Becker (1973), Gilmore (1990), Herdt (1982), and Herzfeld (1985).
5. See Brain (1988), Buckley and Gottlieb (1988), Cassel (1882), Delaney et al. (1988), Devereux (1950), Durkheim (1897), Frazer (1911), Lévy-Bruhl (1935), Lidz and Lidz (1977), Montgomery (1974), Róheim (1949), and Strack (1900).
6. See Bettelheim (1954), Mead (1947), Dundes (1976), Knight (1991), Lewis (1980), and Brain (1988).
7. See Ortner and Whitehead (1981).
8. See Bourdieu (1977).
9. See, for instance, Beidelman (1963), Eliade (1958a), Evans-Pritchard (1933), Jay (1985), Raum (1907), Robinsohn (1896), Róheim (1945), Shapiro (1988, 1989), Tegnaeus (1952), and Trumbull (1885, 1896).
10. See Binford (1962), Deetz (1977), Hodder (1982), McGhee (1977), and Miller and Tilley (1984).
11. See Benveniste (1969), Friedrich (1978), and Szemerényi (1977).

12. See Bender (1987), Conkey and Spector (1984), Gibbs (1987), Gimbutas (1982), Hodder (1984), Marshall (1985), Miller and Tilley (1984), and Moore (1990).

13. See Linke (1985, 1986, 1989).

14. See Childe (1926), Gimbutas (1963, 1970, 1973, 1980, 1982), and Mallory (1989).

15. See Gimbutas (1973, 1980, 1982).

16. See Ammerman and Cavalli-Sforza (1984) and Renfrew (1979, 1988, 1989).

17. See Sherratt and Sherratt (1988: 584–95).

18. See Zvelebil and Zvelebil (1988).

19. See Pulgram (1958), Jackson (1955), Krahe (1936), and Meillet (1964).

20. See Benveniste (1969), Díakonov (1985), Friedrich (1979), Gamkrelidze and Ivanov (1985a, 1985b), Mallory (1989: 114–42), Renfrew (1988), and Skomal and Polomé (1987).

21. See Friedrich (1979: 207–8).

22. See Dumézil (1958, 1977).

23. See Puhvel (1978).

24. The etymology of "blood" corresponds to that of "fire." Indo-European terms for "fire" can be derived from two roots (Pokorny 1959: 293): the first proto-term (e.g., Greek *pŷr* and others), regularly neuter, referred to the realistic household fire, the hearth, while the second proto-term (e.g., Latin *ignis*), usually masculine, denoted the fire of religious cult (Meillet 1920: 249–56; Thass-Thienemann 1973: 312–13). Implicitly attested by such reconstructive efforts is the concept of an outside fire associated with male ritual (collective) action, in contrast to the inside fire, the domestic domain of womanhood. Proto-Indo-European "fire" thus has a linguistic and metaphorical pattern comparable to that of "blood," although it is constituted as a complementary opposition or inversion (dry/wet, male/female, outside/inside). This observation gains further significance when one considers the close symbolic proximity of "blood" and "fire" in mythology, magic, and ritual (La Barre 1984: 82; Bachelard 1968; Bettelheim 1962: 162; Bötticher 1899: 58; Freeman 1968; Needham 1967).

25. My research has uncovered only one case that closely corresponds to the proto-Indo-European linguistic situation: the standard Chinese term for "blood" (*xúe* or *xie*, no. 5877) is a radical whose meaning is modified by two suffixes (*ye* and *beng*). It seems likely that *xúeye* (nos. 5877/3210) refers to blood inside the body, for the suffix *ye* signifies that the term it qualifies is a liquid or fluid (McGraw-Hill Editors 1963: 32, 1485, 1527). The term is semantically opposed to *xúebeng* (nos. 5877/1514), which refers to blood from the uterus, blood from a wound, denoting "outside" blood. The multiple meanings of *beng* extend the semantic field of the external blood to the destruction of the body, as indicated by denotations like crash, collapse, ruin, disintegration, break, fall, avalanche (McGraw-Hill Editors 1963: 54–56, 1481). The close correspondence of Chinese with Indo-European semantic and linguistic markers of blood may lend further support to the current hypothesis of a common prehistoric origin attested here through language (Mallory 1989; Renfrew 1988).

26. Examples can be found among some of the African languages: the Yao in Nyasaland (Sanderson 1954: 304, 190–91), and Zulu (Dent and Nyembezi 1969: 23, 352, 447; Doke et al. 1958: 43, 44, 289, 568).

27. On the chance that the etymology is correct, de Vries (1961: 263) may be cited on his discussion of a parallel semantic development. He suggests that Old Norse *hrae*, corpse (i.e., Norwegian *rae*, Old English *hraew*, Old High Ger-

man *hrēo*), derived from Germanic **hraiwa-*, is not only related to proto-Indo-European **kreu̯-*, blood from a wound, raw flesh. It may also be derived from the roots **(s)kerei-*, to cut, and turn, twist, thereby becoming a cognate of Old Norse *hrøkkva* with an extension or misappropriation of meaning from bend > fall > corpse!

28. See Ashley-Montagu (1937), Herdt (1981), Hiatt (1971), and Turner (1965).

29. See Freud (1925).

30. See Loeb (1923), Róheim (1945), Devereux (1950), Lévi-Strauss (1966), Lévy-Bruhl (1935:285–91), and Mead (1977).

31. See Doke et al. (1958: 44, 289, 568) and Dent and Nyembezi (1969: 23, 352).

32. Schultz-Lorentzen (1927: 35).

33. McGraw-Hill Editors (1963, no. 1481, pp. 54–56).

34. Montgomery (1974: 143).

35. See Bettelheim (1962), Brain (1988), and Lidz and Lidz (1977).

36. See Durkheim (1897: 1–70), Turner (1965), and Lévi-Strauss (1966: 51).

37. See Turner (1967: 41–43).

38. See Onians (1973: 271–72).

39. See Maringer (1976: 226–48) and Timm (1964: 39–55).

40. Wunderlich (1925: 46–58) and Latte (1960: 379–93).

41. See Mallory (1989: 191, 223), Duhn (1906), and Sonny (1906). Red is generally interpreted as a symbol of blood, which likewise carries both positive and negative connotations: it alludes to life and death as well as good and evil (Baum 1922: 520–29; Duhn 1906; Wunderlich 1925: 4–72; Gonda 1980: 45). Even outside the Indo-European context, red is on the one hand the color of fertility, sexual love, reproduction, and childbirth; on the other hand, as the color of blood, flesh, menstruation, and murder, it is considered dangerous and tends to accompany rites with malevolent purposes (Turner 1965: 59–60, 68–69, 79–83).

42. See McCarthy (1969: 169–72, 175).

43. See Gonda (1980: 97, 275, 434) and McCarthy (1969: 172).

44. See McCarthy (1973: 206–8).

45. The association of blood with death is not only confined to the Indo-European world view; it is prevalent also among the early Semites (Buttenwieser 1919: 309–10, 311; McCarthy 1969: 176; Wiedemann 1892a: 113–14; 1923/24: 72–86). The only exception to this pattern is provided by the ancient Hebrews, whose ritual use of blood was connected with a series of prohibitions, based on the idea that blood was sacred and belonged to the realm of the divine (Rüsche 1930: 308–40; Smith 1972: 233–34, 313–14, 342, 344, 379; Steinmueller 1959: 558).

46. Rüsche (1930: 362, 404–5) and Linke (1985: 362).

47. For instance, Dundes (1980).

48. See Onians (1973: 256), Lloyd (1964), and Casalis (1976).

49. Schwartz (1982).

50. It has been suggested that **ēs-r̥-* is a typical *r/n* stem neuter; the /-*r*/ in **ēs-r̥-* alternates morphophonemically with /-*n*/ (Buck 1949: 206; Friedrich 1979: 343). It is therefore likely that the term for inside blood is either a cognate of or identical with the word for spring, summer, which has been reconstructed as proto-Indo-European **(w)ēs-r̥-* with a loss of the initial /*w-*/ by sentence sandhi (Buck 1949: 1014). The Greek term for spring has been derived from proto-Indo-European **wēs-r̥-*, while the root for blood is **ēs-r̥-* (Onians 1973: 177, n. 9; Frisk 1960: 432–33; Pokorny 1959: 1174). Here is a possible case where two dif-

ferent words have merged phonetically and are subsequently regarded as identical by folk etymology.

51. See Kirk and Raven (1957: 234–35), Schöner (1964: 46–50), and Siegel (1968: 216–17).

52. See Friedrich (1979: 229–41).

53. See Benveniste (1973) and Friedrich (1979: 222, 231).

54. The Indo-European terms are Sanskrit *vṛṣṭi, vṛšan-,* and *v̂ŕsa-;* Old Norse *úr* or *úrr;* Latin *verres;* and Greek *érsē* (Benveniste 1973: 13; O'Flaherty 1980: 20; Onians 1973: 177, n. 9; Pokorny 1959: 81).

55. This term has been reconstructed as proto-Indo-European **sū-/*sw-.* For an elaboration of the idea of male unilateral creativity, see Bowler (1971) and Dundes (1983: 35–42).

56. See Friedrich (1979: 209–10).

57. See Benveniste (1973: 191) and Friedrich (1979: 210).

58. See Eliade (1958b: 301).

59. See Lechler (1937: 370).

60. See Kammeyer (1941: 79–80).

61. Eliade (1958b: 271–73, 309) and Frazer (1955: 153).

62. Bauschatz (1982), Butterworth (1970: 7–11), Holmberg (1922–23: 62–77), Weniger (1919), and Wünsche (1905).

63. Kāthaka Upanishad 6.1 in Lechler (1937: 380).

64. See Cook (1974: 11–30) and Eliade (1958b: 281).

65. See Bauschatz (1982: 5), Holmberg (1922/23: 62–77), Lechler (1937: 371), and Rappaport (1943: 264–69).

66. See Bächtold-Stäubli (1929: 462, 998).

67. See Schröder (1931: 94–95).

68. See Arens (1943: 70–80, 1948: 259–65), Butterworth (1970: 32), Frank (1978: 173–76), Marzell (1929: 79–85; 1931: 277; 1932:166–67; 1934; 1935), and Rappaport (1943: 263–72).

69. See Arens (1943: 268).

70. See Friedrich (1970: 156, n. 1; 1979: 85–93).

71. See Cook (1974: 18–30).

72. See Onians (1973: 216).

73. Compare Balys (1942: 172, 175–76), Bolte and Mackensen (1930: 199, 278–79), Marzell (1926: 78; 1927: 77; 1930: 180–81, 184; 1935: 198–99), Neugebauer (1953: 12), and Lauffer (1937: 220).

74. Ovid, *Metamorphoses* 8: 743, passim.

75. See Eliade (1958b: 301), Balys (1942: 172), and Marzell (1933: 147–48).

76. Eliade (1958b: 303) and Mannhardt (1904: 34–43).

77. Compare Taylor (1979: 85–93).

78. Virgil, *Aeneid* 3: 23–49. Very similar is Dante's prose account of "the bleeding trees of suicide" in his *Inferno* (Canto 13.1–54).

79. See Barthes (1972: 128–31).

80. See Friedrich (1979: 231).

81. The list of terms includes Sanskrit *jánas,* Greek *génos,* Latin *genus,* and common Slavic *koleno.*

82. Examples are Greek *gónu* or *kolen,* Latin *genu,* Sanskrit *jánu,* and so forth.

83. See Bunker and Lewin (1951: 363–67), Friedrich (1979: 230–32), and Onians (1973: 174–80).

84. See Hall (1975).

85. See Onians (1973: 119, 174–78).

86. See O'Flaherty (1980: 28–29).
87. Bellows (1923: 7).
88. See Eliade (1961: 40–43) and Cook (1974: 25).
89. See Cook (1974: 8, 15–24), Eliade (1964), Latynin (1933), Toporov (1973: 153, 167–79), and Holmberg (1922–23).
90. See Eliade (1961: 30).
91. See Butterworth (1970: 46) and Eliade (1964: 261–64).
92. Linke (1989, 1992).
93. See Goody (1983).
94. O'Flaherty (1980: 33) and Onians (1973: 119, 121).
95. Proto-Indo-European *swesōr- is represented by Sanskrit svasá, Avestan xᵛanhar-, Latin soror, Tocharian A ṣar and B ṣer, Gothic svistar, Old English sweostor; the Greek correspondent (given in a psilotic dialect) is ĕor-, daughter, cousin, a probable cognate form of ĕar, inside blood (Benveniste 1973: 172–73; Buck 1949: 107–8; Delbrück 1889: 468; Friedrich 1979: 212–13; Pokorny 1959: 1051).
96. Friedrich (1979: 213, 236) and Szemerényi (1977: 33).
97. See Benveniste (1973: 174, 271), Delbrück (1889: 462, 385), Friedrich (1979: 209, 212), and Schrader (1904: 20): proto-Indo-European *sw-/*swe-.
98. See Benveniste (1973: 269–70).
99. This is reflected in the presumed Homeric cognate ŏar, woman, wife; in the first syllable of Avestan har-iš-i female; and in the feminine numeral forms like Sanskrit ti-šrah, three (e.g., Benveniste 1934: 104–6; 1973: 167, 174, 270; Szemerényi 1977: 34–35, 37–40, 42).
100. Mayrhofer (1952); Pisani (1951: 7–8).
101. Linke (1985: 254–56). A schematic summary of the relevant etymological connections, which illustrates how this derivation might occur, appears in Linke (1985: 354–56). For a different view, see Szemerényi (1977).
102. See Benveniste (1973: 173, 179).
103. See Benveniste (1973: 269–70).
104. See Benveniste (1973: 18), Delbrück (1889: 535), and Pokorny (1959: 1043). Proto-Indo-European *swekrū- is reflected in, for example, Latin socrus, Russian svekrov, Gothic swaíhrō, Sanskrit švašrú-, Greek hékurá, and German Schwieger (Benveniste 1973: 180; Delbrück 1889: 535; Friedrich 1979: 216; Pokorny 1959: 1043).
105. That is, *swe- and *krū-; see Schrader (1904: 753), Friedrich (1979: 216), and Szemerényi (1977: 65–66).
106. See Friedrich (1979: 215–16), Buck (1949: 122, 124–5), Benveniste (1973: 201, 269), Krahe (1958: 75), and Delbrück (1889: 516, 528, 537).
107. See Friedrich (1979: 216) and Szemerényi (1977: 67).
108. Hettrich (1985: 15–17).
109. Szemerényi (1977: 67).
110. Benveniste (1973: 193–95).
111. O'Flaherty (1980: 20).
112. For instance, Dundes (1980: 120–24).
113. See O'Flaherty (1980: 17).
114. Rüsche (1930: 363).
115. O'Flaherty (1980: 33, 42, 47).
116. Friedrich (1979: 213–14); Szemerényi (1977: 86–87).
117. Rüsche (1930: 362).
118. O'Flaherty (1980: 40).
119. See Benveniste (1973: 200) and Friedrich (1979: 227).

120. See Rüsche (1930: 404–5) and Siegel (1968: 232).

121. Sarnvarodaya Tantra 2.23 in O'Flaherty (1980: 40, 53).

122. See Dundes (1983: 44–45) and O'Flaherty (1980: 27).

123. See Friedrich (1979: 213), Delbrück (1889: 442), and Szemerény (1977: 86).

124. For instance, Schneider (1968).

125. Benveniste (1973: 19, 1969: 169–72).

126. See Barthes (1972).

127. For example, Brandes (1980), Dundes (1976), Goody (1983), Herdt (1981), O'Flaherty (1980), Friedrich (1978), Linke (1989, 1992), Ortner (1974), and Shapiro (1989).

128. See Durkheim (1897, 1963) and Knight (1991).

129. "Daughter" is derived from a verb "to milk," perhaps expressive of the function of young women as milkmaids in the cattle-breeding cultures of Eastern Europe and Central Asia (Friedrich 1979: 211).

Chapter 2. Artifacts of Race

1. See Smith (1995: 726) and Herzfeld (1992: 26–44).

2. See Jolly (1993) and Davin (1978).

3. For example, Koonz (1987), Allen (1991), and Moeller (1996).

4. See Mallory (1989: 23).

5. See Renfrew (1988), Mallory (1989), and Friedrich (1978).

6. See Hachmann (1971), Krüger (1976), and Todd (1975).

7. See Mallory (1989: 84–85).

8. For instance, Thompson (1965) and Hachmann, Kossack, and Kuhn (1962).

9. See Mallory (1989: 85).

10. See Hachmann et al. (1962) and Krüger (1976).

11. See Polomé (1987).

12. See Klein (1967: 180–81), Kluge (1960: 87), and Ranke (1978: 77).

13. See Kluge (1951: 89) and Grimm and Grimm (1860: 170).

14. See Trier (1973: 92).

15. See Kligman (1988: 102–5), O'Flaherty (1980: 345), and Delaney et al. (1988: 149).

16. See Grimm (1870: 592), Kelle (1881: 166), and Thass-Thienemann (1973: 182, 305).

17. See Müller (1854: 217–18) and Kluge (1960: 87).

18. See Pokorny (1959: 122), Kluge (1960: 87), and Kelle (1881: 55).

19. See Grimm (1870: 544) and Müller (1854: 217–18).

20. See Kelle (1881: 55).

21. Lexer (1959: 24–25) and Müller (1854: 217–19).

22. See Franck (1536, 3: 457).

23. Spalding (1957: 354–55).

24. See Grimm and Grimm (1860: 171–73), Lexer (1959: 24), and Spalding (1957: 358).

25. Dürer's diary has not been preserved in the original script but only in the form of two transcriptions. The older document is in the library at Bamberg, Germany, and dates to the sixteenth century. It is for this reason that the original statements made by Dürer appear in different versions either as *Blüter* or *blütter* (cf. Dürer 1970: 98).

26. Dürer (n.d.: 62).
27. See Foucault (1979: 1–69).
28. See Bächtold-Stäubli (1929: 1438) and Feilberg (1892: 1).
29. Dürer (n.d.: 62, n. 3.10), Apocalypse VI: 9.
30. See Grimm and Grimm (1860: 181).
31. The first edition of the Spanish play appeared in 1500 under the title *Celestina, tragicomedia de Calisto y Melibea,* written by the otherwise unknown Baccalaureus Fernando de Rojas. The early Spanish editions were lost, and the German version was apparently translated from the Italian edition by Alfonso de Ordonez, *Tragi commedia di Calisto e Meliba,* Venezia, 1505 (Penney 1954: 118–19).
32. Kish and Ritzenhoff (1984).
33. See de Rojas (1966: 48).
34. See Grimm and Grimm (1860: 110) and Spalding (1957: 355).
35. The blood symbolism of the dying flower need not always be suggestive of female sexuality or maternal reproduction: it might refer to the loss of life and innocence in a more general sense. For instance, bleeding flowers appear as a central motif in a passage from Old Norse poetry (dating to the thirteenth century), where the images are suggestive of wasted potential, the termination of childhood and youth (*Guðrúnarkvida* II, str. 40). This image of blood-stained flowers, as the organizing motif in a premonitory dream, alludes to the anticipated murder of children. The dreamer, Atli, tells us: "Of plants I dreamed in the garden drooping / That fain would I have full high to grow / Plucked by the roots and red with blood / They brought them hither and bade me eat" (Bellows 1923: 463). The dream foreshadows the death of Atli's two sons, whose flesh Gudrun, his wife, tempts him to eat. The imagery of withering, uprooted, and bleeding flowers here serves as a metaphorical locution for infanticide, a premonition permeated by a father's fears of cannibalism.
36. See Grimm and Grimm (1860: 110) and Spalding (1957: 355–56).
37. See Delaney et al. (1988: 130).
38. See Bolte and Mackensen (1930: 281).
39. See Grimm and Grimm (1812–15, no. 47).
40. See Delaney et al. (1988: 167–68).
41. Ibid., 130.
42. See Grimm and Grimm (1860).
43. Ibid.
44. Ibid.
45. See Grimm (1878: 358).
46. See Friend (1891: 11, 147).
47. See Söhns (1904: 144).
48. Ibid., 145.
49. See Haase (1898: 61).
50. See Friend (1891: 11, 17, 191).
51. See Friend (1889: 432) and Söhns (1904: 16–17).
52. See Friend (1891: 11).
53. See Hecker (1931: 9).
54. See Bachmann (1953: 23).
55. Bötticher (1899: 2), Waltharius, stanza 1405.
56. See Bircher (1970, 1971).
57. Bircher (1971: ii, iii).
58. See Bircher (1971).
59. See Bendix (1978: 23–25) and de Vries (1956: 174).

60. See Bloch (1961: 123–24).
61. See de Vries (1956, 1: 178).
62. See Bloch (1961: 137).
63. See Rosenthal (1966: 138–39).
64. See Bloch (1961: 138).
65. See de Vries (1956: 186).
66. See Bendix (1978: 26–28).
67. Brodeur (1929:259–60). *Heita ok mágar, sifjungar, hleytamenn* (Jónsson 1900:235–36), *Skaldskaparmál,* str. 67.

68. Examples include Old Norse *magr,* Gothic *megs or magan,* Old English *máeg or magas,* and Old High German *mag or maga* (see Buck 1949: 1317, 132; Bosworth 1882: 654; and Pokorny 1959: 707).

69. For specific references regarding the Germanic terms consult the works by Buck (1949: 137, 1317), Bosworth (1882: 654), Pokorny (1959: 695, 707), Kuhn (1968: 138, 158), de Vries (1956: 276–78, 281; 1961: 392), Skeat (1882: 369), and Klein (1967: 982, 925, 990).

70. See *Hávamál* 137 and de Vries (1956: 281).

71. For examples of specific narratives about the binding power of blood, consult the following sources: Bächtold-Stäubli (1929: 1434–36); Bell (1922: 17–26); Bolte and Mackensen (1930: 279–81); Spalding (1957: 360); de Vries (1956: 286); and Strack (1909: 53–54). The thickness of blood as a trope of kinship solidarity is also articulated proverbially: "blood is not water" (Wander 1964: 410); "blood is thicker than water," and "blood is never so thin, it is always thicker than water" (Düringsfeld and Reinsberg-Düringsfeld 1872: 127, no. 252; Grimm 1974: 105, no. 266; and Franck 1896: 584–85). These proverbs allude to the cultural perception that the blood of relatives (*sippebluot*) acts as a strong or powerful adhesive that cannot be severed (Büchmann 1907: 584).

72. Höfler (1934: 223).

73. See de Vries (1961: 45) and Jónsson (1900: 235).

74. de Vries (1961: 45). See Old High German *bluotagón,* and Old Norse *blóðga, blóðiða, blóðrisa, blóðugr.*

75. When investigating the linguistic question of possible connections between words used for blood and terms used for the blood covenant, the following observation can be made: as in early Germanic, elsewhere terms denoting "to cut" seem to prevail. Among the Zande of southwest Sudan, *kure* or *kule* means blood; when speaking of the blood brother, the common term is *gbakule,* which is derived from *gba,* to cut, and *kule,* blood. A more usual form is *bakure,* to cut blood (Evans-Pritchard 1933: 370, n. 2; Tegnaeus 1952: 160). The matrilineal Kaguru of east-central Tanganyika refer to their blood brother as *lusale,* cuts. This word usually refers to the cuts made on the face or chest in order to apply magical medicine. Another term is *soga,* to apply something as to a cut (Beidelman 1963: 324).

76. Bellows (1923: 155), *Lokasenna* 9.

77. See Bellows (1923: 155, n. 9).

78. Bellows (1923: 409), *Brot af Sigurðarqviðo* 17.

79. See Róheim (1945: 17).

80. The metaphorical significance of blood and footprints is embodied in the more explicit symbolism of blood and shoes (de Vries 1956: 292). In a number of tales, shoes stand as a symbol of womanhood (Dundes 1983: 111). The German variant of Cinderella (tale type no. 21) is exemplary: the ash-girl loses one of her golden slippers at the ball, and the prince claims for his bride that girl

whose foot shall be the perfect fit. In the course of his search, the girl's stepsisters try it on, each in turn, but one must cut off her toe, the other slice her heel. And the prince riding off (first with one, then with the second) is warned by two doves that the shoe is a misfit and that blood is streaming forth from their mutilated feet. The prince learns that the true bride still sits at home. This, however, he discovers only when he tries to "ride" with them (Ussher 1983: 198–99). The blood of the shoe is in this tale clearly a female sexual symbol. And while here it is equated with vaginal or uterine blood, in the rite of brotherhood it may represent the blood of birth: siblinghood.

81. Johnston (1963: 7–8).

82. See Grimm (1868: 136), Johnston (1963: 69), and de Vries (1928: 113–15; 1956: 294–95).

83. Alliances based on the exchange of blood have been recorded from many parts of the world, particularly from Africa (Tegnaeus 1952; Trumbull 1885, 1896; Raum 1907; Róheim 1945; Beidelman 1963; Evans-Pritchard 1933). The covenant is contracted either between individuals or groups, and usually for political reasons. In some cultures, the participants drink one another's blood directly from incisions made on their bodies, while in others blood is swallowed with a piece of meat or groundnut.

84. Brodeur (1929: 21), *Gylfaginning* 9.

85. Jónsson (1900: 83), *Gylfaginning* 52.

86. For different versions of this narrative, see Bächtold-Stäubli (1930: 419–22), Greenhill (1954), Lauffer (1936), Marzell (1925–33), Schell (1893), and Simrock (1878).

87. See Finch (1965: 4), *Vǫlsunga Saga*, chap. 2.

88. The first element in the compound, *liuti* (modern German *Leute*), consists of a metaphorical allusion to an organic community: it is derived from proto-Indo-European **leudh-*, grow, originate, and cognate to Gothic *liudan*, grow, and Old Norse *ljóða*, rise, grow (Kluge 1963: 437). The second element *stam* has been derived from proto-Indo-European **sta-*, to stand, to be rooted in place (Kluge 1963: 737).

89. See Kluge (1963: 437, 737).

90. Translation adapted from Brodeur (1916: 235–36).

91. See Grimm (1844: 466).

92. See Bourdieu (1977).

93. See Goody (1983: 273).

94. Bouquet (1996: 47–48).

95. See Bouquet (1996: 46) and Gifford-Gonzalez (1993).

96. Bouquet (1996: 63, n. 5).

97. Bouquet (1996: 61).

Chapter 3. The Theft of Blood, the Birth of Men

1. See Baumann (1986), Dundes (1983), Friedrich (1978), Herdt (1981), Hugh-Jones (1979), O'Flaherty (1980), and Lévi-Strauss (1978).

2. For instance, Lévi-Strauss (1966: 16–22).

3. See Lindow (1985: 21–22).

4. See Leach (1956).

5. For example, Moore (1988).

6. See Godelier (1988: xi–xii).

7. For a reading of the Old Norse prose texts, I have used the normalized edition by Finnur Jónsson (1900). I relied on Neckel (1962) and Kuhn (1968) for my reading of the poetic verses. All translations are mine, in consultation with Bellows (1923), Brodeur (1916, 1929), Detter and Heinzel (1903), Hollander (1928, 1962), Nordal (1978), and other standard reference works.

8. See *Völuspá*, st. 3.

9. See *Gylfaginning*, chap. 4.

10. See de Vries (1930/31: 65–66) and Schier (1963: 309–10).

11. Schier (1963: 310). Comparative material can be found in Stith Thompson's *Motif Index of Folk Literature* (1955/58), under A605 "Primeval chaos"; A605.2 "Primeval cold"; A875.2 "Well in the middle of the earth from which eleven rivers originate"; A621.1 "Creation from vapor produced primeval giant"; A622 "Universe created out of fire world"; and A623 "Universe out of ice and mist."

12. See Schröder (1931: 3–5, 1960: 222, 235).

13. See *Völuspá*, st. 52, and Brodeur (1929: 17).

14. This figuration of fire is a thematic representation of a characteristic motif from solar mythology and reflects early European notions about the sun god and the god of fire (e.g., Jones 1971: 285; O'Flaherty 1980: 205). In the Norse myth, the sun or fire, anthropomorphized by *Surtr*, is equated with life, royalty, and power, while the primeval female fluid (as we shall see) is identified with lechery, sexual danger, and brute appetite.

15. See Schröder (1931: 3–5, 1960: 222, 235).

16. See Baumann (1986: 310–11), La Barre (1984), O'Flaherty (1980: 33), Schier (1963: 303–34), and Schröder (1960: 221–64).

17. Translation adapted from Brodeur (1929: 17). See *Gylfaginning*, chap. 5.

18. For instance, see Goody (1983) and Miller (1990: 139–78).

19. See *Gylfaginning*, chap. 5.

20. See Delaney et al. (1976: 146, 207).

21. Linke (1992, 1985) and Chapter 1, above.

22. Delaney et al. (1976: 129). Examples from German folk narratives, specifically the *Household Tales*, compiled by Jacob and Wilhelm Grimm (1812–15), contain images that reveal the mythological origins of these tales: "Snow White's mother pricks her finger while embroidering on an ebony frame at a snowy window. As the drops of blood fall on the snow, she wishes for a daughter with skin as white as snow, lips as red as blood, and hair as black as ebony. The mother of the little boy in 'The Juniper Tree' stands under a dark tree in white snow, peeling a red apple. She, too, cuts her finger and bleeds on the snow; she, too, wishes for a child as white as snow and as red as blood" (Delaney et al. 1976: 129).

23. See Bettelheim (1962: 107).

24. See Lévy-Bruhl (1935: 319–24).

25. See Linke (1985, 1992) and Chapter 1, above.

26. See Rüsche (1930) and O'Flaherty (1980: 40, 53).

27. See Friedrich (1979: 229–41).

28. See La Barre (1984).

29. See Eliade (1961: 40–43).

30. For instance, Goody (1983) and Miller (1990: 139–78).

31 See *Gylfaginning*, chap. 5.

32. See Buckley and Gottlieb (1988), Delaney et al. (1976), and Lévy-Bruhl (1935: 301–11).

33. See Bettelheim (1962).

34. See Delaney et al. (1976: 1–21, 205–11) and Montgomery (1974: 137–50).

35. Consult de Vries (1961) and Neckel (1962) for details of the specific terms.
36. See Delaney et al. (1976: 61–64)
37. Freud (1959: 198–99).
38. *Gylfaginning*, chap. 6.
39. Ibid., chap. 6.
40. Bede (1969: 91).
41. See Goody (1983: 34–36).
42. Ibid.
43. See Schröder (1931: 7), de Vries (1961: 678), and Meletinskij (1974: 52).
44. See Eliade (1965: 114–15).
45. See Meletinskij (1973: 52).
46. Outside the northern European context, very few of the mythical androgynes owe their existence to a liquid source, although Vedic texts propose that if equal quantities of semen and uterine blood merge inside a woman's womb, the child will be born as a hermaphrodite (O'Flaherty 1980: 48). Most mythological androgynes seem to be the result of the fusion of separate male and female bodies. Others are born in a fused form and subsequently split (often vertically) into distinct sexual bodies for purposes of procreation (284, 295–96, 309). In the Icelandic narrative, the primeval giant remains sexually fused and does not split in half to create offspring.
47. *Vafþrúðnismál*, st. 31.
48. *Gylfaginning*, chap. 5.
49. Ibid.
50. See O'Flaherty (1980: 39–40) and La Barre (1984: 114).
51. See O'Flaherty (1980: 40).
52. Meissner (1921: 206).
53. *Vafþrúðnismál*, st. 33.
54. Bachelard (1964: 24–35).
55. See O'Flaherty (1980: 293–94).
56. See Frye (1957: 148).
57. In other mythological traditions, outside northern Europe, male androgynes by far outnumber female androgynes and are generally regarded as positive, while female androgynes are generally perceived as negative, as in Hindu or Greek mythology (e.g., O'Flaherty 1980: 284).
58. *Gylfaginning*, chap. 6.
59. Ibid.
60. See Brodeur (1916: 18–19) and Meletinskij (1973: 52–53).
61. See Meletinskij (1973: 46–47; 1974: 63–70).
62. However much this particular text might have been influenced by the biblical version of the Great Flood, it retained its unique characteristics through the exclusive focus on a *blood flood*, a deluge generated by excessive amounts of blood, not water (cf. Thompson 1955/58: motif A1012.3.1 "Flood from slain giant's blood"). There exists no corresponding version of this mythological episode elsewhere. Remotely related may be the text of Muspilli, a Bavarian poem about the Day of Judgment, which has been dated to A.D. 800 (Bötticher 1899: 58): the devil fights with the angel Elias for the soul of a dying person and is defeated. The angel is merely wounded but his dripping blood sets fire to trees and mountains: everything wet dries up; the sky melts in the blazing heat; the moon falls down; the world is in flames. In this poetic narrative about the end of the world, blood is a destructive agent that turns into "fire," a purging, nonliquid element. One can perhaps discern a similar motif (i.e., "the raising of the earth

out of a primordial liquid chaos") in the opening stanzas of another Norse poem (*Völuspá*, st. 3). We are told that chaos ruled "Until the sons of Borr lifted the land / out of the sea, middle earth there they made." The earth's origin is attributed to the sons of Borr (Oðinn, Vilji and Vé), who lifted the world out of the primeval deluge. Then they gave it the shape that made it habitable (Nordal 1978: 14–15). Since the earth was hoisted from water, the poet seems to have imagined the surface of chaos as liquid (Detter and Heinzel 1903: 10, n. 3⁵⁻⁶). Liquidation, and the surge of blood, thus appears as a necessary prelude to transformation.

63. Alan Dundes (1988: 167–82) has made the same point in analyzing the flood motif as a "male myth of creation": outside the Scandinavian and northern European realm, the deluge is usually created from male genital fluids (i.e., semen or urine) rather than (menstrual) blood.

64. See Brain (1988) and Dundes (1976: 220–38).

65. *Gylfaginning*, chap. 7.

66. Martin (1981: 367).

67. Similar myths about the origin of the world from body parts of a murdered primal being are known from other regions of the world, although "blood" is rarely mentioned as a creative agent (Geldner 1951: 288–90; Schröder 1931: 14–19, 92–93; Leach 1956).

68. *Gylfaginning*, chap. 7.

69. *Vafþrúðnismál*, st. 21, and Bellows (1923: 74).

70. *Grímnismál*, st. 40, and Bellows (1923: 100).

71. See Jochens (1989: 253–54, 261).

72. See Shapiro (1988) and Linke (1986: 239–72).

73. *Gylfaginning*, chap. 6, and Young (1964: 41).

74. See Meletinskij (1973: 47–48; 1974: 58, 73).

75. *Gylfaginning*, chap. 14.

76. *Völuspá*, st. 9–10.

77. The text suggests that the dwarfs were created from blood and another nonliquid element, *leggr*. The English verse by Bellows proposes "leg" as the appropriate translation (Bellows 1923: 6). I chose to follow other interpretations, which claim that *leggr* also means *Knochen, Knochenröhre*, that is "bone" (de Vries 1961: 349; Kuhn 1968: 125). This choice seems more accurate in light of the fact that Old Norse poetry followed the rules of alliteration, the repetition of an initial sound cluster, usually a consonant, in two or more words in a line of poetry. In this poem, the use of *leggiom* instead of *beinom* avoids placing a fourth alliterating syllable at the end of the second half-line, perhaps a conscious stylistic decision.

78. See de Vries (1967: 42, 56–57), Bellows (1923: 6, n. 9), and Detter and Heinzel (1903: 19, n. 9).

79. See *Gylfaginning*, chap. 10.

80. Hollander (1987: 322, n. 1); also see *Völuspá*, st. 11–16.

81. *Völuspá*, st. 17 and 18.

82. See Polomé (1969: 265–66).

83. *Gylfaginning*, chap. 8–9.

84. See Doht (1974), Frank (1981), and Stübe (1924).

85. Brodeur (1929: 92–93), *Skaldskaparmál*, chap. 57–58.

86. Faulkes (1987: 62).

87. See Stephens (1972: 259).

88. Brodeur (1929: 92–93) and Jónsson (1900: 71).

89. See Clover (1978: 68–69).

90. Faulkes (1987: 64).

91. In striking contrast, male symbolic creativity elsewhere remains focused on the female body and on women's physiological procreativity. The attempt to rival women's "natural" procreativity is usually accomplished by means of the symbolic manipulations of body parts and substances: men "give birth" through their mouth or anus and through the metaphorical conveyance of this creative act in terms of vomit, blood, saliva, feces (e.g., Dundes 1976: 220–38; Róheim 1949; Ashley-Montagu 1937: 307). These concepts are made plausible by a system of metaphors that equate oral incorporation and digestion with processes of female reproduction (Gillison 1983; Hiatt 1975; O'Flaherty 1980: 264).

92. See Keesing (1982) and Hiatt (1971) for comparative evidence.

93. See Hiatt (1975: 156).

94. See Shapiro (1989: 75).

95. In northern European folk narratives, prophetic knowledge often issues from severed (male) heads. See Ross (1962) and Simpson (1962, 1963/64).

96. For example, Karras (1992).

97. See Bottigheimer (1987).

98. See Bloch (1986: 87).

Chapter 4. Sanguine Visions, Sacred Blood

1. By "organic" I mean sanguine and fleshly (i.e., of bodily substance). Durkheim, in later works, reserved this term to describe modern forms of social organization, which he saw as distinguished by the structural division (and interdependence) of labor relations.

2. Voragine (1900: 34); the text dates from 1483.

3. Steinberg (1983: 50–106).

4. Bede (n.d., col. 54); Translation adapted from Steinberg (1983: 52).

5. See Denzinger (1957: 160).

6. Pseudo-Bonaventure (1961: 43–44).

7. Voragine (1900: 34).

8. See O'Malley (1979: 138).

9. See Campano (1495: fols. 85v, 87) and Steinberg (1983: 62).

10. See Lollio (1485: fols. 1, 2, 5v) and Steinberg (1983: 62).

11. Bynum (1987: 33).

12. See Browe (1938), Steinberg (1983), and Schiller (1971–72).

13. This idea of bleeding and bloodshed as a means to restore and heal the world can be historically attested in pre-Christian Europe. Some of the evidence has been preserved in verbal references and early linguistic markers for blood. There exists reliable documentation for sacrificial bloodletting in most northern European languages. Thus modern Germanic terms for bleeding, e.g., *blotan* (Gothic and Old English), *blota* (Old Norse), and *bluozan* (Old High German), also denote sacrifice, venerate, and curse (de Vries 1961: 45; Kuhn 1968: 30; Pokorny 1959: 154). Equating blood with ritual power, these terms for blood offerings are etymologically and historically related to other Old Norse, Old English, Old High German, and Gothic words like *blot, bluostar, bluostari, plozhus,* and *guplostreis,* which refer to the sacrificial priest, his act of sanctification, and his temple or literally "the house of (blood) sacrifice" (de Vries 1956: 399, 414–

15). While the exact etymological origin of these words is uncertain, the textual sources suggest that they were used primarily with reference to rituals of bloodshed and blood spillage.

Moreover, in medieval northern Europe, certain seasons—autumn, winter, late spring, and the middle of summer—were designated as appropriate times for conducting the important blood rites (de Vries 1956: 446–48, 1957: 286, n. 1; Grimm 1868: 77). Each ritual act involved the use of blood. In summer, fresh blood was shed to obtain victory as well as peace. A famous Scandinavian text from the thirteenth century contains a brief mention of such an event: "The next spring King Granmar went to Upsala to the blood offering, which was usually held about summer's day in order that the peace should last" (*Ynglinga saga*, str. 38; in Monsen 1932: 29–30; de Vries 1956: 446; and Kristjánsson 1992: 168). In the text, blood ritual and the fate of kings are closely linked.

Late autumn and the beginning of winter marked the beginning of several other blood-related celebrations. As indicated by the name for this season, the "month of sacrifice" (Old English *blotmonad*), the ceremonies probably relied on actual blood offerings. This notion is rendered plausible by a later reference to this phase of the annual cycle as the "month of slaughter." This same designation is attested in several northern European languages: *slachtmoane* (Old Frisian), *slachtmonet* (Middle High German), *slachtmanet* (Dutch), and *slagtmanad* (Swedish) (see Grimm 1868: 57–59, 61, 63, 65). The textual evidence, drawn from a late medieval Icelandic source, confirms the ritual reliance on bloodshed at least until the tenth century: "There was prepared a feast around the beginning of winter, and a blood sacrifice for the disir [*disablot*] and everyone was supposed to participate in the festivities" (*Víga-Glúms saga*, str. 6; in Doht 1974: 28; see Kristjánsson 1992: 203–23 for attempts at dating the cited source material). In northern Europe, this annual celebration was part of a fertility cult, central to which was the god Frey and the *disir* or female fecundity spirits, who were accompanied and guided by the goddess Freyja. The ritual event was among the most important of the annual feasts, because it coincided with the autumn slaughtering of cattle (Johnston 1963: 73; Ström 1954; de Vries 1956: 455). Blood was offered to these deities during domestic cult celebrations for growth and good harvest.

Occasionally, during the times of public temple worship, human blood was spilled for similar reasons. In German-speaking lands, sacrificial blood offerings were made of tribal chiefs, and sometimes kings, when their power was no longer deemed sufficient to make the crops prosper, when age or illness had robbed them of their fertile powers or a bad harvest proved that they had already been greatly reduced (see Höfler 1952a/b). Among Germanic peoples, "[a]ncient pantheistic beliefs attributed supernatural powers to nature and within society to a kin group or clan (*Sippe*) endowed with special capacities that were attributed to blood" (Bendix 1978: 25): Chieftains or rulers, distinguished by the singular blood potency of their kindred clan, were thought to possess a god-descended power or *mana* which ensured good crops, victory in battle, and the power to heal certain diseases (de Vries 1957, 2: 76–80, 348–52). The fate of Germanic kings was thus directly tied to the fecundity of the soil. The growth of crops or the success of a harvest were read as signs of a leader's blood potency.

The connection between sanguine power and soil was strengthened by the ritual use of blood at the beginning of a king's rule. According to one source from c. 1390 (although probably composed in pagan times), "when Svein became king of Sweden, the sacrificial trees were sprinkled with horses' blood"

(*Hyndluljóð*, str. 10; Ranke 1978: 79). When a king lost his virile powers, the end of his reign was likewise marked by bloodshed. According to an Icelandic legend, dated back to the tenth century, a prolonged famine resulted in a king's death: "they gave him to Odin and made blood offerings in order to have a good season (*Ynglinga saga*, str. 43; Monsen 1932: 32). In pagan northern Europe, kings were held accountable for the outcome of the harvest; their blood potency was believed to affect the fecundity of the land. Political rulers thus often suffered death during a famine, when their blood and body were offered to the gods (Dumézil 1973: 26, 31). After the killing, a king's blood was collected and sprinkled onto the fields to make them fruitful and fecund (Schröder 1953: 172–73). Such ritual deaths are attested in a tenth-century Icelandic text, where the king is killed to "dye the altars with his blood" (*Ynglinga saga*, str. 14; Monsen 1932: 10–11). These images of blood sacrifice and fertility typify northern European attitudes toward the dying body: ritualized bloodshed and blood effusion were regarded as positive occurrences, not as terror-inspiring events. The slain body of the king assumed significance within this semantic field of blood and power. The king's death, like Christ's suffering on the cross, was a redemptive sacrifice of flesh and blood that provided the means to restore and heal the world.

14. See Brown (1981).

15. Late medieval preoccupations with dead bodies, although a theological novelty, attest to the infusion of Christian doctrine by local cultural concerns; see below, note 44. In northern Europe, in German-speaking territories, the cult of blood and body and the veneration of the corpse existed as an integral part of late medieval folklore and folk culture.

16. See Rubin (1991: 63, 82, 108–39).

17. Andrieu (1950: 399–408).

18. See Eynsham (1961: 170) and Finucane (1977: 28).

19. Vitry (1867: 551–56).

20. Clairvaux (1886: 362–72).

21. On stigmatization see Imbert-Gourbeyre (1894), Thurston (1952), Amman (1939), and Debongnie (1936).

22. Clairvaux (1886: 363, 378).

23. Bollandus and Henschenius (1863: 349–53).

24. Colledge and Walsh (1978: 181, 285–98).

25. These collective biographies, or *Nonnenbücher* (nuns' books), were composed in the early fourteenth century; they contain contributions from the nuns of Unterlinden, Töss, and Engelthal (Stagel 1906; Schröder 1871).

26. See Ancelet-Hustache (1930: 340–42).

27. Bynum (1987: 211).

28. Vauchez (1981: 408).

29 Laurent (1940: 127–28).

30. See Albert the Great (1916: 682).

31. Bynum (1987: 23).

32. Rollins (1921: 363–64).

33. Leiden (1865: 272–75).

34. See Bynum (1987: 148).

35. Perusinus (1866: 188).

36. Ibid.: 217.

37. Bosco-Gualteri (1865: 737, 739–40).

38. Bollandists (1899: 313–15, 314–17, 353).

39. Reypens (1964: 105).

40. Birlinger (1881: 281–83).

41. Vaux (1865: 554–55, 560–62).

42. Bynum (1987: 274).

43. Ibid.

44. Late medieval notions of unusual or extraordinary bleeding were reinforced by local cultural images and practices. In northern Europe, even before Christianization, blood was a central ritual symbol; according to thirteenth-century textual sources, it assumed a variety of symbolic functions in pagan fertility rites. Blood and bloodshed were used to appease the gods, to ensure good crops, and to influence fate. Control over blood or blood-related matters was thus a crucial signifier of power. Such a symbolics of blood had been established as an important element in pagan rituals of divination. Here the interpretation of sanguine visions and unusual flows had become a means for revealing supernatural intent or presence.

Such a preoccupation with blood is attested by several medieval Icelandic texts. A mythological passage, written in Old Norse poetic verse, tells us that once upon a time, when the gods intended to hold a feast, they used blood magic to find out where they could best meet (*Hymiskviða*, chap. 1): "Of old the gods made feast together. And drink they sought ere sated they were. Twigs they shook and blood they tried: Rich fare in Aegir's hall they found" (Bellows 1923: 139). The poem alludes to an act of divination, a ritualized practice of acquiring knowledge about the future by using blood as a portent. The rite required dipping a bundle of chips or twigs into a kettle containing blood and then shaking the blood off (Bellows 1923: 139, n. 1). The procedure itself was only briefly described as *hristu teine ok a hlaut sa*, which has been interpreted to mean "they sprinkled the blood and read the prophecy from the splashes" (Nordal 1978: 115).

Such a ritual use of blood is also attested in other texts. One short mention of the rite exists in an Old Norse passage that describes King Thorolf's construction of a temple: "On the top of the hill, next to the temple, [stood] the blood kettle and in[to] it were . . . dipped the bundled twigs for sprinkling the blood . . . called *hlaut*. It was the blood from slaughtered animals that had been sacrificed to the gods" (Golther 1895: 599). The passage informs us that a blood sacrifice initiated the act of divination: animals were slaughtered and offered to the gods in order to obtain a favorable reading. The sacrificial blood (called *hlaut*) was later used for purposes of foretelling the future. The augur was thus based on a blood offering. Poured into a kettle, the blood was scattered about by a bundle of twigs. These ritual instruments had been officially termed *hlaut vior* or *hlautteinn*, "the sprinkler for scattering sacrificial blood" (Nordal 1978: 115). The act of divination itself was called *fella blotspan*, "to cast the blood (twigs) and pronounce fate" (Golther 1895: 633–64). In medieval northern Europe, pagan peoples would offer a blood sacrifice and then proceed to divine the future.

There exists some linguistic evidence for this connection: the term *hlaut* "sacrificial blood" is in Old Norse related to *hliota* "cast the dice" and "decide fate" (Ranke 1978: 79). The assumption was that the gods would reveal to the ritual participants their future destiny through the medium of the blood offering. This interpretation is supported by several other sources. Classical authors documented that the Cimbri, a Germanic people, had among their possessions a kettle, which they used for the collection of sacrificial human blood. Human blood from this cauldron played an important role in the rites of divination (de Vries 1956: 392–93; Ranke 1978: 79). Prisoners of war, once chosen as an appropriate offering, were prepared for the event by gray-haired and barefoot women. These women, dressed in white linen gowns, led the men to a large metal kettle: they then cut their throats and foretold the future from the blood spillage.

Several Old Norse texts mention, in the context of sacrifice, a kettle or cauldron that was designated for the collection and storage of blood from slaughtered animals. One source describes a famous celebration in *Lade*, where horse blood was poured into large cauldrons (*Heimskringla*, chap. 14, p. 149): during the festivities, this blood was sprinkled onto the images of the gods, the temple walls, and the participants of the sacrifice (Ranke 1978: 79). This act of blood-dousing was intended as a blessing. Another example describes a similar occurrence, at which sacrificial blood was splashed about, probably for good luck and perhaps blessing: "All farmers came together for the sacrifice at the place of worship. All received beer; also several small animals and horses were killed — the blood was called *hlaut*, and the kettles in which it was collected were named *hlautbollar* . . . The blood was sprinkled onto the temple walls inside and onto the participants outside. In the center of the hall were fires, above which the (blood) kettles were swinging from the ceiling" (de Vries 1956: 416; *Hakornamál* I [Hakon inn goði], st. 186–87). As in late medieval Christianity, the thematic images of bloodshed and sacrifice were intimately connected and linked to assumptions of divine presence: controlled forms of bleeding were perceived as expressions of supernatural forces.

45. See Rubin (1991: 14).

46. Macy (1984: 21).

47. Walpole (1922: 350–51).

48. Ibid.: 345–46.

49. Denzinger (1967: 260).

50. From "Pange, lingua," in Byrnes (1943: 168), Gaselee (1937: 144), and Connelly (1957: 120).

51. From "Verbum supernum prodiens," in Gaselee (1937: 145) and Connelly (1957: 123).

52. From "Lauda, Sion, Salvatorem," in Gaselee (1937: 146–47), Byrnes (1943: 180–88), and Connelly (1957: 126).

53. See Bynum (1987: 60).

54. See Bosco-Gualteri (1865: 44).

55. Hildegard of Bingen (1978: 225–306).

56. Cavallini (1968: 331–34).

57. Hart (1980: 260).

58. Kieckhefer (1984: 171).

59. Bosco-Gualteri (1865: 737, 729–40).

60. See Fathers of St. Bonaventure's College (1897: 445).

61. See Eynsham (1961: 93–94).

62. See Vaux (1865: 558).

63. These visions resonated with already existing superstitions and cultural assumptions about blood. It was widely believed that dramatic events revealed themselves through visual or perceptual manifestations of blood. In northern Europe, in the Icelandic sagas of the late Middle Ages, blood and bloody objects that appeared in dreams were recorded as omens: Glum sees two women sprinkle blood over the whole land in his dream; Njal envisions that his table and food are bloody; Gisli, in his dream, is washed with blood by a woman (Ranke 1978: 79). In all these instances, visions of blood were interpreted as concrete portents of danger. Equally persistent was the cultural assertion that natu-

ral catastrophes were divinely foretold, in particular through frightful visions of blood and the cross. The sixteenth-century theologian Sebastian Franck von Wörd documented the existence of European legends of this sort in his *Chronica zeitbuch vnnd geschicht bibell* (Franck 1536). Visions of blood were interpreted as god-sent forebodings of destruction, famine, and death. But these miraculous blood signs, the physical manifestations of the suffering man/God, also attested to the tangible presence of the divine.

64. See Steinberg (1983).

65. See Bynum (1987: 161).

66. Reypens (1964: 152–53).

67. Ibid.: 137–40.

68. Bosco-Gualteri (1865: 734–44).

69. Guy-l'Evêque (1866: 516–17).

70. Bollandists (1899: 313).

71. Bollandus and Henschenius (1894: 167–209).

72. Bynum (1987: 134).

73. Bollandus and Henschenius (1894: 167).

74. Stachnik et al. (1978: 214, 277).

75. See Bollandists (1884: 439–41, 425).

76. See Humbert of Romans (1603, fol. 59rb)

77. See Gellrich (1985: 22) and Berthold of Regensburg (1968: 63–67).

78. Bollandus and Henschenius (1863: 341–44).

79. Doyere (1968: 303–7).

80. Consult Bynum (1987: 59, 327–28, nn. 115–17), who discusses these cases and offers a wide array of textual and bibliographic references.

81. Bynum (1987: 53).

82. Ibid.: 51.

83. Dumoutet (1942) and Aquinas (1964, 58: 52–122).

84. Gy (1983: 82–83), Vitry (1972: 234–36), and Megivern (1963).

85. Aquinas (1964, 58: 52–122).

86. Macy (1984: 30–31).

87. From "Lauda, Sion, Salvatorem," in Gaselee (1937: 146–47, Byrnes (1943: 180–88), and Connelly (1957: 126).

88. Dumoutet (1943: 217–18).

89. Dumoutet (1942: 109–10).

90. This point was succinctly made by Bynum (1987: 51).

91. See Geary (1978: 39–40).

92. Franz (1963: 87–92) and Niedermeyer (1974).

93. See Braun (1924) and Dumoutet (1926: 38–41, 50–53). Miri Rubin (1991: 45–48, 251–58) discusses these changes at length.

94. See Dendy (1959: 38).

95. Corblet (1885), Bertaud (1961: 1621), and Hamman et al. (1961).

96. See Trexler (1974: 122–23).

97. See Gougaud (1923: 86–87).

98. See Bynum (1987: 54).

99. Ibid.: 56.

100. See Klauser (1979: 98–103, 120), Jungmann (1951: 374–80), and Brooke (1967).

101. Brinton (1954: 212–17) and Audelay (1931: 67).

102. Baix and Lambot (1964: 67).

103. Kennedy (1946) and Hontoir (1946).

104. Heuser (1948: 94–95) and Rubin (1991: 58–59).

105. Browe (1933) and Jungmann (1951: 119–21).

106. Rothkrug (1979: 36) and Mayer (1971: 34–36).

107. Marienwerder (1884: 409).

108. See Browe (1933) and Rubin (1991).

109. See Dumoutet (1926: 25).

110. Mansi (1759, col. 140).

111. Ibid.: col. 149.

112. See Rubin (1991: 292).

113. See King (1965: 104–8).

114. See Jungmann (1951: 381–85, 412–14), King (1955: 129–30, 372), and Aquinas (1964, 58: 96–100; 59: 84–85).

115. Baix and Lambot (1964: 113–23), Gougaud (1927), and Bynum (1982).

116. Browe (1933: 82).

117. The intimate connection of the Christian altar (i.e., the center of worship) to images of blood sacrifice and bloodshed was deeply rooted in European pagan culture. While many of the important northern European rituals made use of blood in sacrifice and divination, blood was deemed necessary for the consecration of the altar. During pagan times, in German-speaking lands and in the northern parts of Europe, the altar consisted of a simple mount of stones, called *horgr* in Old Norse and *harug* in Old High German (de Vries 1956: 378). Blood is mentioned in several descriptions of such a place of worship. One late medieval text informs us that a copper kettle stood directly on the altar: all blood, which was offered to the god Thor in sacrifice, was collected in this vessel (*Kjalnesinga saga*, str. 2; Ranke 1978: 79). Another thirteenth-century source reveals that King Heidrekr reddened the altar with the blood of Harolds and his son Hálfdan (*Heidrekr saga*; Ranke 1978: 79). Elsewhere we learn that such a place of worship acquired sacrality by "redden(ing) the altar (walls) with blood" (*Hakornamál* II, 219; de Vries 1956: 418). Other medieval texts allude to the presence of blood in the altar's initial consecration (*Hyndluljoð* 10): "He made me an altar out of layered stones. Now the rock has turned to glass. He reddened it in the fresh blood of an ox. And Ottar consecrated it to the gods" (de Vries 1956: 392). After being built from a heap of stones, the altar was reddened with the blood of cattle and glazed by fire.

Such ritual procedures are attested in language: Old English *bloedsian* or *bletsian*, bless, consecrate, is related to Old English *blot*, blood offering, and it thus alludes to the former existence of human or animal blood sacrifices (Klein 1967: 179). The original meaning of "to bless" was probably as in Germanic **blodison*, "consecrate by sprinkling or reddening the altar with blood" (de Vries 1961: 45; Klein 1967: 179; Ranke 1978: 78). Given these meanings in Germanic, blood was assumed to bestow sacrality or sanctification, in the sense of "blessing" or "good fortune."

118. See Gougaud (1927: 114).

119. Gougaud (1927: 104–10) and Coletti (1953: 100–101).

120. Thomas á Kempis (1956: 225).

121. In Powicke and Cheney (1964: 77).

122. Peter of Poitiers (1841: cols. 789–1280), my emphasis.

123. See Schlette (1959).

124. Alexander of Hales (1957, 4: 204–5).

125. Quoted in Bodenstedt (1944: 133, n. 94).

126. See Wenzel (1978).

127. Heuser (1948: 94–95).
128. Ibid.
129. See Gray (1963: 87–88).
130. On these devotional images, see Gougaud (1925: 99–100), Heuser (1948: 169–80), Assion and Wojciechowski (1970), and Dolan (1897).
131. See Gougaud (1927: 82–83).
132. Gray (1963: 88), Gougaud (1925: 99–100), and Pfaff (1970: 62–83).
133. See Gougaud (1927: 164–65).
134. See Steinberg (1983).
135. See Rubin (1991: 305).
136. See Bühler (1964: 273–74).
137. See Rubin (1991: 305).
138. See Robbins (1939: 419–20).
139. See Dolan (1897).
140. See Louis (1980: 152).
141. See Haubst (1958: 545).
142. Heuser (1948: 34, 49–56) and Maltzahn (1908: 9, 17).
143. See Breest (1881: 137–43) and Hildburgh (1908: 205–6).
144. Perusinus (1866: 162, 159).
145. See Gougaud (1927: 89).
146. Hontoir (1946: 134–35, 137), Rothkrug (1979: 41) and Deutz (1841).
147. See Tubach (1969).
148. See Bauerreis (1958: 545) and Heuser (1948: 1–34).
149. See Bynum (1987: 63). Several centuries later, these frightful images of bleeding and blood flow as accusation or a pronouncement of violation had become firmly embedded in northern European folk culture. Several sixteenth-century warning tales describe how a dead man's wounds began to bleed to reveal his murderer (Grimm 1854; Cassel 1882: 24–25). In a number of German cases, we are told that a "blood test" (termed *Bahrrecht* or *Bahrprobe*) was used whenever a murder had been committed: the suspect was forced to approach and even touch the corpse. Then, if the dead man's wounds began to bleed, the accused was held responsible for the crime. However, if the corpse remained dry, and no blood appeared, the suspect was acquitted. The earliest documentation of these blood accusations can be found in thirteenth-century German epic poems (Bartsch 1866: 192; 1880: 158; Fehr 1955: 148; 1930; Benecke and Lachmann 1877). In one instance, we learn, "the closer [the murderer] came, the more [the corpse] threw up a scum, and when [the man] approached it and was supposed to pledge his oath, [the body] paled and began to bleed [so much] that the blood seeped through the stretcher" (Grimm 1854: 930). Although none of the medieval or early modern laws ever made mention of this procedure, the "test of blood" seems to have been deeply rooted in the religiosity and culture of the late Middle Ages and was thus considered an acceptable practice by the courts (Heinemann 1922: 32; Grimm 1854: 930). Such readings of the corpse or blood testimony was still current in Lower Saxony as late as 1750, where folk narratives insisted that the suspect place his fingers three times on the severed hand of the murdered man (Grimm 1854: 931): if the severed limb bled, the suspect was convicted; if no blood appeared, he was declared innocent.

Visions of threatening flows of blood can be found in modern European folk narratives. In nineteenth-century tales of "the bleeding bone" (motif no. D1318.5), we are told how a gruesome murder is revealed and avenged through the blood that issued from the victim's remains (Bächtold-Stäubli 1929: 1434–

35; Mackensen 1923; Fehr 1955: 149; Wyss 1917: 12; Sprenger 1893). Although known throughout Europe, the tale type takes on a peculiar form in the German and Swiss variants (Kessler 1915; Mackensen 1923: 100–105). When the physical remains of a victim were accidentally unearthed, the generic European version of the tale describes how the victim's bones were made into a musical instrument by the perpetrator: the murderer was thus revealed by sound (Bolte and Polívka 1913; Krohn 1931). In the German versions, by contrast, the bones or skull of the slain victim begin to bleed profusely when the murderer stumbles upon the corpse or touches the skeletal remains. These examples suggest that the flow of blood, as an accusation or a proclamation of transgression, became an integral part of German folk culture after the late Middle Ages.

150. See Browe (1933: 104). This motif of the child in the host is very common: the image reveals the transubstantiated eucharist as the real Christ in one of his suffering personas: a glorious youth, a sacrificed child, or a bleeding infant (Rubin 1991: 135–39).

151. See Browe (1933: 124).

152. See Vitry (1890, n. 270: 113) and Little (1908: 8).

153. See Browe (1933: 119). Other boundary-enforcing blood miracles can be found in Corblet (1885: 447–515) and Eynsham (1961: 93–94).

154. Heisterbach (1901: 4–6; 1851). For the use of the host as magical charm, see Browe (1930).

155. See Müller (1961: 177–84).

156. See Heuser (1948: 20–21) and Dumoutet (1926: 81).

157. See Fliege (1977) and Breest (1881: 137–43).

158. See Zika (1988: 49–59).

159. See Heuser (1948: 17).

160. In Assion and Wojciechowski (1970: 147).

161. See Browe (1933: 115–16) and Jungmann (1951: 119).

162. Vitry (1867: 547–50, 562–63, 565–66).

163. See Dumoutet (1926).

164. See MacCulloch (1932: 159).

165. Endres (1917), Bollandus and Henschenius (1865b: 133–34, 152), and Westfeling (1982).

166. See Eynsham (1961: 93–94).

167. See Browe (1933: 72–83).

168. See Zingerle (1891: 505–6).

169. Ibid.: 505.

170. Ibid.

171. See Rubin (1991: 122).

172. See Hsia (1992) and Dundes (1991).

173. See Heuser (1948: 20).

174. Rothkrug (1979: 29); also Browe (1933: 128).

175. Gibson (1978: 81, n. 1) and Lanfranc (1841, chap. 2, cols. 410–11).

176. See Jungmann (1951: 381–82).

177. Klauser (1979: 110), Baix and Lambot (1964: 40–41), and Browe (1938: 97–98).

178. See Wilkins (1737, 3: 11).

179. Vitry (1972: 219), Pontal (1983: 326), Rubin (1991: 37–49, 294–97, 340).

180. Powicke and Cheney (1964: 27).

181. Aquinas (1964, 3: 153).

182. See Gietl (1891: 232) and Vitry (1972: 214).

183. Bynum (1987: 64).
184. See Doyere (1968: 102–4).
185. See Celano (1898: 250–51).
186. See Bynum (1987: 64).
187. Hildegard of Bingen (1978: 272–76).
188. See Klauser (1979: 98–103) and Jungmann (1951, 2: 374–80).
189. See Brown (1988: 146, 433).
190. See Browe (1932: 376) and Rubin (1991: 147–50).
191. See Jungmann (1951, 2: 381–85, 412–14) and King (1955: 129–30, 372).
192. Aquinas (1964, 59: 84–85, and vol. 3).
193. Jungmann (1951, 2: 364). See Rubin (1991: 70–72) and Bynum (1987:56–58) for a more extensive discussion.
194. Congar (1973: 159).
195. Assisi (1949: 102–3); also Habig (1973: 105).
196. See Brooke (1967).
197. Albert the Great (1894: 378–80).
198. See Bynum (1987: 140).
199. Vitry (1867, 5: 568). Translation adapted from Bynum (1987: 59); also Bynum (1982).
200. See Bollandus and Henschenius (1863), vol. 2 (June), "Life of Alice," 473–74; vol. 13 (October), "Life of Ida of Léau," 113–14; vol. 1 (April), "Life of Juliana," 445–46; vol. 2 (April), "Life of Ida of Louvain," 164, 182–83.
201. See Ferré and Baudry (1927: 16, 138).
202. Bollandus and Henschenius (1866: 474).
203. Hildegard of Bingen (1978: 228).
204. Cantimpré (1866: 192–94).
205. See Bosco-Gualteri (1865: 734–44).
206. Drane (1915: 271) and Fawtier and Canet (1948: 230–32, 238). The descriptions regarding Catherine of Siena are taken from Bynum (1987: 177–78); consult her text for greater elaboration of these passages.
207. Female hunger or craving for blood was a cultural motif that existed in northern Europe before the onset of Christianity. In folklore, myth, and magical incantations, female spirits of blood and fate appeared in the form of *Norns* and *Valkyrs*. Linked to ideas of predestination and foreknowledge, the Norns gave souls to newborn humans, protected deliveries, and functioned as midwives and donors of fate (Meletinskij 1977: 253; Hollander 1928: 4–5; Brodeur 1929: 28–29). The Norns, intimately linked with female blood and chthonic knowledge, controlled the course of human events: they chose life, presided at birth, laid down laws, and pronounced fate (Turville-Petre 1964: 280; Bauschatz 1982: 4, 8, 11–13). Moreover, the image of three women who were somehow associated with blood effusion was so deeply rooted in folk belief that there is no doubt about the Germanic origin of this motif (Ebermann 1903: 83).

Under the influence of Christian missionaries, the concept of the Norns as guardians of blood, and thereby human fate, was gradually transformed into images of blood contained and boiled in kettles kept by female demons or evil spirits. Several Finnish incantations describe how blood is boiled in a kettle in hell and how to obtain such a vessel from the devil (Hästesko 1914: 11; Christiansen 1914: 162). Other Scandinavian versions of these magical spells allude to the "little devils" of hell, who are supposed to possess a kettle in which blood is cooked. But even in the pre-Christian era, not all of the activities of the three Norns were beneficent and generative. Some incantations seem to suggest a blood craving as the distinguishing attributes of these female fates (Ebermann 1903: 86–88). The first Norn desires blood: she is called a "greedy drinker of blood"; the second Norn lets the blood run forth and pours it out—she is named "the spiller of blood"; the third contains or stops the blood flow (88). The earliest written German incantation, in which the Norns seek or hunger for blood, can be dated to 1349 (81, 91).

The main motif in these magical spells revolved around the simultaneous giving and taking of blood. Ultimately, these female spirits of fate were connected to ideas of birth, death, and the shedding of blood. Some appeared as warrior women, the *Valkyries*, or "choosers of the slain," who marked the victims of battle and decided victory and defeat. Valkyrs were the armed shield-maidens of Odin, the god of war; they were warrior women who scoured the battlefield for the bodies and blood of the slain (Hollander 1928: 7; Brodeur 1929: 48). These images of women's lust (or need) for blood surfaced as an important motif in German folklore, where it gave rise to ideas about bloodthirsty witches and demonic spirits of blood.

In any case, assumptions regarding the female hunger for blood were a familiar cultural theme by the twelfth and thirteenth centuries, and probably reinforced (and made plausible) the emergent images of holy women's cravings or thirst for Christ's blood during the later Middle Ages.

208. See Fawtier and Canet (1948: 268–73) and Gougaud (1927: 75–130).

209. Misciattelli (1913: 337–38).

210. See Cavallini (1968: 37–42, 50–55, 274–86) and Misciattelli (1913, 1: 115–24).

211. Cavallini (1968: 37–38, 51–53, 276–78, 352–54) and Drane (1915: 261).

212. Noffke (1980: 215).

213. See Cavallini (1968: 313–14).

214. Ibid.: 51–56.

215. Misciattelli (1913, 4: 217–24).

216. Bynum (1987: 376, n. 135).

217. See Hart (1980, no. 15: 350–52).

218. Bynum (1987: 292).

219. Capua (1865: 902–3).

220. Misciattelli (1913, 1: 135–42; 2: 341–42).

221. Ibid., 1: 81–82; Cavallini (1968: 225–30, 440); and Noffke (1980: 52).

222. Bynum (1987: 269).

223. See Wood (1981), Needham (1959: 37–74), and Preus (1977).

224. See Bynum (1987: 265).

225. See Hildegard of Bingen (1978: 11–12, 147–48).

226. See Oingt (1965: 98–99).

227. See Dronke (1984).

228. See Pelphrey (1982).

229. See Bradley (1976).

230. See Bynum (1987: 266).

231. See McLaughlin (1974: 115–18) and Wood (1981: 719).

232. See Stählin (1936: 104–21).

233. Bynum (1982: 151–54).

234. See Magdeburg (1869: 11–13, 29–30).

235. Bynum (1987: 271).

236. See Bollandus and Henschenius (1866: 474).

237. See Schiller (1971–72: 205–206).

238. See Bynum (1987: 274, 122).
239. Ibid.
240. See Sanday (1986) and Gillison (1983).
241. See Brown and Tuzin (1983), Sanday (1986), Sahlins (1983), Conklin (1995), and Battaglia 1992).
242. See Sanday (1986: 59–82).
243. Ibid.: 65.
244. See Arens (1979) and Adams (1990: 31–32).
245. See Rappaport (1991) and Schuster (1970).
246. See Dundes (1991: 354).
247. See Bynum (1987: 281).
248. Ibid.: 278.
249. Description adapted from Rappaport (1991: 309, 331–32).
250. See Steinberg (1983).
251. See Mintz (1985: 244, n. 52).
252. See Dundes (1991: 354).
253. See Gillison (1983).
254. Ibid.: 35.
255. See Strathern (1982: 125).
256. See Gillison (1980: 150).
257. For instance, Bell (1985).
258. See Dundes (1976), Róheim (1949), Ashley-Montagu (1937), Bettelheim (1954), and Hiatt (1971, 1975).
259. See Bettelheim (1954).
260. See Hiatt (1975: 156)
261. Ibid.: 152.
262. See Freud (1950), Rank (1959), and Jones (1971), among others.
263. See Gillison (1980: 148).
264. Bloch (1982); Bloch and Parry (1982: 28–32).
265. See Dundes (1991).
266. Ibid.: 339. There is an immense literature on the blood libel legend. For scholarly and critical introductions to the subject, see *Ritualmordbeschuldigung* (1934), Chwolson (1901), Delitzsch (1883), Hayn (1906), Hellwig (1914), Holmes (1981), Hsia (1988, 1992), Peuckert (1935), Stern (1893), Strack (1909), and Roth (1934), among others. For an especially insightful analysis regarding the iconographic and symbolic aspects of the legend, see Jeggle (1993).
267. Jews allegedly used Christian blood for religious and secular purposes: in preparing matzo; for annointing rabbis; for circumcision; in curing eye ailments; in stopping menstrual and other bleedings; in preventing epileptic seizures; for removing bodily odors; to ward off the evil eye; to make amulets, love potions, and magical powder; and to paint the bodies of the dead (see Peuckert 1935: 734).
268. Poliakov (1974: 60).
269. See Rappaport (1975: 95).
270. Holmes (1981: 266).
271. Rappaport (1975: 95).
272. Ibid.
273. Ibid.: 96.
274. See Holmes (1981: 266).
275. See Rappaport (1975: 96).
276. See Holmes (1981: 266–67).

277. In the earliest subtype of the legend, attested before 1200, the dead boy's voice (not his blood) issued miraculously from the well (Dundes 1991: 338-39). These early versions are related to the "blood test" (see n. 149 above on *Bahr-recht* and the *Singing Bone*).

278. See Dubnov (1926, n. 18) and Strack (1909: 179).

279. Documente (1882: 159).

280. Strack (1909: 191, 180, 183-84).

281. Known as "Sir Hugh or The Jew's Daughter" in ballad form (Child 1962: 240-41, n. 155), the tale circulated under the title of "Little Sir Hugh" and "Hugh of Lincoln" in the European oral tradition (e.g., Brunvand 1984: 90; and Dundes 1991: 338, n. 8).

282. This tale passed into common circulation through its place in Geoffrey Chaucer's Prioress's Tale in the *Canterbury Tales* (composed from about 1387 until his death in 1400), which relates "the mutilated boy" legend as a religious miracle and proclaims in the concluding stanza: "yonge Hugh of Lyncoln, slayn also with cursed Jewes . . . but a litel while ago" (Brunvand 1984: 91; also Archer 1984).

283. Child (1962: 240-41, n. 155).

284. See Brunvand (1984: 90-91).

285. Rappaport (1975: 96).

286. See Hsia (1988: 200).

287. See Dundes (1991: 357).

288. See Rappaport (1975: 102-3).

289. See Róth (1964: 192-93).

290. Ibid.: 197.

291. Examples include Frankfurt (1241), Ortenburg (1245), Meiningen (1243), Pforzheim (1244), Sinzig (1265), Koblenz (1265), Mainz (1283), Bacharach (1283), Sinzig (1287), Cochem (1287), Lahnstein (1287), and Bonn (1288). For additional sources regarding late medieval pogroms in the German Rhineland, consult Aronius (1902), Berliner (1900), Kober (1931), Liebe (1903), Róth (1964: 200-201, 210-11), Salfeld (1898), and Stobbe (1866), among others.

292. This example, like those which follow, is taken from Rappaport (1975: 96).

293. Strack (1909: 178, 261).

294. Hsia (1988: 202).

295. See Róth (1964: 213-14).

296. Ibid.: 216.

297. Ibid.: 217.

298. See Roth (1934), Stern (1893), Dundes (1991: 344), and *Päpstlichen* (1900). Only two purported victims of ritual murder were to be officially recognized by the papacy: Andreas of Rinn and Simon of Trent.

299. See Stern (1893: 14-17) and Roth (1934: 21).

300. See Dundes (1991).

301. See Hsia (1992).

302. "Persistence" (1975: 283).

303. See Hsia (1988: 218).

304. See Dundes (1991: 341).

305. Hsia (1988: 222).

306. In fact, the cult continued until 1985 (Hsia 1988: 22, n. 76; Dundes 1991: 342-43; Rappaport 1975). Under National Socialism, the legend of Judenstein was used for racial anti-Semitic propaganda. In 1984, Reinhold, bishop of Inns-

bruck, ordered the suppression of the cult. This led to confrontations between the clergy and the parishioners, who rallied to a defense of their "Anderl of Rinn" (Riedl 1985: 74). Additional modern cases were reported elsewhere (e.g., Rappaport 1975; Roth 1934; Hsia 1988; *Ritualmordbeschuldigung* 1934; "Persistence" 1975; and Balaban 1930).

307. See Anderson (1964: 14).
308. See Hauser (1969: 123).
309. See Dundes (1991: 342).
310. See Hsia (1988: 210–13).
311. See Shachar (1974) and Dundes (1984) for a more extended discussion of this motif of scatology and feces in German anti-Semitism during the Reformation.
312. See Roth (1934: 17).
313. See Rappaport (1975: 108).

Chapter 5. Mapping the Modern Body

1. See Duden (1991: 4).
2. See Rothman et al. (1995: 3) and Bynum (1987).
3. Duden (1991: 8).
4. See Delumeau (1978), Bynum (1987), and O'Neill (1984).
5. See Accati (1979).
6. See Foucault (1979).
7. Muchembled (1985: 248).
8. See Camporesi (1984: 16–18).
9. See Duden (1991: 9).
10. See Temkin (1977), Ackerknecht (1971), and Mann (1984).
11. See Haeser (1971: 280) and Linebaugh (1975).
12. Strack (1909: 92).
13. Ibid.: 93.
14. Ibid.: 95.
15. Ibid.: 101–2, 115.
16. Ibid.: 100–101.
17. Ibid.: 97–100.
18. On the magical uses of blood, see Achelis (1892), Ankert (1918), Herrmann (1969), Jahn (1886, 1888), Lammert (1869), and Schrenk (1971, 1974).
19. See Grimm (1884: 1125).
20. Ibid.
21. Strack (1909: 86–87). Consult Strack (1909: 85–88) for additional examples of the specific regional and local articulations of this blood ethos.
22. Bächtold-Stäubli (1929: 1437).
23. Ibid.: 1438.
24. See Dölger (1926: 208–9) and Hsia (1988: 8).
25. See Bächtold-Stäubli (1929: 1438)
26. See Stemplinger (1927: 1430).
27. Strack (1900: 30–31).
28. See Bächtold-Stäubli (1929: 1436) and Hertz (1862).
29. See Hsia (1988: 9).
30. See Benz (1977: 81–83).
31. See Bächtold-Stäubli (1929: 1437).

32. Ibid.: 1437–38.
33. See Zimmels (1956).
34. See Strack (1909: 163)
35. See Stemplinger (1927).
36. See Strack (1909: 56–57).
37. See Hsia (1988, chap. 7).
38. See Franz (1902) and Browe (1933).
39. Franz (1902: 730).
40. Franz (1902: 32) and Browe (1933: 36–38).
41. See Browe (1930: 135–37).
42. See Browe (1930: 137–40) and Hsia (1988: 10).
43. See Browe (1930: 140).
44. Ibid.: 141–42.
45. See Hsia (1988: 126–28). For a synopsis of Eck's publication, *Ains Juden-büchlins Verlegung*, see Graetz (1897) and Hsia (1988).
46. See Hsia (1988: 127).
47. See Stemplinger (1927: 1140).
48. See Hsia (1988).
49. See Trachtenberg (1943).
50. See Dörfler (1892), Marzell (1929, 1932, 1936), Haase (1897, 1898), and Mannhardt (1904).
51. See Köhler (1891: 27), Marzell (1929: 81; 1932: 171; 1936: 175), Mannhardt (1904: 21–22), and Strack (1909: 66–67).
52. These examples are taken from Strack (1909: 66–69).
53. Strack (1909:65).
54. *Curieuse* (1700: 40), and Strack (1909: 57).
55. Quoted in Strack (1909: 52–53, 30).
56. *Curieuse* (1700: 45), in Strack (1900: 30–31).
57. See Strack (1909: 55).
58. Consult Strack (1909: 50–61, 70–84) and Dölger (1926: 207–8).
59. Strack (1909: 50–61, 70–84), Bächtold-Stäubli (1929: 1437–38), and Stemplinger (1927).
60. Strack (1900: 30).
61. Strack (1909: 70).
62. Ibid.
63. See Ur-Quell (1893: 99).
64. Strack (1909: 71).
65. Ibid.: 70.
66. See Ankert (1918: 131).
67. See Tannahill (1975: 64) and Strack (1909: 71).
68. See Strack (1909: 71–72).
69. In Rochholz (1862: 40).
70. In Strack (1900: 44).
71. Ibid.: 45.
72. See Payer (1984).
73. In *Vallicellian Penitential*, vol. 1, p. 97, Capitula Pseudo-Romanum 11. See Wiedemann (1892b: 182), Schmitz (1958, 1: 318–20, 480), and Wasserschleben (1851: 369, 121, 147, 160, 175, 316–17, 415, 677).
74. In *Penitential of Cummean*, Capitula iudiciorum 23. See Wasserschleben (1851: 137, 153, 180, 254, 300, 446) and Schmitz (1958, 1: 3812, 668; 1958, 2: 184, 541).

75. In *Parisian Penitential* 18. See Schmitz (1958, 1: 617, 748) and Wasserschleben (1851: 137, 446, 466).

76. In *Cummean Penitential* III. 3, b. 32. See Wasserschleben (1851: 468, 158, 317, 446), Schmitz (1958, 1: 480, 531, 562, 691), and Wiedemann (1892b: 183).

77. See Wiedemann (1892b: 183).

78. In the *Paenitentiale ad Heribaldum* (853 A.D.). See Payer (1984: 68).

79. Tale type motif D 1335.3.1.

80. See Bolte and Polivka (1923: 281).

81. See Grimm (1884: 1125).

82. See Rochholz (1856: 22).

83. Ibid.: 64.

84. Strack (1909: 64).

85. Cassel (1882: 184–85).

86. Simrock (1865: 237).

87. See Strack (1909: 64–65).

88. Cassel (1882: 197–214) and Grimm and Grimm (1815: 172).

89. Strack (1909: 89).

90. This metaphorical linkage of blood sacrifice and cleansing persists in contemporary German idioms: for instance, to prepare a blood bath (*ein Blutbad anrichten*) means, in a figurative sense, to slaughter a large number of people; but in a literal sense it refers to a bathing or washing of the dirt-stained body with blood (Grimm 1860: 175; Götze 1939: 376).

91. See Hsia (1988: 6).

92. See Delumeau (1978).

93. See Strack (1909: 89–91).

94. These same images appear in a recent German publication on blood (Nössler and Flocke 1997), which celebrates female vampirism, lesbianism, and the erotic consumption of blood by women.

95. Ury (1700: 34).

96. See Carter (1982: 223).

97. Ibid. The text derives from a thirteenth-century Latin manuscript that was translated into English verse in 1608.

98. See Rothman et al. (1995: 4).

99. In Page (1981: 22).

100. See Peters (1900: 41).

101. Peters (1900: 41–42).

102. As suggested by the index of Forbes et al. (1832–1835); cf. Carter (1982: 223).

103. See the entry in *Lancet* 10 (1827): 624.

104. Ury (1700: 34, 44).

105. In Peters (1900: 41).

106. Ibid.

107. Ibid.: 56a (enclosure 2).

108. Ibid.: 40.

109. See Ury (1700: 36–45); my summary.

110. Page (1981: 22).

111. See Ury (1700: 46–63).

112. Ibid.: 74.

113. Ibid.: 75.

114. See Carter (1982: 229)

115. Forbes et al. (1832: 518).

116. Forbes et al. (1834: 62).
117. Forbes et al. (1832: 52, 92, 159, 468).
118. Forbes et al. (1833: 369).
119. Forbes et al. (1832: 98, 100).
120. For instance, Bettelheim (1954).
121. See Carter (1982: 228).
122. Ibid.: 229.
123. See Page (1981: 24) and Peters (1900: 40).
124. See Carter (1982: 224).
125. Peters (1900:40).
126. See Bullough (1973: 486).
127. See Temkin (1973: 102).
128. See Sennett (1994: 163).
129. In Temkin (1973: 103).
130. See Sennett (1994: 163–64).
131. See Tannahill (1975: 62).
132. Ibid.
133. Kant (1800 [1974]: 153–57).
134. Duden (1991: 11).
135. See Calvi (1989).
136. See Duden (1991: 71)
137. See Farge (1979).
138. See Duden (1991: 108).
139. Ibid.: 108–9.
140. Ibid.: 111.
141. Ibid.
142. Ibid.: 112.
143. See Zedler (1745: 526).
144. For specific cultural histories of menstruation in northern Europe, see Showalter and Showalter (1970), Hirsch (1922), Crawford (1981), Fischer-Homburger (1979), and Lupton (1993).
145. See Duden (1991: 113).
146. Ibid.: 113–14. The translations of Storch's texts have been adapted from Duden (1991).
147. Storch (1747b: 548).
148. Ibid.: 549.
149. Ibid.: 553.
150. Ibid.: 114.
151. Ibid.: 547.
152. See Juncker (1724: 752).
153. Storch (1747b: 547).
154. Ibid.: 74.
155. See Storch (1747b: 99; 1752: 165; 1751a: 577; 1752: 99; 1752: 319).
156. Zedler (1737: 1643).
157. See Duden (1991: 115, n. 11).
158. See Storch (1752: 277).
159. Ibid.: 279.
160. Duden (1991: 115).
161. Ibid.
162. See Höfler (1899: 4).
163. See Zedler (1735: 123).

164. Duden (1991: 116).
165. See Stahl (1730) and Alberti (1702).
166. Alberti (1722, part 2: 3).
167. Duden (1991).
168. Ibid.: 117.
169. See Schurig (1744: 275).
170. Ibid., and Duden (1991: 117).
171. Additional categories of flux discharge were distinguished in general medical practice, among them catarrh, wound secretion, intestinal and bowel flux, apopleptic fit, rheumatism, fontanel, menses, and lochia (Höfler 1899:159–64). The term was used until the end of the eighteenth century, by humoral pathologists as well as in popular medicine. But in everyday German usage, the term persists in the twentieth century. Thus in October 1997, I was informed by my mother (a seventy-year-old retired teacher) that she had experienced a sudden loss of hearing in her right ear, a condition that was diagnosed by her sister, an educated pharmacist, as a violent attack of "flux" (*Blutsturz*), a dangerous accumulation and "stagnation" of blood in the inner ear that required immediate medical attention and the prescription of purgatory (blood-liquifying) remedies. The German physician commenced treatment, which included the use of eardrops and blood-thinning curatives!
172. Duden (1991: 120).
173. Ibid.
174. Storch (1748: 439).
175. Storch (1747b: 154).
176. Ibid.: 333.
177. Storch (1751a: 756).
178. Storch (1747a: 19).
179. Juncker (1725: 83–84).
180. Duden (1991: 122).
181. See Storch (1747b: 452, case 125).
182. See Storch (1747b: 249, case 58).
183. Duden (1991: 124).
184. Ibid.: 227, n. 43.
185. Ibid.
186. Storch (1747b: 220).
187. Duden (1991: 125).
188. Storch (1747b: 222).
189. Storch (1751a: 190).
190. Storch (1752: 454).
191. Storch (1748: 112).
192. Duden (1991: 126).
193. Ibid.: 127.
194. Storch (1747b: 246).
195. See Duden (1991: 128).
196. Storch (1747b: 248, case 56).
197. Storch (1752: 456, case 131).
198. Ibid.: 457.
199. Ibid.: 458.
200. These concepts of blood "stagnation" persist in modern German medical practice. In November 1997, I came across an advertisement for a salve for treating "heavy legs"; it was printed on the enclosing cover of my German train

ticket, and used the following language: "For application in cases of swelling and stagnation [*Stauungen*], . . . and blood accumulations," resulting in "tired, heavy, and aching legs"; "available only in your apothecary."

201. Storch (1751b: 1, case 1, no. 1).
202. Duden (1991: 134).
203. Storch (1751b: 175).
204. Duden (1991: 137).
205. Storch (1752: 435).
206. Ibid.: 556, 438.
207. Ibid.: 107.
208. Ibid.: 438.
209. Duden (1991: 138).
210. See Storch (1752: 328, case 80).
211. See Storch (1751a: 623, case 297).
212. Storch (1752: 582).
213. Duden (1991: 139).
214. Storch (1749b: 32).

Chapter 6. Between Blood and Soil

1. See Leonhardt (1934: 188).
2. Burke (1984: 76).
3. See Müller-Freienfels (1936: 77) and Braatz (1971: 166).
4. See Cassirer (1946) and Mosse (1975).
5. See Kamenetsky (1977: 168–69).
6. Such statements, often accompanied by visual images, were typical of the texts published in the anthropological journal *Volk und Rasse* during the 1930s.
7. See Berning (1960: 82–83).
8. See Roberts (1938: 54).
9. Darré (1936: 12). Also see Wiegand (1937: 39) and *Völkischer Beobachter* (7 April 1944), 1.
10. Rechenbach (1937: 219).
11. See Hitler (1939: 754–55).
12. Ibid.: 760.
13. See Bidiss (1975: 16) and Cassirer (1946: 245).
14. See Burke (1984: 64, 67).
15. Hitler (1939: 357).
16. Ibid.: 751–52.
17. See Strack (1909) and Dundes (1991).
18. In *Der Völkische Beobachter* (9 May 1944), 2.
19. Ibid. (17 April 17 1943), 1.
20. Ibid. (11 March 1943), 1.
21. Ibid. (17 April 1943), headline.
22. Ibid. (15 August 1933), 3.
23. Hitler (1939: 269, 339, 739).
24. See Bidiss (1975: 16).
25. Rosenberg (1935: 461).
26. For instance, Dundes (1984: 119–53).
27. See Mieder (1982: 442).
28. Translated by Mieder (1982: 442).

29. See Kamenetsky (1977: 168).

30. See, for instance, Bausinger (1965), Berning (1960), Ehlich (1989), Glunk (1966), Kamenetsky (1972), Linke (1995), Lixfeld (1994), Sauers (1978), and Voigt (1967, 1974).

31. See especially Kamenetsky (1977), Kecskemeti and Leites (1947), Seidel and Seidel-Slotty (1961), Frind (1964, 1966), Mieder (1983), and Betz (1955).

32. See Domarus (1962, 1: 86, 205).

33. See Mieder (1982: 441).

34. See Bergmann (1936a: 296–97).

35. Mieder (1982: 450).

36. Bergmann (1936b: 367).

37. Ibid.

38. See Vondung (1979: 399).

39. Hitler (1938).

40. See Mosse (1975: 26).

41. Ibid.: 23.

42. In Domarus (1962, 1: 533).

43. See Kecskemeti and Leites (1948: III, 244–45; 1948: IV, 15; 1947: I, 145, 151–52; 1948: II, 91–93), and Bosmajian (1979: 7).

44. In Rauschning (1939: 237).

45. Hitler (1939: 278).

46. See Braatz (1971: 169).

47. In Kotze and Krausnick (1966: 126–27).

48. See Schwab (1937: 19–20) and Gütt et al. (1937).

49. See Gross (1937: 83) and Schröder (1934: 155).

50. See Berning (1960: 96, 100) and Frind (1964: 104).

51. See Wülker (1937: 234–41).

52. See Schwanitz (1937: 249–52).

53. Gütt (1936a: 325). Also see *Völkischer Beobachter* 15, no. 1 (1940), 10.

54. In Kotze and Krausnick (1966: 156–57).

55. See Mosse (1975: 3).

56. The "blood banner" (*Blutfahne*) refers to the swastika that was carried in Hitler's abortive Beerhall putsch on 18 November 1923. Under National Socialism, the participants in this event were integrated into an "order of the blood" as a symbol of their early membership in the Nazi movement (cf. Paechter 1944: 22; Spalding 1957: 359; Götze 1939: 376; and Kogon 1958: 49).

Chapter 7. Gendered Difference, Violent Imagination

1. See Linke (1995:57). For an expanded discussion, see Schrep (1983: 72–73) and Lange-Feldhahn et al. (1983: 207, 209).

2. See Elias (1939) and Weber (1947).

3. For instance, Durkheim (1933), Sorel (1941), Foucault (1979), Girard (1979), Freud (1961), and Canetti (1973).

4. Fein (1979) and Melson (1992).

5. See Hilberg (1985), Lifton (1986), Friedlander (1995), Bartov (1996), and Herzfeld (1992).

6. See Feldman (1991), Kuper (1981), Malkki (1995a), and Tilly (1970).

7. See Brubaker (1992) and Borneman (1992b: 48–52).

8. See Williams (1995).

9. See Handler (1988), Herzfeld (1987), Hobsbawm and Ranger (1983), and Linke (1997).

10. See Heitmeyer (1992), Held and Horn (1992), Hoffmeister and Sill (1993), Marx (1994), and Linke (1995).

11. See Feldman (1991) and de Lauretis (1989).

12. See Proctor (1988), Lifton (1986), Aly et al. (1994), Friedlander (1995), Mosse (1985: 133–52), and Müller-Hill (1988).

13. See Gilman (1992: 178).

14. See Linke (1995), Herzfeld (1992: 17–70), and Theweleit (1987).

15. See Brubaker (1992).

16. See Lidtke (1982: 174, 182–83, 185) and Theweleit (1987: 234, nn. 26, 27).

17. See Bächtold-Stäubli (1917: 3).

18. See Theweleit (1987: 236–37).

19. See Ebermann and Trampert (1991: 10).

20. Ibid.: 12.

21. Ibid.

22. See Otto (1988: 14) and Jhering (1988: 79).

23. See Mattson (1995: 72–73).

24. According to Minkenberg (1994), a preoccupation with hierarchy, order, continuity of tradition, and status quo defines the agenda of the political right. A concern with secular and egalitarian issues, discontinuity, and revolutionary or futuristic transformations designates the agenda of the political left. Minkenberg examines the dualism or political polarization of "left" and "right" from a historical perspective, tracing the shifting articulations of this polarization from the French Revolution to the German post-cold war era. He argues that despite ideological changes based on religion, class, income, and post-materialist concerns (i.e., the "new" left), the dichotomization of German political parties into left and right has been meaningfully maintained.

25. The working dinner (on 11 January 1989) was organized by Ministerial Counsellor Götz Freiherr von Groll (i.e., the representative of the Federal Foreign Ministry in West Berlin). The aim of the evening was to bring together German politicians with American academics, in this case Bosch and SSRC Fellows resident in Berlin, to discuss issues of relevance to the still divided city and its role in Western European politics. Since the event was scheduled a few weeks before the upcoming Berlin Senate elections, the political representatives took the opportunity to present their official party platforms. In addition to the Green/Alternative representative, the Christian Democrats, the Free Democrats, and the Social Democrats each had one delegate.

26. Vonnekold's remark here refers to the citizenship law of the Federal Republic of Germany, which defines "national belonging" and citizenry through the idiom of descent, as expressed by the Latin term *jus sanguinis*, "power/law of blood" (Article 116, Basic Law; see Senders 1996).

27. The event, sponsored by Die Gruppe Grüne Panther, a splinter group of the Green/Alternative Party in Berlin, was scheduled for 3 February 1989. The second in a series of discussions, the meeting revolved around the adoption of federal laws by West Berlin and the possible opposition to such a "nationalization" or legal incorporation of the city by a potential Green/Alternative and Social Democratic coalition ("Veranstaltung 2: Übernahme von Bundesgesetzen—eine Hürde für Rot-Grün?" Discussants: H. Gassner, Dr. E. Körting, R. Künast).

28. See Gruhl (1990: 148).

29. See Senders (1996).
30. See Brubaker (1992).
31. See Wildenthal (1994a, 1994b).
32. See Archiv für Sozialpolitik (1993a: 31; 1993b: 16).
33. See Linke (1992), and Chapter 1, above.
34. See Gilman (1986, 1987).
35. See Dundes (1991), Hsia (1988), and Geller (1992).
36. See Gallagher and Laqueur (1987), Poovey (1988), and Foucault (1973).
37. See Foucault (1978) and Turner (1984).
38. See Gilman (1992).
39. See Mosse (1985) and Herzfeld (1992).
40. Friedrich Ebert (1870–1925) was the first president of the German Republic. The son of a tailor, he became a harness maker, joined the Social Democratic Party, was elected to the Reichstag in 1912, and assumed leadership after Bebel's death, representing henceforth the extreme rightist wing of the Social Democratic Party (e.g., Lowie 1945: 117).
41. Rabinbach and Benjamin (1989: xv).
42. Dwinger (1939: 296). In Theweleit (1987: 177).
43. Dwinger (1939: 276ff). In Theweleit (1987: 179–80).
44. Theweleit (1987: 191).
45. See Salomon (1930: 180, 184). In Theweleit (1987: 65).
46. Theweleit (1987: 191–92) makes this point by relying heavily on Sigmund Freud, who argued in his *Interpretation of Dreams* (1976) that the equation betwen mouth and vagina/womb was not a mere product of unconscious thinking but could be attested in linguistic usage by drawing a parallel between the *labia* and the *lips* that frame the aperture of the mouth. Therefore, the secretions of the human body emerging from the two body parts can, in some contexts, function as symbolic replacements. Emily Martin (1990) offers a feminist interpretation of the connection between the female mouth and the vagina/womb. She argues that the link is one of control, that is, the attempts in modern Western history by medical/political interests to take control of women's bodies and sexuality.
47. Interestingly, Theweleit himself rarely uses the term *rape*, which appears twice in the entire volume. Instead, he applies the image of "sexual intercourse" to these violent encounters, although he does acknowledge that "the penis is also put to use in nonsymbolic ways as a weapon" (1987: 192, n.). The notion of rape seems more appropriate to these instances.
48. See Dwinger (1935: 141, 144). In Theweleit (1987: 187–89).
49. Theweleit (1987: 229).
50. Ibid.
51. Ehrenreich (1987: xv).
52. See Bartov (1996).
53. See Nordstrom (1996) and Feldman (1995).
54. See Enloe (1993), Nordstrom (1991), Olujic (1995), Stiglmayer (1994), and Sutton (1995).
55. See Schwerdtfeger (1980) and Senders (1996).
56. For instance, Linke (1982).
57. See Klee (1975) and Linke (1982).
58. See Borneman (1992a), Linke (1982), and Senders (1996).
59. See Birkenmaier (1980: 3).
60. See Fromme (1980a: 1).
61. See Birkenmaier (1980: 3).

62. Alfelder Zeitung (1980a: 1).
63. Frankfurter Allgemeine Zeitung (1980h: 1).
64. Spiegel (1980a: 17).
65. Spiegel (1980b: 32).
66. Rhein-Zeitung (1980c).
67. Spiegel (1980b: 34).
68. Fromme (1980a: 1).
69. Frankfurter Allgemeine Zeitung (1980j: 2).
70. Fromme (1980b: 10).
71. Alfelder Zeitung (1980b).
72. Philipp (1980).
73. Frankfurter Allgemeine Zeitung (1980d: 1).
74. Klein (1980).
75. Fluid metaphors also appear in the American media, but without the corresponding expressions of repugnance and nationwide catastrophe. For example, descriptions of the influx of Haitian refugees into the United States abound with references to "the tide," "the flood," "the flow," which "comes," "surges," "rises," and "swamps" (Greenhouse 1994a: 1, 6; 1994b: 3). But an earlier analysis of American media images and political metaphors of Cuban refugees in 1980 suggests that such liquid metaphors and underlying fears of immigrant "waves" were linked to perceived threats of sexual attack (Borneman 1986). Although regarded as a "male threat" at this time, such a gendered perception of Cuban refugees was grounded in fears of feminization: an implosion of "the Cuban gay male threat," the "red (Cuban/Communist) invasion," and "the erosion of American masculinity." These were images framed by political fears of disorder, loss of control, perversion, illegality, and criminality. Other regimes of representation and corporeality are pertinent in transnational media images of refugees and transborder populations elsewhere (Seremetakis 1996; Malkki 1996b).
76. Frankfurter Allgemeine Zeitung (1980c).
77. Rhein-Zeitung (1980b).
78. Birkenmaier (1980: 3).
79. Edinger (1986: 56–57).
80. Frankfurter Allgemeine Zeitung (1980e: 1–2).
81. Spiegel (1980a: 17).
82. Frankfurter Allgemeine Zeitung (1980f).
83. Spiegel (1980a: 18).
84. See, for instance, Philipp (1980). The reference to "over-foreignization" appeared continually in most media reports from January through July of 1980. The term was popularized once again in the early 1990s. The initial use of this word can be traced to the 1930s and 1940s, when it carried anti-Semitic connotations.
85. Frankfurter Allgemeine Zeitung (1980i: 1).
86. Frankfurter Allgemeine Zeitung (1980k).
87. See Schütt (1981: 65).
88. Archiv für Sozialpolitik (1994b: 38).
89. Archiv für Sozialpolitik (1993d: 23).
90. Archiv für Sozialpolitik (1994a: 35).
91. Archiv für Sozialpolitik (1994a: 32).
92. Spiegel (1980a: 18).
93. Frankfurter Allgemeine Zeitung (1980d: 2).

94. Birkenmaier (1980: 3).

95. Spiegel (1980b: 32).

96. For additional examples, see Frankfurter Allgemeine Zeitung (1980a: 4; 1980e: 2; 1980g: 1), and Alfelder Zeitung (1980a). In a technical sense, the word *Sammellager* should be translated as "assembly camp": German *sammeln* means gather together, assort, collect, assemble. But *Sammellager* can be read, I believe, as a postwar locution for *Konzentrationslager* (concentration camp), a Nazi term whose usage is categorically taboo except as a historical signifier. Yet this insertion of *Sammellager* into political language conveys something more than a convenient terminological displacement. It also points to a profound denial of history, a muting of collective memory. In German (as of course in English, too), *Konzentration* means "to focus," "to fix one's attention upon something," and "to gather one's thoughts or efforts to accomplish a matter." These are meanings that disclose the Nazis' programmatic use of camps for physical annihilation, a murderous campaign semantically disguised as a concentrated mental effort: that is, the political conception of a "final solution" for the "Jewish problem." But unlike the corresponding English terms, *Konzentration* or *konzentrieren* lacks connotations of internment: in German, "concentration camps" are semantically, and linguistically, configured as death camps. The current German use of *Sammellager* represses this nexus to murder entirely. By a shift of meaning to "rounding up" or "amassing" people," it prevents the disturbing evocation of the past. Nevertheless, the intent behind such camps is not entirely benign. As suggested by the semantic field of *Sammellager*, the internment of refugees is perceived as a means to "regain composure," to achieve "a state of tranquility or repose," and to become "self-possessed" (e.g., *sich sammeln*), meanings that hint at a cultural desire to purge the troublesome and foreign.

The move to house refugees in so-called concentration camps (*Sammellager*), an idea first suggested in Bavaria in the late 1970s, had a decided impact both on the public perception and on the public identity of the refugees (Mattson 1995: 74–75). Initially intended as one of the measures designed to scare away refugees (Münch 1992: 73) and later justified as necessary to simplify public assistance for the asylum applicants, these steps ironically were also defended as crucial to ensuring the safety of the refugees from attacks by right-wing extremists (Wassermann 1992: 16). Of course, it also became much easier for right-wing terrorists to find and attack the refugees that the government had brought together in large groups (Mattson 1995: 75). Thereby the "concentration" camps in fact facilitated the political goal to get rid of unwanted foreign populations.

97. Frankfurter Allgemeine Zeitung (1980b).

98. Spiegel (1980a: 18).

99. Fromme (1980b: 10).

100. See Lutz (1988) and Stewart (1993).

101. Frankfurter Allgemeine Zeitung (1980d: 1).

102. Spiegel (1980a: 17, 18).

103. Klein (1980).

104. Frankfurter Allgemeine Zeitung (1980d: 4).

105. Fromme (1980a: 1).

106. See Lutz and Collins (1993: 153).

107. For instance, Steward (1993).

108. For a closer reading of the legal semantics, see *Grundgesetz und Landesverfassung* (1971), a publication of the Institut für Staatsbürgerliche Bildung in Rheinland-Pfalz, which I consulted. In German legal rhetoric, basic rights are

typically granted through the invocation of phrases like *"Anspruch auf," "Recht auf," "hat das Recht"*—has a right to or can insist on (28, 32, 120–21). The term *geniessen* or "to enjoy" appears infrequently, and only in connection with certain types of "privileges": geographical mobility, freedom of residence and trade, political asylum and protection from extradition (see Basic Law [GG], articles 16.2 and 11.1, etc.). This vision of the consumption of rights probably emerged in response to the symbolic requirements of Germany's postwar capitalist economy.

109. See Borneman (1992a, 1992b).

110. See Fehrenbach (1995).

111. See Mattson (1995: 69).

112. See, for instance, Klein (1980), Philipp (1980), and Fromme (1980b). For a more extensive discussion of the negative connotations of terms like "refugee" and "asylum seeker" in German, see Gerhard and Link (1991), Jäger (1993), and Link (1983).

113. Rhein-Zeitung (1980a).

114. Spiegel (1980b: 35).

115. Douglas (1980).

116. Spiegel (1988b: 35).

117. Ibid.

118. See Fromme (1980a: 1).

119. See Mattson (1995: 80–81).

120. Quoted in (and translated by) Mattson (1995: 80).

121. See Fromme (1980a: 1).

122. See Heutgen (1980).

123. See Spiegel (1980a: 17).

124. See Linke (1997).

125. Anderson (1983); Linke (1990); Malkki (1995a/b).

126. Offe (1987: 2).

127. See Bhabha (1990) and Sedgwick (1992).

128. See Anthias and Yuval-Davis (1994).

129. See Yuval-Davis and Anthias (1989) and Martin (1990).

130. See Connell (1990).

131. See Parker et al. (1992: 6).

132. See Mosse (1985) and Theweleit (1987, 1989).

133. See Taussig (1992).

134. Allen Feldman (16 June 1996), personal communication.

Epilogue

1. Konkret (1994:42).

Bibliography

Accati, Louisa. 1979. "Lo spirito della Fornicazione." *Quaderni Storici* 41: 650.

Achelis, Thomas. 1892. "Über den Zauber mit Blut und Körperteilen von Menschen und Tieren." *Am Ur-Quell* 3: 81–86.

Ackerknecht, Ernst. 1971. "Primitive Autopsies and the History of Anatomy." In his *Medicine and Ethnology*. Vienna: Hans Huber.

Adams, Carol J. 1990. *The Sexual Politics of Meat*. New York: Continuum.

Albert the Great. 1894. *Opera omnia* (A. Borgnet, ed.). Vol. 29. Paris: Ludovicus Vivès.

———. 1916. *De animalibus libri XXVI nach der Cölner Urschrift*. Vol. 1. Münster: Aschendorff.

Alberti, Michael. 1702. *Dissertatio inauguralis medica, de haemorrhoidibus secundam et praeter naturam* (Erfurt). Reprinted in *Dissertationes academicae de haemorrhoidibus in peculiare volumen collectae*. Halle: Christian Henckel, 1719.

———. 1722. *Tractatus de haemorrhoidibus . . . pathologice et practice*. Halle: Impensis Orphanotropei.

Alexander of Hales. 1951–57. *Glossa in quatuor libros sententiarum* (Past and Present of the College of St. Bonaventure, eds.). 4 vols. Quaracchi: Collegium S. Bonaventurae.

Alfelder Zeitung. 1980a. "Kabinett stoppt Vorschlag zur Eindämmung der Asylbewerber." *Alfelder Zeitung* 129/130 (12 June): 1.

——— 1980b. "Asylverfahren wird beschleunigt." *Alfelder Zeitung* 152 (3 July).

Allen, Ann Taylor. 1991. *Feminism and Motherhood in Germany, 1800–1914*. New Brunswick, N.J.: Rutgers University Press.

Allen, Warner H. (ed.). 1908. *Celestina; or, the Tragic Comedy of Calisto and Meliba* (M. Jones, trans., 1631). London: Routledge.

Aly, Goetz, Peter Chroust, and Christian Pross. 1994. *Cleansing the Fatherland* (B. Cooper, trans.). Baltimore: Johns Hopkins University Press.

Amman, E. 1939. "Stigmatisation." In *Dictionnaire de théologie catholique* (A. Vacant et al., eds.). Vol. 14, pt. 1, cols. 2617–19. Paris: Letouzey et Ané.

Ammerman, A. J., and L. L. Cavalli-Sforza. 1984. *The Neolithic Transition and the Genetics of Population in Europe*. Princeton: Princeton University Press.

Ancelet-Hustache, Jeanne (ed.). 1930. "Les 'Vitae Sororum' d'Unterlinden." *Archives d'histoire doctrinale et lettéraire du moyen âge* 5: 317–509.

Anderson, Benedict. 1983. *Imagined Communities*. London: Verso.

Anderson, M. D. 1964. *A Saint at Stake: The Strange Death of William of Norwich, 1144*. London: Faber and Faber.

Andrieu, M. 1950. "Aux origines du culte du saint-sacrement." *Analecta Bollandiana* 68: 397–418.

Ankert, Heinrich. 1918. "Menschenblut als Medizin." *Österreichische Zeitschrift für Volkskunde* 24: 131.

Anthias, Floya, and Nira Yuval-Davis. 1994. "Women and the Nation-State." In *Nationalism* (J. Hutchinson and A. D. Smith, eds.), 312–16. Oxford: Oxford University Press.

Aquinas, Thomas. 1964. *Summa theologiae* (Blackfriars, eds.). 61 vols. New York: McGraw-Hill.

Archer, J. 1984. "The Structure of Anti-Semitism in the 'Prioress Tale.'" *Chaucer Review* 19: 46–54.

Archiv für Sozialpolitik. 1993a. "Jeder ist uns der Nächste." *Konkret* 1 (Jan.): 28–31.

———. 1993b. "Jeder ist uns der Nächste." *Konkret* 2 (Feb.): 14–17.

———. 1993c. "Jeder ist uns der Nächste." *Konkret* 10 (Oct.): 28–32.

———. 1993d. "Jeder ist uns der Nächste." *Konkret* 11 (Nov.): 23–24.

———. 1994a. "Jeder ist uns der Nächste." *Konkret* 3 (March): 32–36.

———. 1994b. "Jeder ist uns der Nächste." *Konkret* 5 (May): 38–39.

Ardener, Sheryl. 1975. *Perceiving Women.* New York: Wiley.

Arendt, Hannah. 1964. *Eichmann in Jerusalem.* Munich: R. Pieper.

Arens, W. 1979. *The Man-Eating Myth.* New York: Oxford University Press.

Arens, Wilhelm. 1943. "Der Baum als Symbol der Frau." *Volkswerk* (Berlin) 3: 259–66.

———. 1948. "Baum und Frau im Glauben des deutschen Volkes." *Österreichische Zeitschrift des Vereins für Volkskunde* (Vienna) 51: 70–80.

Aronius, Julius. 1902. *Regesten zur Geschichte der Juden im fränkischen und deutschen Reiche bis zum Jahre 1273.* Berlin: L. Simion.

Ashley-Montagu, M. F. 1937. *Coming into Being Among the Australian Aborigines.* London: Routledge.

Assion, Peter, and Stefan Wojciechowski. 1970. "Die Verehrung des heiligen Blutes von Wallduern bei Polen und Tschechen." *Archiv für Mittelrheinische Kirchengeschichte* 22: 141–67.

Assisi, Francis of. 1949. *Opuscula sancti patris Francisci Assisiensis.* 2d ed. Quaracchi: Collegium S. Bonaventurae.

Audelay, John. 1931. *The Poems of John Audelay* (E. K. Whiting, ed.). Early English Text Society, no. 184. London: Oxford University Press.

Bachelard, Gaston. 1964. *The Psychoanalysis of Fire* (A. C. M. Ross, trans.). Boston: Beacon Press.

Bachmann, Heinrich (ed.). 1953. *Ekkehards Waltharius.* Paderborn: Ferdinand Schöningh Verlag.

Bächtold-Stäubli, Hanns. 1917. *Deutscher Soldatenbrauch und Soldatenglaube.* Strasbourg: K. J. Trübner.

———. 1929. *Handwörterbuch des deutschen Aberglaubens.* Berlin: Walter de Gruyter.

———. 1930. "Geburtsbaum." In his *Handwörterbuch des deutschen Aberglaubens.* Vol. 1, no. 3, 419–22. Berlin: Walter de Gruyter.

Baix, F., and C. Lambot. 1964. *La Dévotion à l'eucharistie de le VIIe centenaire de la Fête-Dieu.* Gembloux: Duculot.

Balaban, Majer. 1930. "Hugo Grotius und die Ritualmordprozesse in Lublin (1636)." In *Festschrift* (Ismar Elbogen et al., eds.), 87–112. Berlin: Jüdischer Verlag.

Balys, J. 1942. "Baum und Mensch im litauischen Volksglauben." *Deutsche Volks-kunde* (Berlin) 13: 171–77.

Barthes, Roland. 1972. *Mythologies*. New York: Noonday Press.

Bartov, Omer. 1996. *Murder in Our Midst*. New York: Oxford University Press.

Bartsch, Karl. 1866. *Das Nibelungenlied*. Leipzig: Brockhaus.

———. 1880. *Das Nibelungenlied*. 2d ed. Leipzig: Brockhaus.

Battaglia, D. 1992. "The Body in the Gift." *American Ethnologist* 19 (1): 3–18.

Bauerreis, R. 1958. "Bluthostien." In *Lexikon für Theologie und Kirche* (J. Hofer and K. Rahner, eds.). Vol. 2. Freiburg: Herder Verlag.

Baum, P. F. 1922. "Judas's Red Hair." *Journal of English and German Philology* 21 (1): 520–29.

Bauman, Zygmunt. 1989. *Modernity and the Holocaust*. Ithaca: Cornell University Press.

Baumann, Hermann. 1986. *Das Doppelte Geschlecht*. Berlin: Dietrich Reimer Verlag.

Bauschatz, Paul C. 1982. *The Well and the Tree*. Amherst: University of Massachusetts Press.

Bausinger, Hermann. 1965. "Volksideologie und Volksforschung." *Zeitschrift für Volkskunde* 61: 177–204.

Becker, Ernest. 1973. *The Denial of Death*. New York: Free Press.

Bede. 1969. *Ecclesiastical History of the English People* (B. Colgrave and R. A. B. Mynors, eds.). Oxford: Oxford University Press.

———. N.d. "In die festo circumcisionis domini, homiliae genuinae." In *Patrologiae cursus completus: series latina* (J.-P. Migne, ed.). Vol. 94. Paris: Migne.

Beidelman, T. O. 1963. "The Blood Covenant and the Concept of Blood in Ukaguru." *Africa* 33 (4): 321–41.

Bell, C. H. 1922. "The Call of Blood in the Medieval German Epic." *Modern Language Notes* (Baltimore) 37 (1): 17–26.

Bell, Rudolph. 1985. *Holy Anorexia*. Chicago: University of Chicago Press.

Bellows, Henry Adams. 1923. *Edda Saemundar* (The Poetic Edda, Icelandic). 2 vols. New York: American-Scandinavian Foundation.

Bender, Barbara. 1987. "The Roots of Inequality." In *Domination and Resistance* (D. Miller, M. Rowlands, and C. Tilley, eds.). Cambridge: Cambridge University Press.

Bendix, Reinhard. 1978. *Kings or People*. Berkeley: University of California Press.

Benecke, G. F., and K. Lachmann (eds.). 1877. *Iwein, eine Erzählung von Hartmann von Aue*. 4th ed. Berlin: Ferdinand Dümmlers Verlagsbuchhandlung.

Benjamin, Jessica, and Anson Rabinbach. 1989. Foreword to *Male Fantasies*, by Klaus Theweleit. Vol. 2, ix–xxv. Minneapolis: University of Minnesota Press.

Benveniste, Emile. 1934. "Un nom indoeuropéen de la 'femme.'" *Bulletin de la Société de Linguistique de Paris* 35: 104–6.

———. 1969. *Le vocabulaire des institutions indo-européennes*. 2 vols. Paris: Éditions de Minuit.

———. 1973. *Indo-European Language and Society* (E. Palmer, trans.). Miami Linguistics Series, no. 12. Coral Gables: University of Miami Press.

Benz, Richard E. (ed.). 1977. *Historia von D. Johann Fausten, dem weitbeschreyten Zauberer und Schwarzkünstler*. Reprint. Stuttgart: Reclam.

Bergmann, Karl. 1936a. "Lebendige Rassenhygiene im deutschen Sprichwort." *Volk und Rasse* 11: 296–97.

———. 1936b. "Völkisches Gedankengut im deutschen Sprichwort." *Zeitschrift für deutsche Bildung* 12: 363–73.

Berliner, Abraham. 1900. *Aus dem inneren Leben der deutschen Juden im Mittelalter.* Berlin: M. Poppelauer.

Berning, Cornelia. 1960. "Die Sprache des Nationalsozialismus." *Zeitschrift für deutsche Wortforschung* 16 (1960): 71–149, 178–88; 17 (1961): 83–121, 171–82; 18 (1962): 108–18, 160–72; 19 (1963): 92–112. (All preceding references reflect article as published in parts.)

Bertaud, Emile. 1961. "Dévotion eucharistique." In *Dictionnaire de spiritualité, ascétique et mystique, doctrine et histoire* (M. Viller et al., eds.). Vol. 4, pt. 2. Paris: Beauchesne.

Berthold of Regensburg. 1968. *Deutsche Predigten* (D. Richter, ed.). Munich: W. Fink.

Bettelheim, Bruno. 1954. *Symbolic Wounds.* New York: Free Press.

———. 1962. *Symbolic Wounds.* Rev. ed. New York: Free Press of Glencoe/Collier Books.

Betz, Werner. 1955. "The National-Socialist Vocabulary." In *The Third Reich* (M. Baumont, J. Fried, and E. Vermeil, eds.), 784–96. New York: Praeger.

Bhabha, Homi K. (ed.). 1990. *Nation and Narration.* New York: Routledge.

Bidiss, Michael D. 1975. "European Racist Ideology, 1850–1945: Myths of the Blood." *Patterns of Prejudice* 9 (5): 11–9.

Binford, Lewis. 1962. "Archaeology as Anthropology." *American Antiquity* 28 (2): 217–25.

Bircher, Martin (ed.). 1970. *Die Fruchtbringende Gesellschaft: Quellen und Dokumente in vier Bänden.* Reprint from 1646. Munich: Kösel Verlag.

———. 1971. *Fürst Ludwig von Anhalt-Köthen: Der Fruchtbringenden Gesellschaft Nahmen, Vorhaben, Gemählde und Wörter (Frankfurt 1646).* Munich: Kösel Verlag.

Birkenmaier, Werner. 1980. "Das Asylrecht im Härtetest." *Deutsches Allgemeines Sonntagsblatt* 7 (17 Feb.): 3.

Birlinger, Anton. 1881. "Leben heiliger alemannischer Frauen des XIV–XV Jahrhunderts." *Alemannia* 9: 275–92.

Bloch, Ernst. 1990. *Heritage of Our Times.* Cambridge: MIT Press.

Bloch, Maurice. 1961. *Feudal Society.* Chicago: University of Chicago Press.

———. 1982. "Death, Women, and Power." In *Death and the Regeneration of Life* (M. Bloch and J. Parry, eds.), 211–30. Cambridge: Cambridge University Press.

Bloch, Maurice, and Jonathan Parry (eds.). 1982. *Death and the Regeneration of Life.* Cambridge: Cambridge University Press.

Bloch, R. Howard. 1986. "Medieval Misogyny." In *Continuity and Change* (E. Vestergaard, ed.). Odense: Odense University Press.

Bodenstedt, Mary Immaculate. 1944. *The "Vita Christi" of Ludolphus the Carthusian.* Washington, D.C.: Catholic University of America Press.

Bollandists (eds.). 1884. "Septilium B. Dorotheae, treatise 3: De eucharista." *Analecta Bollandiana* 3. Brussels: Société des Bollandistes.

———. 1899. "Life of Lukardis." In *Analecta Bollandiana* 18, chap. 6. Brussels: Société des Bollandistes.

Bollandus, J., and G. Henschenius. 1863. "Life of Gertrude van Oosten." In *Acta sanctorum . . . editio novissima* (J. Carnandet et al., eds.). Vol. 1, 349–53. Paris: Palmé.

———. 1865a. "Life of Margaret of Cortona." *In Acta sanctorum . . . editio novissima* (J. Carnandet et al., eds.). Vol. 3, 304–63. Paris: Palmé.

———. 1865b. *Acta sanctorum . . . editio novissima* (J. Carnandet et al., eds.). Vol. 3. Paris: Palmé.

————. 1866. "Life of Alda of Siena." *In Acta sanctorum . . . editio novissima* (J. Carnandet et al., eds.). Vol. 3. Paris: Palmé.

————. 1894. "Life of Alpaïs of Cudot." In *Acta sanctorum . . . editio novissima* (J. Carnandet et al., eds.). Vol. 2 (Nov.), pt. 1, 167–209. Brussels: Palmé.

Bolte, Johannes, and Lutz Mackensen. 1930. *Handwörterbuch des deutschen Märchens.* Vol. 1. Berlin: Walter de Gruyter.

Bolte, Johannes, and Georg Polivka (eds.). 1913. "28. Der Singende Knochen." In their *Anmerkungen zu den Kinder- und Hausmärchen der Brüder Grimm,* 260–76. Leipzig: Dieterichsche Verlagsbuchhandlung.

————. 1913–31. *Anmerkungen zu den Kinder- und Hausmärchen der Brüder Grimm.* 5 vols. Leipzig: Dieterichsche Verlagsbuchhandlung.

Borneman, John. 1986. "Emigres as Bullets: Immigration as Penetration." *Journal of Popular Culture* 20 (3): 73–92.

————. 1992a. *Belonging in the Two Berlins.* Cambridge: Cambridge University Press.

————. 1992b. "State, Territory, and Identity Formation in the Postwar Berlins, 1945–1989." *Cultural Anthropology* 7 (1): 45–62.

Bosco-Gualteri, Martin of. 1865. "Life of Jane Mary of Maillé." In J. Bollandus and G. Henschenius, *Acta sanctorum . . . editio novissima* (J. Carnandet et al., eds.). Vol. 3 (March), 734–44. Paris: Palmé.

Bosmajian, Hamida. 1979. *Metaphors of Evil.* Iowa City: University of Iowa Press.

Bosworth, Joseph. 1882. *An Anglo-Saxon Dictionary* (T. Northcote Toller, ed.). Oxford: Clarendon Press.

Bötticher, Gotthold. 1899. *Hildenbrandlied und Waltharilied nebst den 'Zaubersprüchen' und 'Muspilli' als Beigaben.* Halle: Verlag der Buchhandlung des Waisenhauses.

Bottigheimer, Ruth. 1987. *Grimms' Bad Girls and Bold Boys.* New Haven: Yale University Press.

Bouquet, Mary. 1996. "Family Trees and Their Affinities: The Visual Imperative of the Genealogical Diagram." *Journal of the Royal Anthropological Institute,* n.s., 2: 43–66.

Bourdieu, Pierre. 1977. *Outline of a Theory of Practice* (R. Nice, trans.). New York: Cambridge University Press.

Bowler, Peter J. 1971. "Preformation and Pre-Existence in the Seventeenth Century." *Journal of the History of Biology* 4: 221–44.

Braatz, Werner E. 1971. "The Völkisch Ideology and Anti-Semitism in Germany." *Yivo Annual of Jewish Social Sciences* 15: 166–87.

Bradley, Ritamary. 1976. "The Motherhood Theme in Julian of Norwich." *Fourteenth-Century English Mystics Newsletter* 2 (4): 25–30.

Brain, James L. 1988. "Male Menstruation in History and Anthropology." *Journal of Psychohistory* 15 (3): 311–23.

Brandes, Stanley. 1980. *Metaphors of Masculinity.* Philadelphia: University of Pennsylvania Press.

Braun, J. 1924. *Der christliche Altar in seiner geschichtlichen Entwicklung.* 2 vols. Munich: Koch.

Breest, Ernst. 1881. "Das Wunderblut von Wilsnack (1383–1552). Quellenmäßige Darstellung seiner Geschichte." *Märkische Forschungen* 16: 130–302.

Brinton, Thomas. 1954. *The Sermons of Thomas Brinton, Bishop of Rochester (1373–1389)* (M. A. Devlin, ed.). Camden 3d ser., 85–86. London: Offices of the Royal Historical Society.

Brodeur, Arthur Gilchrist (trans.). 1916. *The Prose Edda by Snorri Sturluson.* New York: American-Scandinavian Foundation.

―――. 1929. *The Prose Edda by Snorri Sturluson.* 2d ed. New York: American-Scandinavian Foundation.

Brooke, C. N. L. 1967. "Religious Sentiment and Church Design in the Later Middle Ages." *Bulletin of the John Rylands Library* 50 (1): 13–33.

Browe, Peter. 1930. "Die Eucharistie als Zaubermittel im Mittelalter." *Archiv für Kulturgeschichte* 20: 134–54.

―――. 1932. "Die Kommunionvorbereitung im Mittelalter." *Zeitschrift für Kirchengeschichte* 20: 134–54.

―――. 1933. *Die Verehrung der Eucharistie im Mittelalter.* Munich: Hueber.

―――. 1938. *Die Eucharistischen Wunder des Mittelalters.* Breslauer Studien zur historischen Theologie, n.s., 4. Breslau: Müller and Seifert.

Brown, Paula, and Donald Tuzin (eds.). 1983. *The Ethnography of Cannibalism.* Washington, D.C.: Society for Psychological Anthropology.

Brown, Peter. 1981. *The Cult of the Saints.* London: SCM.

―――. 1988. *The Body and Society: Men, Women, and Sexual Renunciation in Early Christianity.* New York: Faber.

Brubaker, Rogers. 1992. *Citizenship and Nationhood in France and Germany.* Cambridge: Harvard University Press.

Brunvand, Jan Harold. 1984. *The Choking Doberman and Other "New" Urban Legends.* New York: Norton.

Büchmann, Georg. 1907. *Geflügelte Worte.* (E. Ippel, ed.). 23d rev. ed. Berlin: Haude Verlag and Spenersche Buchhandlung.

Buck, Carl Darling. 1949. *A Dictionary of Selected Synonyms in the Principal Indo-European Languages.* Chicago: University of Chicago Press.

Buckley, Thomas, and Alma Gottlieb (eds.). 1988. *Blood Magic.* Berkeley: University of California Press.

Bühler, C. F. 1964. "Prayers and Charms in Certain Middle English Scrolls." *Speculum* 39: 270–78.

Bullough, Vern L. 1973. *The Subordinate Sex.* Urbana: University of Illinois Press.

Bunker, Henry Alden, and Bertram D. Lewin. 1951. "A Psychoanalytic Notation on the Root GN, KN, CN." In *Psychoanalysis and Culture* (G. B. Wilbur and W. Muensterberger, eds.), 363–67. New York: International Universities Press.

Burke, Kenneth. 1984. "The Rhetoric of Hitler's 'Battle.'" In *Language and Politics* (M. J. Shapiro, ed.), 61–80. New York: New York University Press.

Buttenwieser, Moses. 1919. "Blood Revenge and Burial Rites in Ancient Israel." *Journal of the American Oriental Society* 39: 303–21.

Butterworth, E. A. S. 1970. *The Tree at the Navel of the Earth.* Berlin: Walter de Gruyter.

Bynum, Caroline Walker. 1982. *Jesus as Mother.* Berkeley: University of California Press.

―――. 1987. *Holy Feast and Holy Fast.* Berkeley: University of California Press.

Byrnes, Aquinas (ed.). 1943. *The Hymns of the Dominican Missal and Breviary.* St. Louis: Herder.

Calvi, Giulia. 1989. *Histories of a Plague* (D. Bocca and B. T. Rogan, Jr. trans.). Berkeley: University of California Press.

Campano, Giovanni Antonio. 1495. *De circumcisione oratio.* Rome: E. Silber.

Camporesi, Piero. 1984. *Il sugo della vita: Simbolismo e magia del sangue.* Milan: Edizioni di Comunita.

Canetti, Elias. 1973. *Crowds and Power* (C. Stewart, trans.). New York: Continuum.

Cantimpré, Thomas of. 1866. "Life of Lutgard." In J. Bollandus and G. Henschenius, *Acta sanctorum . . . editio novissima* (J. Carnandet et al., eds.). Vol. 4. Paris: Palmé.

Capua, Raymond of. 1865. "Life of Catherine of Siena: Legenda maior," In J. Bollandus and G. Henschenius, *Acta sanctorum . . . editio novissima* (J. Carnandet et al., eds.). Vol. 3, 861–967. Paris: Palmé.

Carter, Codell K. 1982. "On the Decline of Blood-Letting in Nineteenth Century Medicine." *Journal of Psychoanalytic Anthropology* 5 (3): 219–34.

Casalis, Matthiew. 1976. "The Dry and the Wet: A Semiological Analysis of Creation and Flood Myths." *Semiotica* 17: 35–67.

Cassel, Paulus D. 1882. *Die Symbolik des Blutes*. Berlin: A. Hoffmann.

Cassirer, Ernst. 1946. *The Myth of the State*. New Haven: Yale University Press.

Cavallini, Giuliana (ed.). 1968. *Catherine of Siena*. Rome: Edizioni Cateriniane.

Celano, Thomas of. 1898. "Second Life of Francis." In *Analecta franciscana, sive Chronica aliaque varia documenta ad historiam Fratrum minorum spectantia* (Fathers of St. Bonaventure's College, eds.). Vol. 10. Quaracchi: Collegium S. Bonaventurae.

Child, Francis James. 1962. *The English and Scottish Popular Ballads*. New York: Cooper Square Publishers.

Childe, V. G. 1926. *The Aryans: A Study of Indo-European Origins*. London: Kegan Paul.

Christenfeld, Timothy. 1996. "Wretched Refuse Is Just the Start: Alien Expressions." *New York Times* (10 Mar.): 4.

Christiansen, Reidar T. 1914. "Die finnischen und die nordischen Varianten des zweiten Merseburger Spruches." *Folklore Fellows Communications* 18: 77–218.

Chwolson, Daniel. 1901. *Die Blutanklage und sonstige mittelalterliche Beschuldigungen der Juden*. Frankfurt am Main: J. Kaufmann.

Clairvaux, Philip of. 1886. "Life of Elizabeth [of Spalbeek], 'Nun of Herkenrode.'" In *Catalogus codicum hagiographicorum bibliothecae regiae Bruxellensis, subsidia hagiographica* I (Bollandists, eds.). Vol. 1, pt. 1. Brussels: Typis Polleunis Ceuterick and Lefébure.

Clauss, L. F. 1936. *Rasse und Seele: Eine Einführung in den Sinn der leiblichen Gestalt*. Munich: Lehmann.

Clover, Carol. 1978. "Skaldic Sensibility." *Arkiv för Nordisk Filologi* 93: 63–81.

Cohen, Abner. 1969. "Political Anthropology." *Man* 4: 215–35.

Coletti, Luigi. 1953. *Pittura Veneta del Quattrocento*. Novara: Instituto Geografico de Agostini.

Colledge, Edmund E., and James Walsh (eds.). 1978. *Julian of Norwich: A Book of Showings to the Anchoress Julian of Norwich*. Studies and Texts 35, pt. 2: Long Text. Toronto: Pontifical Institute of Medieval Studies.

Congar, Yves. 1973. "Modèle monastique et modèle sacerdotal en Occident de Grégoire VII (1073–1085) à Innocent III (1198)." In his *Etudes de civilisation médiévale*. Poitiers: CESCM.

Conkey, Margaret, and Janet Spector. 1984. "Archaeology and the Study of Gender." *Advances in Archaeological Method and Theory* 7: 1–38.

Conklin, Beth. 1995. "'Thus Are Our Bodies, Thus Was Our Custom': Mortuary Cannibalism in an Amazonian Society." *American Ethnologist* 22 (1): 75–101.

Connell, R. W. 1990. "The State, Gender, and Sexual Politics." *Theory and Society* 19 (5): 507–44.

Connelly, Joseph. 1957. *Hymns of the Roman Liturgy*. Westminster, Md.: Newman Press.

Cook, R. 1974. *The Tree of Life: Symbol of the Center*. London: Thames and Hudson.

Corblet, Jules. 1885–86. *Histoire dogmatique, liturgique, et archéologique du sacrament de l'eucharistie*. 2 vols. Paris: Société Générale de Librairie Catholique.

Crawford, Patricia. 1981. "Attitudes to Menstruation in Seventeenth-Century England." *Past and Present* 91: 2–20.

Curieuse. 1700. *Curieuse . . . verwunderungswürdige Hauss-Apothec . . . von einem Liebhaber der Medicin*. Frankfurt am Main: Friedrich Knochen.

Dante Alighieri. 1969. *Divina commedia. Inferno* (A. Gilbert, trans.). Durham, N.C.: Duke University Press.

Darré, Walther. 1931. "Das Zuchtziel des deutschen Volkes." *Volk und Rasse* 6 (3): 138–44.

———. 1936. "Blut und Boden: ein Grundgedanke des Nationalsozialismus." *Schriftenreihe des Reichsausschusses für Volksgesundheitsdienst*. Heft 3. Berlin: Reichsdruckerei.

Davin, Anna. 1978. "Imperialism and Motherhood." *History Workshop* 5: 9–65.

Debongnie, Pierre. 1936. "Essai critique sur l'histoire des stigmatisations au moyen âge." *Etudes carmélitaines* 21 (2): 22–59.

Deetz, James. 1977. *In Small Things Forgotten*. Garden City, N.Y.: Doubleday.

Delaney, Janice, Mary Jane Lupton, and Emily Toth. 1976. *The Curse: A Cultural History of Menstruation*. Urbana: University of Illinois Press.

———. 1988. *The Curse: A Cultural History of Menstruation*. Rev. ed. Urbana: University of Illinois Press.

de Lauretis, Teresa. 1988. "Sexual Indifference and Lesbian Representation." *Theater Journal* 40 (2): 151–77.

———. 1989. "The Violence of Rhetoric." In *The Violence of Representation* (N. Armstrong and L. Tennenhouse, eds.), 239–58. London: Routledge.

Delbrück, Berthold. 1889. *Die indogermanischen Verwandtschaftsnamen*. Abhandlungen der philologisch-historischen Classe der königlichen sächsischen Gesellschaft der Wissenschaften. Vol. 11, no. 5. Leipzig: S. Hirzel Verlag.

Delitzch, Franz J. 1883. *Schachmatt den Blutlügnern*. Erlangen: A. Deichert.

Delumeau, Jean. 1978. *La peur en Occident, XVIe-XVIIIe siècles*. Paris: Fayard.

deMause, Lloyd. 1981. "The Fetal Origins of History." *Journal of Psychoanalytic Anthropology* 4 (1): 1–92.

Dendy, D. R. 1959. *The Use of Lights in Christian Worship*. Alcuin Club Collections, no. 41. London: SPCK.

Dent, G. R., and C. L. S. Nyembezi. 1969. *Scholar's Zulu Dictionary*. Pietermaritzburg: Shuter and Shooter.

Denzinger, Henry. 1957. *The Sources of Catholic Dogma* (Roy J. Deferrari, trans.). St. Louis: Herder.

———. 1967. "Decrees of the Fourth Lateran Council." In *Enchiridion symbolorum* (A. Schönmetzer, ed.). 34th ed. Freiburg: Herder.

de Rojas, Fernando. 1966. *La Celestina* (Editorial M + S). Barcelona: Exclusiva Euro Liber.

Detter, F., and R. Heinzel 1903. *Saemundar Edda*. 2 vols. Leipzig: Verlag von Georg Wigand.

Deutz, Rupert of. 1841. "De divinis officiis." In *Patrologiae cursus completus: series latina* (J.-P. Migne, ed.). Vol. 170. Paris: Migne.

Devereux, George. 1950. "The Psychology of Female Genital Bleeding." *International Journal of Psychoanalysis* 31: 237–57.

de Vries, Jan. 1928. "Der altnordische Rasengang." *Acta Philologica Scandinavia* 3 (2): 106–35.

———. 1930/31. "Ginnungagap." *Acta Philologica Scandinavia* 5: 41–66.

———. 1956. *Altgermanische Religionsgeschichte.* Vol. 1. 2d rev. ed. Berlin: Walter de Gruyter.

———. 1957. *Altgermanische Religionsgeschichte.* Vol. 2. 2d rev. ed. Berlin: Walter de Gruyter.

———. 1961. *Altnordisches etymologisches Wörterbuch.* Leiden: E. J. Brill.

———. 1967. *The Study of Religion* (R. W. Bolle, trans.). New York: Harcourt, Brace and World.

Díakonov, I. M. 1985. "On the Original Home of the Speakers of Indo-European." *Journal of Indo-European Studies* 13 (1–2): 92–174.

Distel, T. 1888. *Neues Archiv für sächsische Geschichte und Alterthumskunde.* Vol. 9. Dresden.

Documente. 1882. "Simon von Trient: Die Blutbeschuldigung gegen die Juden." *Documente zur Aufklärung* 32 (2): 158–88.

Doht, Renate. 1974. *Der Rauschtrank im Germanischen Mythos.* Wiener Arbeiten zur germanischen Altertumskunde und Philologie, no. 3. Vienna: Karl M. Halosar.

Doke, C. M., D. McK. Malcolm, and J. M. A. Sikakna (eds.). 1958. *English-Zulu Dictionary.* Johannesburg: Witwatersrand University Press.

Dolan, G. 1897. "Devotion to the Sacred Heart in Medieval England." *Dublin Review* 120: 373–85.

Dölger, Franz J. 1926. "Gladiatorenblut und Martyrerblut." *Vorträge der Bibliothek Warburg* (F. Saxl, ed.). Leipzig: B. G. Teubner.

Domarus, Max. 1962. *Hitler, Reden und Proklamationen 1932 bis 1945.* 2 vols. Neustadt a.d. Aisch: Schmidt.

Dörfler, A. F. 1892. "Das Blut im magyarischen Volkglauben." *Am Ur-Quell: Monatschrift für Volkskunde* 3 (9): 267–71.

Douglas, Mary. 1973. *Natural Symbols.* New York: Pantheon Books.

———. 1980. *Purity and Danger.* London: Routledge.

Doyere, Pierre (ed.). 1968. *Gertrude the Great: Oeuvres spirituelles.* Vol. 2, *Le Héraut.* Paris: Editions du Cerf.

Drane, Augusta T. 1915. *The History of St. Catherine of Siena and Her Companions.* 4th ed. 2 vols. London: Burns Oates and Washbourne.

Dronke, Peter. 1984. *Women Writers of the Middle Ages.* Cambridge: Cambridge University Press.

Dubnov, S. M. 1926. *Die Geschichte des jüdischen Volkes in Europa.* Vol. 4. Berlin.

Duden, Barbara. 1991. *The Woman Beneath the Skin* (T. Dunlap, trans.). Cambridge: Harvard University Press.

Duhn, Friedrich von. 1906. "Rot und tot." *Archiv für Religionswissenschaft* 9: 1–24.

Dumézil, Georges. 1958. *L'idéologie tripartie des Indo-Européens.* Brussels: Latomus.

———. 1973. *Gods of the Ancient Northmen* (E. Haugen, ed.). Berkeley: University of California Press.

———. 1977. *Les dieux souverains des Indo-Européens.* Paris: Gallimard.

Dumoutet, Edouard. 1926. *Le désir de voir l'hoste et les origines de la dévotion au saint-sacrement.* Paris: Beauchesne.

———. 1942. *Corpus Domini: Aux sources de la piété eucharistique médiévale.* Paris: Beauchesne.

———. 1943. "La Théologie de l'eucharistie à la fin du xiie siècle." *Archives d'histoire doctrinale et littéraire du moyen-âge* 18–20: 181–262.

Dundes, Alan. 1976. "A Psychoanalytic Study of the Bullroarer." *Man,* n.s., 11: 220–38.

————. 1980. "Wet and Dry, the Evil Eye: An Essay on Indo-European and Semitic Worldview." In his *Interpreting Folklore*, 93–133. Bloomington: Indiana University Press.

————. 1983. "Couváde in Genesis." In *Studies in Aggadah and Jewish Folklore* (I. Ben-Ami and J. Dan, eds.), 35–53. Jerusalem: Magnes Press.

————. 1984. *Life Is Like a Chicken Coop Ladder*. New York: Columbia University Press.

————. 1988. "The Flood as Male Myth of Creation." In his *The Flood Myth* (ed.), 167–82. Berkeley: University of California Press.

————. 1991. "The Ritual Murder or Blood Libel Legend." In his *The Blood Libel Legend* (ed.), 336–76. Madison: University of Wisconsin Press.

———— (ed.). 1983. *Cinderella: A Casebook*. New York: Wildman Press.

Dürer, Albrecht. N.d. *Tagebuch der niederländischen Reise* (F. Bergemann, ed.). Leipzig: Insel Verlag.

————. 1970. *1520–21. Das Tagebuch der niederländischen Reise* (J.-A. Goris and G. Marlier, eds.). Brussels: La Connaissance.

Düringsfeld, Ida von, and Otto Freiherr von Reinsberg-Düringsfeld. 1872. *Sprichwörter der germanischen und romanischen Sprachen vergleichend zusammengestellt*. Leipzig: Hermann Fries Verlag.

Durkheim, Emile. 1897. "La prohibition de l'inceste et ses origines." *L'Année Sociologique* 1: 1–70.

————. 1933. *The Division of Labor in Society* (G. Simpson, trans.). Glencoe, Ill.: Free Press.

————. 1963. *Incest: The Nature and Origin of the Taboo* (E. Sagarin, trans.). New York: Lyle Stuart.

Dwinger, Edwin Erich. 1935. *Die letzten Reiter*. Jena: Eugen Diederichs Verlag.

————. 1939. *Auf halbem Wege*. Jena: Eugen Diederichs Verlag.

Ebermann, Oskar. 1903. *Blut- und Wundsegen in ihrer Entwicklung dargestellt*. Palaestra: Untersuchungen und Texte aus der deutschen und englischen Philologie, no. 24. Berlin: Mayer and Müller.

Ebermann, Thomas, and Rainer Trampert. 1991. "Zum Städele hinaus . . ." *Konkret* 11: 10–14.

Edinger, Lewis J. 1986. *West German Politics*. New York: Columbia University Press.

Ehlich, Konrad. 1989. *Sprache im Faschismus*. Frankfurt am Main: Suhrkamp.

Ehrenreich, Barbara. 1987. Foreword to *Male Fantasies*, by Klaus Theweleit. Vol. 1, ix–xvii. Minneapolis: University of Minnesota Press.

Eliade, Mircea. 1958a. *Rites and Symbols of Initiation*. New York: Harper and Row.

————. 1958b. *Patterns in Comparative Religion* (R. Sheed, trans.). New York: Sheed and Ward.

————. 1961. *Images and Symbols* (P. Mairet, trans.). New York: Sheed and Ward.

————. 1964. *Shamanism*. Rev. and enl. ed. (W. R. Trask, trans.). New York: Bollinger Foundation.

————. 1965. *Mephistopheles and the Androgyne*. New York: Sheed and Ward.

Elias, Norbert. 1939. *Über den Prozess der Zivilisation*. 2 vols. Basel: Haus zum Falken.

————. 1982. *Power and Civility*. Oxford: Basil Blackwell.

Endres, J.-A. 1917. "Die Darstellung der Gregoriusmesse im Mittelalter." *Zeitschrift für christliche Kunst* 30: 146–56.

Enloe, Cynthia. 1993. *The Morning After*. Berkeley: University of California Press.

————. 1995. "Have the Bosnian Rapes Opened a New Era of Feminist Consciousness?" In *Mass Rapes* (A. Stiglmayer, ed.), 219–30. Lincoln: University of Nebraska Press.

Evans-Pritchard, E. E. 1933. "Zande Blood-Brotherhood." *Africa* 6 (4): 369–401.

Eynsham, Adam of. 1961. *The Life of St. Hugh of Lincoln* (D. L. Douie and H. Farmer, eds.). 2 vols. London: Nelson.

Farge, Arlette. 1979. "Signe de vie, risque de mort: Essai sur le sang et la ville au XVIIIe siècle." *Urbi* 2: 15–22.

Fathers of St. Bonaventure's College (eds.). 1897. "Life of John of Alverna." In *Analecta franciscana, sive Chronica aliaque varia documenta ad historiam Fratrum minorum spectantia.* Vol. 3. Quaracchi: Collegium S. Bonaventurae.

Faulkes, Anthony (trans.). 1987. *Snorri Sturluson Edda.* London: J. M. Dent.

Fawtier, Robert, and Louis Canet. 1948. *La double expérience de Catherine Benincasa.* Paris: Gallimard.

Fehr, Hans. 1930. "Die Bahrprobe." In his *Das Recht in der Dichtung,* 117–19. Bern: A. Francke Verlag.

———. 1955. "Altes Strafrecht im Glauben des Volkes." *Deutsches Jahrbuch für Volkskunde* 1–2: 148–56.

Fehrenbach, Heide. 1995. *German Body Politics.* Rutgers Center for Historical Analysis. New Brunswick: Rutgers University Press.

Feilberg, H. F. 1892. "Totenfetische im Glauben nordgermanischer Völker." *Am Ur-Quell* 3 (1): 1–7.

Fein, Helen. 1979. *Accounting for Genocide.* New York: Free Press.

Feldman, Allen. 1991. *Formations of Violence.* Chicago: University of Chicago Press.

———. 1995. "Violence and the Gendered Gaze." International Conference on (En)Gendering Violence, Zagreb (Croatia). 27–28 October 1995.

Ferré, M.-J., and L. Baudry (eds.). 1927. *Angela of Foligno: Le livre de l'expérience des vrais fidèles* (M.-J. Ferré, and L. Baudry, trans.). Paris: Droz.

Finch, R. G. (ed. and trans.). 1965. *The Saga of the Volsungs.* London: Thomas Nelson.

Finucane, Ronald C. 1977. *Miracles and Pilgrims.* Totowa, N.J.: Rowman and Little-field.

Fischer-Homberger, Esther. 1979. "Krankheit Frau—aus der Geschichte der Menstruation." In her *Krankheit Frau und andere Arbeiten zur Medizingeschichte der Frau,* 49–84. Bern: Huber.

Fliege, Jutta. 1977. "Nikolaus von Kues und der Kampf gegen das Wilsnacker Wunderblut." In *Das Buch als Quelle historischer Forschung* (J. Dietze et al., eds.), 62–70. Leipzig: V.E.B. Bibliographisches Institut.

Forbes, John, et al. (eds.). 1832–35. *Cyclopaedia of Practical Medicine.* 4 vols. London: Sherwood.

Foucault, Michel. 1973. *The Order of Things* (A. M. S. Smith, trans.). New York: Random House.

———. 1975. *The Birth of the Clinic.* New York: Vintage Books.

———. 1978. *History of Sexuality* (R. Hurley, trans.). New York: Random House.

———. 1979. *Discipline and Punish.* New York: Vintage Books.

Fox, William Sherwood. 1916. *Greek and Roman Mythology.* Boston: Marshall Jones.

Franck, J. 1896. "Blut ist dicker als Wasser." *Preussische Jahrbücher* 85: 584–94.

Franck, Sebastian von Wörd. 1536. *Chronica zeitbüch vnnd geschichtbibell von anbegyn bis in die gegenwertig M.D. xxxvi. iar verlengt.* Ulm: J. Varnier.

Frank, Roberta. 1978. *Old Norse Court Poetry: The Drøttkvaet Stanza* (Islandica 42). Ithaca: Cornell University Press.

———. 1981. "Snorri and the Mead of Poetry." In *Speculum Norroenum* (U. Dronke et al., eds.), 155–70. Odense: Odense University Press.

Frankfurter Allgemeine Zeitung. 1980a. "Länder bei der Lösung des Asylproblems im Stich gelassen." *Frankfurter Allgemeine Zeitung* 40 (16 Feb.): 4.

———. 1980b. "Bonn sorgt sich über die steigende Zahl von Asylbewerbern." *Frankfurter Allgemeine Zeitung* (1 Mar.).

———. 1980c. "Der Bundesrat will allem zustimmen 'was ein Stück weiter führt.' " *Frankfurter Allgemeine Zeitung* (29 May).

———. 1980d. "Änderung des Asylrechts gefordert." *Frankfurter Allgemeine Zeitung* 126 (2 June): 1–2, 4.

———. 1980e. "Baum will mit einem Sofortprogramm die Flut der Asyl-Bewerber eindämmen." *Frankfurter Allgemeine Zeitun* 128 (4 June): 1–2.

———. 1980f. "Anarchisches Asylrecht." *Frankfurter Allgemeine Zeitung* 130 (7 June).

———. 1980g. "Wo sich die Koalition mit der Opposition in der Asylanten-Frage einigen könnte." *Frankfurter Allgemeine Zeitung* 134 (12 June): 1.

———. 1980h. "Wehner sieht Einigkeit im Kabinett zum Asylrecht." *Frankfurter Allgemeine Zeitung* 135 (13 June): 1.

———. 1980i. "Soviel Asylbewerber wie Dorfbewohner." *Frankfurter Allgemeine Zeitung* 146 (27 June): 1.

———. 1980j. "Visum-Pflicht für Türken tritt im Oktober in Kraft." *Frankfurter Allgemeine Zeitung* 146 (27 June): 2.

———. 1980k. "Frankfurt will kein Lager für Asylbewerber." *Frankfurter Allgemeine Zeitung* 152 (4 July).

Franz, Adolph. 1902. *Die Messe im deutschen Mittelalter.* Freiburg: Herder.

———. 1963. *Die Messe im deutschen Mittelalter.* Reprint. Darmstadt: Wissenschaftliche Buchgesellschaft.

Frazer, Sir James George. 1911. "Blood Tabooed." In his *Taboo and the Perils of the Soul,* 239–51. New York: Macmillan.

———. 1955 [1936]. *Aftermath: A Supplement to the Golden Bough.* Reprint. London: Macmillan.

Freeman, Derek. 1968. "Thunder, Blood, and the Nicknaming of God's Creatures." *Psychoanalytic Quarterly* 37: 353–99.

Freud, Sigmund. 1925 [1918]. "Contribution to the Psychology of Love: The Taboo of Virginity." In *Collected Papers,* (J. Riviere, trans.). Vol. 4, 216–35. International Psycho-Analytic Library, no. 10. London.

———. 1950. *Totem and Taboo.* New York: Norton.

———. 1959. "Contributions to the Psychology of Love: A Special Type of Choice Object Made by Men." *Collected Papers.* Vol. 4. New York: Norton.

———. 1961. *Civilization and Its Discontents.* (J. Strachey, trans.). New York: Norton.

———. 1976 [1900]. *The Interpretation of Dreams.* Harmondsworth: Penguin Books.

Friedlander, Henry. 1995. *The Origins of Nazi Genocide.* Chapel Hill: University of North Carolina Press.

Friedrich, Johannes. 1952. *Hethitisches Wörterbuch.* Heidelberg: Carl Winter Universitätsverlag.

Friedrich, Paul. 1970. *Proto-Indo-European Trees.* Chicago: University of Chicago Press.

———. 1978. *The Meaning of Aphrodite.* Chicago: University of Chicago Press.

————. 1979. *Language, Context, and the Imagination* (A. S. Dil, ed.). Stanford: Stanford University Press.

Friend, Rev. Hilderic. 1889. *Flowers and Flower Lore.* New York: John B. Alden.

————. 1891. *Flowers and Flower Lore.* New York: Columbian Publishing.

Frind, Sigrid. 1964. "Die Sprache als Propagandainstrument in der Publizistik des Dritten Reiches." Inaugural diss. Philosophische Fakultät der Freien Universität Berlin.

————. 1966. "Die Sprache als Propagandainstrument des Nationalsozialismus." *Muttersprache* 76: 129–35.

Frisk, Hjalmar. 1960. *Griechisches etymologisches Wörterbuch.* Vol. 1. Heidelberg: Carl Winter Universitätsverlag.

————. 1970. *Griechisches etymologisches Wörterbuch.* Vol. 2. Heidelberg: Carl Winter Universitätsverlag.

Fromme, Friedrich Karl. 1980a. "Suchen sie Schutz oder Wohlstand?" *Frankfurter Allgemeine Zeitung* 144 (25 June): 1.

————. 1980b. "Dämme gegen Asylanten-Springflut." *Frankfurter Allgemeine Zeitung* 122 (28 May): 10.

Frye, Northrop. 1957. *Anatomy of Criticism.* Princeton: Princeton University Press.

Gallagher, C., and T. Laqueur (eds.). 1987. *The Making of the Modern Body.* Berkeley: University of California Press.

Gamkrelidze, T. V., and V. V. Ivanov. 1985a. "The Ancient Near East and the Indo-European Question." *Journal of Indo-European Studies* 13 (1–2): 3–48.

————. 1985b. "The Migration of Tribes Speaking the Indo-European Dialects from Their Original Homeland in the Near East to Their Historical Habitations in Eurasia." *Journal of Indo-European Studies* 13 (1–2): 49–91.

Gaselee, Stephen. 1937. *The Oxford Book of Medieval Latin Verse.* Reprint. Oxford: Clarendon Press.

Geary, P. 1978. *Furta sacra: Theft of Relics in the Central Middle Ages.* Princeton: Princeton University Press.

Geldner, K. F. 1951. *Der Rig-Veda.* Vol. 3. Cambridge: Harvard University Press.

Geller, Jay. 1992. "(G)nos(e)ology." In *People of the Body* (H. Eilberg-Schwartz, ed.), 243–82. Albany: State University of New York Press.

Gellrich, J. M. 1985. *The Idea of the Book in the Middle Ages.* Ithaca: Cornell University Press.

Gerhard, Ute, and Jürgen Link. 1991. "Kleines Glossar neorassistischer Feindbild-Begriffe." In *Buntesdeutschland* (H. Boehncke and H. Wittich, eds.), 138–48. Reinbeck: Rowohlt.

Gibbs, Liv. 1987. "Identifying Gender Representation in the Archaeological Record." In *The Archaeology of Contextual Meanings* (I. Hodder, ed.), 79–89. Cambridge: Cambridge University Press.

Gibson, M. 1978. *Lanfranc of Bec.* Oxford: Oxford University Press.

Gietl, Ambrosius M. 1891. *Die Sentenzen Rolands nachmals Papstes Alexander III.* Freiburg: Herdersche Verlagshandlung.

Gifford-Gonzalez, D. 1993. " 'You Can Hide, But You Can't Run': Representations of Women's Work in Illustrations of Palaeolithic Life." *Visual Anthropology Review* 9: 23–41.

Gillison, Gillian. 1980. "Images of Nature in Gimi Thought." In *Nature, Culture, Gender* (C. MacCormack and M. Strathern, eds.), 143–73. Cambridge: Cambridge University Press.

————. 1983. "Cannibalism Among Women in the Eastern Highlands of Papua

New Guinea." In *The Ethnography of Cannibalism* (P. Brown and D. Tuzin, eds.), 33–50. Washington, D.C.: Society for Psychological Anthropology.

Gilman, Sander L. 1986. *Difference and Pathology*. Ithaca: Cornell University Press.

———. 1987. "The Struggle of Psychiatry with Psychoanalysis." *Critical Inquiry* 13: 293–313.

———. 1992. "Plague in Germany, 1939/1989." In *Nationalisms and Sexualities* (A. Parker et al., eds.), 175–200. New York: Routledge.

Gilmore, David. 1990. *Manhood in the Making*. New Haven: Yale University Press.

Gimbutas, Marija. 1963. "The Indo-Europeans." *American Anthropologist* 65: 825–36.

———. 1970. "Proto-Indo-European Culture." In *Indo-European and Indo-Europeans* (G. Cardona, H. M. Koenigswald, and A. Senn, eds.), 155–98. Philadelphia: University of Pennsylvania Press.

———. 1973. "Old Europe, 7000–3500 B.C." *Journal of Indo-European Studies* 1: 1–20.

———. 1980. "The Kurgan Wave Migration (3400–3200 B.C.) into Europe and the Following Transformation of Culture." *Journal of Near Eastern Studies* 8: 273–315.

———. 1982. *The Goddesses and Gods of Old Europe*. Berkeley: University of California Press.

Girard, René. 1979. *Violence and the Sacred* (P. Gregory, trans.). Baltimore: Johns Hopkins University Press.

Glunk, Rolf. 1966. "Erfolg und Misserfolg der nationalsozialistischen Sprachlenkung." *Zeitschrift für deutsche Sprache* 22 (1966): 57–73, 146–53; 23 (1967): 83–113, 178–98; 24 (1968): 72–91, 184–91; 26 (1970): 84–97, 176–83; 27 (1971): 113–23, 177–87. (All preceding references reflect article as published in parts.)

Godelier, Maurice. 1988. *The Making of Great Men*. Cambridge: Cambridge University Press.

Golther, Wolfgang. 1895. *Handbuch der germanischen Mythologie*. Leipzig: S. Hirzel Verlag.

Gonda, Jan. 1980. *Vedic Ritual*. Vol. 4, pt. 1 of *Handbuch der Orientalistic*. Zweite Abteilung: Indien. Leiden: E. J. Brill.

Goody, Jack R. 1983. *The Development of the Family and Marriage in Europe*. Cambridge: Cambridge University Press.

Götze, Alfred A. W. (ed.). 1939. *Trübner's deutsches Wörterbuch*. Berlin: Walter de Gruyter.

Gougaud, Louis. 1923. "Etude sur la reclusion religieuse." *Revue Mabillon* 13: 86–87.

———. 1925. *Dévotions et pratiques ascétiques du moyen-âge*. Collection Pax 21. Paris: J. Gabalda.

———. 1927. *Devotional and Ascetic Practices in the Middle Ages* (G. C. Bateman, trans.). London: Burns Oates and Washbourne.

Graetz, Heinrich H. 1897. *Geschichte der Juden von den ältesten Zeiten bis auf die Gegenwart*. Vol. 9. Leipzig: O. Leiner.

Gray, D. 1963. "The Five Wounds of Our Lord." *Notes and Queries* 208: 50–51, 82–89, 127–34, 163–68.

Greenhill, Eleanor Simmons. 1954. "The Child in the Tree." *Traditio* 10: 323–71.

Greenhouse, Stephen. 1994a. "As Tide of Haitian Refugees Rises . . ." *New York Times* (30 June).

———. 1994b. "Haitians Taking to the Sea in Droves." *New York Times* (28 June).

Grimm, Jacob. 1844. *Deutsche Mythologie.* 2d ed. Vol. 2. Göttingen: Dieterichsche Buchhandlung.

———. 1854. *Deutsche Rechtsalterthümer.* 2d ed. Göttingen: Dieterichsche Buchhandlung.

———. 1860. *Deutsches Wörterbuch.* Vol. 2. Leipzig: S. Hirzel Verlag.

———. 1868. *Geschichte der deutschen Sprache.* 2 vols. 3d ed. Leipzig: S. Hirzel Verlag.

———. 1870. *Deutsche Grammatik.* Pt. 1. Berlin: F. Dümmlers Verlagsbuchhandlung.

———. 1878. *Deutsche Mythologie.* (E. H. Meyer, ed.). 4th ed. Berlin: Ferdinand Dümmler Verlag.

———. 1884. *Deutsche Mythologie.* Vol. 2. Göttingen: Dieterische Buchhandlung.

———. 1974. *Reinhart Fuchs.* Reprint. Hildesheim: Georg Olms Verlag.

Grimm, Jacob, and Wilhelm Grimm. 1812–15. *Kinder- und Haus-Märchen.* Berlin: In der Realschulbuchhandlung.

———. 1815. *Der arme Heinrich von Hartmann von der Aue.* Berlin: Ferdinand Dümmlers Verlagsbuchhandlung.

———. 1860. *Deutsches Wörterbuch.* Vol. 2. Leipzig: S. Hirzel Verlag.

Gross, Walter. 1937. "Das ewige Deutschland: Rede auf der Kundgebung des Reichsbundes der Kinderreichen am 11. Februar 1937 in Berlin." *Volk und Rasse* 12 (3): 81–88.

Grosz, Elizabeth. 1994. *Volatile Bodies.* Bloomington: Indiana University Press.

Gruhl, Herbert. 1990. "Die Grünen habe ihre Chance verpaßt!" *Die Grünen: 10 Bewegte Jahre* (M. Schoeren, ed.), 148. Vienna: Carl Ueberreuter.

Grundgesetz und Landesverfassung. 1971. *Grundgesetz für die Bundesrepublik Deutschland und Verfassung für Rheinland-Pfalz.* Mainz: Hase and Köhler Verlag.

Gütt, Arthur. 1936a. "Gesundheits- und Ehegesetzgebung im Dritten Reich." *Volk und Rasse* 11 (8): 321–30.

———. 1936b. "Die Bedeutung von Blut und Boden für das deutsche Volk." *Schriftenreihe des Reichsausschusses für Volksgesundheitsdienst.* Vol. 4. Berlin: Reichsdruckerei.

Gütt, Arthur, Herbert Linden, and Franz Massfeller. 1937. *Blutschutz- und Ehegesundheitsgesetz.* Munich: J. F. Lehmanns Verlag.

Guy-l'Evêque, Garin of. 1866. "Life of Margaret of Hungary (1340)." In *Acta sanctorum . . . editio novissima* (J. Carnandet et al., eds.). Vol. 3, chap. 4. Paris: Palmé.

Gy, P. M. 1983. "La Relation au Christ dans l'eucharistie selon S. Bonaventure et S. Thomas d'Aquin." In *Sacraments de Jesus-Christ* (J. Doré, ed.), 69–106. Paris: Jesus et Jesus-Christ 12.

Haase, K. E. 1897. "Volksmedizin in der Grafschaft Ruppin und Umgegend." *Zeitschrift des Vereins für Volkskunde* 7: 53–65.

———. 1898. "Volksmedizin in der Grafschaft Ruppin und Umgegend." *Zeitschrift des Vereins für Volkskunde,* n.s., 8: 61.

Habig, Marion A. (ed.). 1973. *St. Francis of Assisi.* 3d ed. Chicago: Franciscan Herald Press.

Hachmann, Rolf. 1971. *The Germanic Peoples* (J. Hogarth, trans.). London: Barrie and Jenkins.

Hachmann, Rolf, G. Kossack, and Hans Kuhn. 1962. *Völker zwischen Kelten und Germanen.* Neumünster: K. Wachholtz.

Haeser, Heinrich. 1971. *Lehrbuch der Geschichte der Medizin und der epidemischen Krankheiten.* 3 vols. Reprint. Hildesheim: G. Olms.

Hall, Thomas S. 1975. "Euripus, or the Ebb and Flow of the Blood." *Journal of the History of Biology* 8 (2): 321–50.

Hamman, Adalbert, E. Longpré, and E. Bertaud. 1961. "Eucharistie." In *Dictionnaire de spiritualité, ascétique et mystique, doctrine et histoire* (M. Viller et al., eds.). Vol. 4, pt. 2, cols. 1553–1648. Paris: Beauchesne.

Handler, Richard. 1988. *Nationalism and the Politics of Culture in Quebec.* Madison: University of Wisconsin Press.

Hart, Columba. 1980. *Hadewijch: The Complete Works.* New York: Paulist Press.

Hartmann, Martin. 1896. "Blut ist dicker als Wasser." *Zeitschrift des Vereins für Volkskunde,* n.s., 6: 442–3.

Hästesko, F. A. 1914. "Motiv Verzeichnis west-finnischer Zaubersprüche nebst Aufzählungen der bis 1908 gesammelten Varianten." *Folklore Fellows Communications* 19: 1–66.

Haubst, R. 1958. "Blut Christie." In *Lexikon für Theologie und Kirche* (J. Höfer and K. Rahner, eds.). Vol. 2, 544–45. 2d rev. ed. Freiburg: Herder Verlag.

Hauser, Jean. 1969. "A propos de l'accusation de meutres rituels: La legende d'Andre de Rinn." *Rencontre: Chrétiens et Juifs* 3: 117–27.

Hayn, Hugo. 1906. *Übersicht der (meist in Deutschland erschienenen) Literatur über die angeblich von Juden verübten Ritualmorde und Hostienfrevel.* Jena: H. W. Schmidt.

Hecker, Jutta. 1931. *Das Symbol der blauen Blume im Zusammenhang mit der Blumensymbolik der Romantik.* Jena: Verlag der Frommanschen Buchhandlung.

Heinemann, Franz. 1922. *Der Richter und die Rechtspflege in der deutschen Vergangenheit.* Leipzig: Offizin W. Drugulin.

Heisterbach, Caesarius of. 1851. *Dialogus miraculorum* (J. Strange, ed.). 2 vols. Cologne: Heberle.

———. 1901. *Die Fragmente der Libri VIII Miraculorum des Caesarius von Heisterbach* (A. Meister, ed.). Römische Quartalschrift für christliche Alterthumskunde und für Kirchengeschichte, supp. Vol. 13. Rome: Spithöver.

Heitmeyer, Wilhelm. 1992. *Die Bielefelder Rechtsextremismusstudie.* 2d ed. Weinheim: Juventa.

Held, Josef, and H. W. Horn. 1992. *Du musst so handeln, dass Du Gewinn machst.* Duisburg: Duisburger Institut für Sprach- und Sozialforschung.

Hellwig, Albert. 1914. *Ritualmord und Blutaberglaube.* Minden: J. C. C. Bruns.

Herdt, Gilbert H. 1981. *Guardians of the Flutes.* New York: McGraw Hill.

———. 1982. *Rituals of Manhood.* Berkeley: University of California Press.

Herrmann, Ferdinand. 1969. "Blutrituale." *Die Kapsel* 25: 973–80.

Hertz, W. 1862. *Der Wehrwolf: Beitrag zur Sagengeschichte.* Stuttgart: A. Kröner.

Herzfeld, Michael. 1985. *The Poetics of Manhood.* Princeton: Princeton University Press.

———. 1987. *Anthropology Through the Looking Glass.* New York: Cambridge University Press.

———. 1992. *The Social Production of Indifference.* New York: Berg.

Hettrich, Heinrich. 1985. "Indo-European Kinship Terminology in Linguistics and Anthropology." Manuscript.

Heuser, J. 1948. "'Heilig-Blut' in Kult und Brauchtum des deutschen Kulturraums." Ph.D. diss. Philosophische Fakultät der Universität Bonn.

Heutgen, Alfons. 1980. "Eine Schutzstätte wird geplündert." *Deutsches Allgemeines Sonntagsblatt,* no. 7 (22 June).

Hiatt, L. R. 1971. "Secret Pseudo-Procreation Rites Among the Australian Aborigines." In *Anthropology in Oceania* (L. R. Hiatt and C. Jaywardene, eds.), 77–88. San Francisco: Chandler.

————. 1975. "Swallowing and Regurgitation in Australian Myth and Rite." In *Australian Aboriginal Mythology* (L. R. Hiatt, ed.), 143–62. Canberra: Australian Institute for Aboriginal Studies.

Hiemer, Ernst. 1942. *Der Jude im Sprichwort der Völker.* Nuremberg: Der Stürmer.

Hilberg, Raul. 1985. *The Destruction of the European Jews.* 3d rev. ed. New York: Holmes and Meier.

Hildburgh, W. L. 1908. "Notes on Some Flemish Amulets and Beliefs." *Folk-Lore* (London) 19: 200–13.

Hildegard of Bingen. 1855. *Libri subtilitatum diversarum natur. creatur.* Paris: Migne.

————. 1978. *Scivias* (A. Führkötter and A. Carlevaris, eds.). 2 vols. Turnhout: Brepols.

Hirsch, Julian. 1922. "Zur Frage nach der Giftigkeit des Menstrualblutes." *Archiv für Frauenkunde, Eugenetik und Vererbungslehre* 8 (1): 24–26.

Hitler, Adolf. 1933. *Mein Kampf.* 2 vols. 52d ed. Munich: Zentralverlag der NSDAP.

————. 1937. *Reden des Führers am Parteitag der Arbeit 1937.* Munich: Zentralverlag der NSDAP.

————. 1938. "Das dichterische Wort im Werke Adolf Hitlers." *Wille und Macht,* special issue on the occasion of 20 April 1938.

————. 1939. *Mein Kampf.* 2 vols. 474–78th ed. Munich: Zentralverlag der NSDAP.

Hobsbawm, Eric, and Terence Ranger (eds.). 1983. *The Invention of Tradition.* New York: Cambridge University Press.

Hodder, Ian (ed.). 1982. *Symbolic and Structural Archaeology.* Cambridge: Cambridge University Press.

————. 1984. "Burials, Houses, Women and Men in the European Neolithic." In *Ideology, Power, and Prehistory* (D. Miller and C. Tilley, eds.), 51–68. Cambridge: Cambridge University Press.

Hoffmeister, D., and O. Sill. 1993. *Zwischen Aufstieg und Ausstieg.* Opladen: Leske and Budrich.

Höfler, Max. 1899. *Deutsches Krankheitsnamen-Buch.* Munich. Reprinted, Hildesheim: G. Olms, 1970.

Höfler, Otto. 1934. *Kultische Geheimbünde der Germanen.* Vol. 1. Frankfurt am Main: Diesterweg.

————. 1952a. *Germanisches Sakralkönigtum.* Vol. 1. Tübingen: Max Niemeyer Verlag.

————. 1952b. "Das Opfer im Semonenhain und die Edda." In *Edda, Skalden, Saga* (H. Schneider, ed.), 1–67. Heidelberg: Carl Winter Universitätsverlag.

Hollander, Lee M. (trans.). 1928. *The Poetic Edda.* Austin: University of Texas Press.

————. 1962. *The Poetic Edda.* 2d ed. Austin: University of Texas Press.

————. 1987. *The Poetic Edda.* 2d rev. ed. Austin: University of Texas Press.

Holmberg, Uno. 1922–23. *Der Baum des Lebens.* Helsinki: Suomalainen Tiedeakatemia.

Holmes, Colin. 1981. "The Ritual Murder Accusation in Britain." *Ethnic and Racial Studies* 4 (3): 265–88.

Hontoir, M. Camille. 1946. "La Dévotion au saint sacrament chez les premiers cisterciens (XIIe–XIIIe siècles)." *Studia eucharistica DCC anni a condito festo sanctissimi Corporis Christi,* 132–56. Antwerp: De Nederlandsche Boekhandel.

Hsia, R. Po-Chia. 1988. *The Myth of Ritual Murder.* New Haven: Yale University Press.

————. 1992. *Trent 1475: Stories of a Ritual Murder Trial.* New Haven: Yale University Press.

Hugh-Jones, Christine. 1979. *From the Milk River.* Cambridge: Cambridge University Press.

Humbert of Romans. 1603. *Beati Umberti sermones.* Venice.

Imbert-Gourbeyre, Antoine. 1894. *La stigmatisation.* 2 vols. Clermont-Ferrand: Librairies Catholique.

Jackson, K. H. 1955. "The Pictish Language." In *The Problem of the Picts* (F. T. Wainwright, ed.), 126–66. Edinburgh: Nelson.

Jäger, Margret. 1993. "Sprache der Angst." *die tageszeitung* (24 Mar.).

Jahn, Ulrich. 1886. *Hexenwesen und Zauberei in Pommern.* Stettin: T. von der Nahmer.

————. 1888. "Zauber mit Menschenblut und anderen Teilen des menschlichen Körpers." *Verhandlungen der Berliner Anthropologischen Gesellschaft* 4: 130–40.

Jay, Nancy. 1985. "Sacrifice as Remedy for Having Been Born of Woman." In *Immaculate and Powerful* (C. W. Atkinson, C. H. Buckanan, and M. R. Miles, eds.), 283–309. Boston: Beacon Press.

Jeggle, Utz. 1993. "Tatorte: Zur imaginären Topographie von Ritualmordlegenden." In *Die Legende vom Ritualmord* (R. Erb, ed.), 239–52. Berlin: Metropol.

Jhering, Barbara von. 1988. "Sprachkünstler auf hohem Seil: Stoiber, Kohl, und die *taz.*" *Die Zeit* 49 (2 Dec.): 79.

Jochens, Jenny. 1989. "Völuspá: Matrix of Norse Womanhood." *Journal of English and Germanic Philology* 88 (3): 344–62.

Johnston, George (trans.). 1963. *The Saga of Gisli.* Toronto: University of Toronto Press.

Jolly, Margaret. 1993. "Colonizing Women." In *Feminism and the Politics of Difference* (S. Gunew and A. Yeatman, eds.), 103–27. Boulder, Colo.: Westview Press.

Jones, E. 1971. *On the Nightmare.* New York: Liveright.

Jónsson, Finnur. 1900. *Snorri Sturluson Edda.* Copenhagen: Universitetsboghandler G.E.C. Gad.

Juncker, Johannes. 1724. *Conspectus medicinae theoretico-practicae.* Halle: Orphanotrophei.

————. 1725. *Conspectus Therapiae generalis cum notis in materiam medicam.* Halle: Orphanotrophei.

Jungmann, Josef A. 1951. *The Mass of the Roman Rite.* 2 vols. New rev., abridged ed. New York: Benziger.

Kamenetsky, Christa. 1972. "Folklore as a Political Tool in Nazi Germany." *Journal of American Folklore* 85: 221–35.

————. 1977. "Folktale and Ideology in the Third Reich." *Journal of American Folklore* 90 (356): 168–79.

Kammeyer, Hans F. 1941. "Lebensbaum und Baumkult der Völker." *Mitteilungen der deutschen dendrologischen Gesellschaft* 54 (Jahrbuch): 73–87.

Kandiyoti, Denize. 1994. "Identity and Its Discontents." In *Colonial and Post-Colonial Theory* (P. Williams and L. Chrisman, eds.), 376–91. New York: Columbia University Press.

Kant, Immanuel. 1800. *Anthropologie in pragmatischer Hinsicht abgefasst.* 2d rev. ed. Königsberg: Friedrich Nicolovius.

————. 1974. *Anthropology from a Pragmatic Point of View* (M. J. Gregor, trans.). The Hague: Martinus Nijhoff.

Karras, Ruth Mazo. 1992. "Servitude and Sexuality in Medieval Iceland." In *From Sagas to Society* (G. Pálsson, ed.), 289–304. Enfield Lock: Hisarlik Press.

Kecskemeti, Paul, and Nathan Leites. 1947. "Some Psychological Hypotheses on Nazi Germany: I." *Journal of Social Psychology* 26 (1947): 141–83; II, 27 (1948): 91–117; III, 27 (1948): 241–70; IV, 28 (1948): 141–64. (All preceding references reflect article as published in parts.)

Keesing, Roger M. 1982. "Toward a Multidimensional Understanding of Male Initiation." In *Rituals of Manhood* (G. Herdt, ed.), 2–43. Berkeley: University of California Press.

Kelle, Johann (ed.). 1881. *Otfrids von Weissenburg Evangelienbuch.* Vol. 3, *Glossar.* Regensburg: G. Joseph Manz.

Kennedy, V. L. 1946. "The Date of the Parisian Decree on the Elevation of the Host." *Medieval Studies* 8: 87–92.

Kessler, Gottfried. 1915. "Wunderbare Äusserungen des Blutes." *Schweizer Volkskunde* 5 (3–4): 28–30.

Kidd, B. J. 1958. *The Later Medieval Doctrine of the Eucharistic Sacrifice.* Reprint. London: SPCK.

Kieckhefer, Richard. 1984. *Unquiet Souls: Fourteenth-Century Saints and Their Religious Milieu.* Chicago: University of Chicago Press.

King, Archdale A. 1955. *Liturgies of the Religious Orders.* London: Longmans.

———. 1965. *Eucharistic Reservation in the Western Church.* London: Longmans.

Kirk, G. S., and J. E. Raven. 1957. *The Pre-Socratic Philosophers.* Cambridge: Cambridge University Press.

Kish, Kathleen V., and Ursula Ritzenhoff (eds.). 1984. *Die Celestina.* Hildesheim: G. Olms Verlag.

Klauser, Theodor. 1979. *A Short History of the Western Liturgy* (J. Halliburton, trans.). 2d ed. Oxford: Oxford University Press.

Klee, Ernst (ed.). 1975. *Gastarbeiter.* 3d ed. Frankfurt am Main: Suhrkamp Verlag.

Klein, Ernst. 1967. *A Comprehensive Etymological Dictionary of the English Language.* 2 vols. New York: Elsevier.

Klein, Heinz Günter. 1980. "Asyl-Sorgen." *Rhein-Zeitung* (25 June).

Kligman, Gail. 1988. *The Wedding of the Dead.* Berkeley: University of California Press.

Kluge, Friedrich. 1951. *Etymologisches Wörterbuch der deutschen Sprache.* 15th ed. Berlin: Walter de Gruyter.

———. 1960. *Etymologisches Wörterbuch der deutschen Sprache.* 18th ed. Berlin: Walter de Gruyter.

———. 1963. *Etymologisches Wörterbuch der deutschen Sprache.* 19th ed. Berlin: Walter de Gruyter.

Knight, Chris. 1991. *Blood Relations.* New Haven: Yale University Press.

Kober, A. 1931. "Aus der Geschichte der Juden im Rheinland." *Rheinischer Verein für Denkmalpflege und Heimatschutz* (Düsseldorf). Heft 1.

Kogon, Eugen. 1958. *The Theory and Practice of Hell* (H. Norden, trans.). New York: Berkley Books.

Köhler, Reinhold. 1891. "Baumseele." *Am Ur-Quell* 2: 27.

Konkret. 1994. "Zusammenfassung der Diskussion von der Arbeitsgruppe Gedenkstätte der Initiative 9. November 1938." *Konkret* 1: 42.

Koonz, Claudia. 1987. *Mothers in the Fatherland.* New York: St. Martin's Press.

Kotze, Hildegard von, and Helmut Krausnick (eds.). 1966. *Es spricht der Führer: 7 exemplarische Hitler-Reden.* Gütersloh: Sigbert Mohn Verlag.

Krahe, Hans. 1936. "Ligurisch und Indogermanisch." In *Festschrift für H. Hirt.* Vol. 2, 241–55. Heidelberg: von H. Hirt and Streitberg.

———. 1958. *Indogermanische Sprachwissenschaft.* Vol. 1. Berlin: Walter de Gruyter.

Krauss, Karl. 1955. *Die dritte Walpurgisnacht* (H. Fischer, ed.). Munich: Kösel.

Kreft, Ursula. 1991. "Alles mit Mass und mit Ziel." *Konkret* 11 (Nov.): 28–29.

Kristjánsson, Jónas. 1992. *Eddas and Sagas* (P. Foote, trans.). 2d ed. Reykjavík: Hið íslenska bókmenntafélag.

Krohn, Kaarle. 1931. "Übersicht über einige Resultate der Märchenforschung: Der singende Knochen." *Folklore Fellows Communications* 96: 74–81.

Krüger, Bruno (ed.). 1976. *Die Germanen.* 2 vols. Berlin: Akademie-Verlag.

Kuhn, Hans. 1968. *Edda: Die Lieder des Codex Regius nebst verwandten Denkmälern.* Vol. 2, *Kurzes Wörterbuch.* 3d ed. Heidelberg: Carl Winter Universitätsverlag.

Kuper, Leo. 1981. *Genocide.* New Haven: Yale University Press.

La Barre, Weston. 1984. *Muelos: A Stone Age Superstition About Sexuality.* New York: Columbia University Press.

Lammert, G. 1869. *Volksmedizin und medizinischer Aberglaube in Bayern und den umliegenden Bezirken.* Würzburg: F. A. Julien.

Lancet. 1827. "Untitled." *Lancet* 10: 26.

Lanfranc of Bec. 1841. "Liber de corpore et sanguine domini." In *Patrologiae cursus completus: Series latina* (J.-P. Migne, ed.). Vol. 150, cols. 407–42. Paris: Migne.

Lange-Feldhahn, Klaus, Claudia Duppel, Axel Pfaff, and Ingrid Reick. 1983. "11. 11. 1981—Ausbruch (?) aus dem Irrenhaus." In *Friedensbewegung* (K. Horn and E. Senghaas-Knobloch, eds.), 202–17. Frankfurt: Fischer Verlag.

Latte, Kurt. 1960. *Römische Religionsgeschichte.* Munich: C. H. Becksche Verlagsbuchhandlung.

Latynin, B. A. 1933. "[The Cosmic Tree and the Tree of Life in the Folklore and Art of Eastern Europe]." *Izvetiia Gosudarstvennoi akademii istori materialnoi kultury*, no. 69. Leningrad: Izdatelstvo GAIMK.

Lauffer, Otto. 1936. "Kinderherkunft aus Bäumen." *Zeitschrift für Volkskunde* 44 (6): 93–106.

———. 1937. "Schicksalsbaum und Lebensbaum im deutschen Glauben und Brauch." *Zeitschrift für Volkskunde* (Berlin), n.s., 7 (3): 215–30.

Laurent, M.-H. 1940. "La Plus Ancienne Légende de la B. Marguerite de Città di Castello." *Archivum Fratrum Oraedicatorum* 10: 125–28.

Leach, Maria. 1956. *The Beginning: Creation Myths Around the World.* New York: Funk and Wagnalls.

Lechler, George. 1937. "The Tree of Life in Indo-European and Islamic Cultures." *Ars Islamica* 4: 369–21.

Leiden, John Walter of. 1865. "Life of Lidwina." In J. Bollandus and G. Henschenius, *Acta sanctorum . . . editio novissima* (J. Carnandet et al., eds.). Vol. 2, 271–301. Paris: Palmé.

Leonhardt, Ludwig. 1934. "Deutsche Rasse oder nordische Rasse im deutschen Volk." *Volk und Rasse* 9 (6): 188–89.

Lévi-Strauss, Claude. 1966. *The Savage Mind.* Chicago: University of Chicago Press.

———. 1969 [1964]. *The Raw and the Cooked.* New York: Harper.

———. 1978. *The Origin of Table Manners.* London: Jonathan Cape.

Lévy-Bruhl, Lucien. 1935. "Blood and Its Magic Virtues," and "Blood and Its Sinister Virtues." In his *Primitives and the Supernatural* (L. A. Clare, trans.), 323–432. New York: Dutton.

———. 1939. *The Notebooks on Primitive Mentality* (P. Riviere, trans.). Oxford: Blackwell.

Lewis, Gilbert. 1980. *Day of Shining Red.* Cambridge: Cambridge University Press.

Lexer, Matthias. 1959. *Mittelhochdeutsches Taschenwörterbuch.* 29th ed. Stuttgart: S. Hirzel Verlag.

Lidtke, Vernon. 1982. "Songs and Nazis." In *Essays on Culture and Society in Modern Germany* (D. King et al., eds.), 167–200. College Station: Texas A&M University Press.

Lidz, R. W., and Theodore Lidz. 1977. "Male Menstruation." *International Journal of Psychoanalysis* 58 (1): 17–37.

Liebe, Georg. 1903. *Das Judentum in der deutschen Vergangenheit.* Leipzig: E. Diederichs.

Lifton, Robert Jay. 1986. *The Nazi Doctors.* New York: Basic Books.

Lindow, John. 1985. "Mythology and Mythography." In *Old Norse-Icelandic Literature* (C. J. Clover and J. Lindow, eds.), 21–67. Islandica 45. Ithaca: Cornell University Press.

Linebaugh, Peter. 1975. "The Tyburn Riots Against the Surgeons." In *Albion's Fatal Tree* (D. Hay et al., eds.), 65–111. New York: Pantheon Books.

Link, Jürgen. 1983. "Asylanten, ein Killwort." *kultuRRevolution* 2 (Feb.): 36–38.

Linke, Uli. 1982. "From Caste to Class in Germany: A Study of the Power Politics of Labor Migration from 1955–1980." *Kroeber Anthropological Society Papers* 61/62: 78–87.

———. 1985. "Blood as Metaphor in Proto-Indo-European." *Journal of Indo-European Studies* 13 (3–4): 333–76.

———. 1986. "Where Blood Flows, a Tree Grows: A Study of Root Metaphors in German Culture." Ph.D. diss. Department of Anthropology, University of California, Berkeley.

———. 1989. "Women, Androgynes, and Models of Creation in Norse Mythology." *Journal of Psychohistory* 16 (3): 231–61.

———. 1990. "Folklore, Anthropology, and the Government of Social Life." *Comparative Studies in Society and History* 32 (1): 117–48.

———. 1992. "Manhood, Femaleness, and Power." *Comparative Studies in Society and History* 34 (4): 579–620.

———. 1995. "Murderous Fantasies: Violence, Memory, and Selfhood in Germany." *New German Critique* 64 (winter): 37–59.

———. 1997. "Colonizing the National Imaginary." In *Cultures of Scholarship* (S. Humphreys, ed.), 97–138. Ann Arbor: University of Michigan Press.

Little, Andrew G. (ed.). 1908. *Liber exemplorum ad usum praedicantium.* British Society of Franciscan Studies 1. Aberdeen: Typis academicis.

Lixfeld, Hannjost. 1994. *Folklore and Fascism* (J. R. Dow, ed., trans.). Bloomington: Indiana University Press.

Lloyd, G. E. R. 1964. "The Hot and the Cold, the Dry and the Wet in Greek Philosophy." *Journal of Hellenic Studies* 84: 92–106.

Loeb, E. M. 1923. *The Blood Sacrifice Complex.* American Anthropological Association Memoir, no. 30. Menasha, Wisc.: Collegiate Press.

Lollio, Antonio. 1485. *Oratio circumcisionis dominicae.* Rome: S. Plannck.

Louis, C. (ed.). 1980. *The Commonplace Book of Robert Reynes of Acle.* Garland Medieval Texts, no. 1. New York.

Lowie, Robert H. 1945. *The German People.* New York: Farrar.

Lupton, Mary Jane. 1993. *Menstruation and Psychoanalysis.* Urbana: University of Illinois Press.

Lutz, Catherine A. 1988. *Unnatural Emotions*. Chicago: University of Chicago Press.

Lutz, Catherine A., and Jane L. Collins. 1993. *Reading the National Geographic*. Chicago: University of Chicago Press.

Maccoby, Hyam. 1982. *The Sacred Executioner*. London: Thames and Hudson.

MacCormack, Carol P., and Marilyn Strathern (eds.). 1986. *Nature, Culture, Gender*. Cambridge: Cambridge University Press.

MacCulloch, John A. 1932. *Medieval Faith and Fable*. Boston: Marshall Jones.

Mackensen, Lutz. 1923. *Der singende Knochen: Ein Beitrag zur vergleichenden Märchenforschung*. Folklore Fellows Communications, no. 49. Helsinki: Suomalainen Tiedeakatemia.

Macy, G. 1984. *The Theologies of the Eucharist in the Early Scholastic Period*. Oxford: Oxford University Press.

Magdeburg, Mechtild of. 1869. *Offenbarungen der Schwester Mechtild von Magdeburg* (G. Morel, ed.). Regensburg: Manz. Reprint, Darmstadt: Wissenschaftliche Buchgesellschaft, 1963.

Malkki, Liisa H. 1995a. *Purity and Exile*. Chicago: University of Chicago Press.

———. 1995b. "Refugees and Exile." *Annual Review of Anthropology* 24: 495–523.

———. 1996. "National Geographic." In *Becoming National* (G. Eley and R. G. Suny, eds.), 434–53. New York: Oxford University Press.

Mallory, J. O. 1989. *In Search of the Indo-Europeans*. London: Thames and Hudson.

Maltzahn, Elisabeth von. 1908. *Das heilige Blut*. 4th ed. Schwerin: F. Bahn Verlag.

Mann, Gunter. 1984. "Exekution und Experiment: Medizinische Versuche bei der Hinrichtung des Schinderhannes." *Lebendiges Rheinland-Pfalz* 21 (2): 11–16.

Mannhardt, Wilhelm. 1904. *Der Baumkultus der Germanen und ihrer Nachbarstämme*. 2d ed. Berlin: Gebrüder Borntraeger Verlag.

Mansi, Giovanni D. (ed.). 1759. *Sacrorum conciliorum nova et amplissima collectio*. Vol. 32. Florence. Reprint, Paris: H. Welter, 1901.

Marienwerder, John. 1884. *Septilium B. Dorotheae, treatise 3* (F. Hipler, ed.). In *Analecta Bollandiana* 3. Brussels: Société des Bollandistes.

———. 1964. *Vita Dorotheae Montoviensis Magistri Johannis Marienwerder* (H. Westpfahl, ed.). Cologne: Böhlau.

Maringer, Johannes. 1976. "Das Blut im Kult und Glauben der vorgeschichtlichen Menschen." *Anthropos* 71 (1–2): 226–53.

Marshall, Yvonne. 1985. "Who Made the Lapita Pots?" *Journal of Polynesian Society* 94: 205–33.

Martin, Emily. 1989. *The Woman in the Body*. Boston: Beacon Press.

———. 1990. "The Ideology of Reproduction." In *Uncertain Terms* (F. Ginsburg and A. L. Tsing, eds.), 300–314. Boston: Beacon Press.

Martin, John Stanley. 1981. "*Ar vas alda*. Ancient Scandinavian Creation Myths Reconsidered." In *Speculum Norroenum* (U. Dronke et al., eds.), 357–69. Odense: Odense University Press.

Marx, Rita. 1994. "Zum Verlieren der Emphatie mit dem Opfer in der Gegenübertragung." International Colloquium, Gewalt: Nationalismus, Rassismus, Ausländerfeindlichkeit. 11 Feb., 1994, Berlin.

Marzell, Heinrich. 1925–36. "Die deutschen Bäume in der Volkskunde: Esche; Eberesche; Erle; Tanne; Lärche; Wacholder; Rotbuche; Birke; Linde." *Mitteilungen der deutschen dendrologischen Gesellschaft* 35: 75–86; 37: 71–78; 38: 76–82; 41: 78–87; 42: 180–86; 43: 270–80; 45: 144–54; 46: 121–31; 47: 196–204. (All preceding references reflect article as published in parts.)

Mattson, Michelle. 1995. "Refugees in Germany." *New German Critique* 64 (winter): 61–85.

Mayer, Anton L. 1971. *Die Liturgie in der Europäischen Geistesgeschichte* (E. von Severus, ed.). Darmstadt: Wissenschaftliche Buchgesellschaft.

Mayrhofer, Manfred. 1952. "Gibt es ein indogermanisches *sor- 'Frau'?" *Studien zur indogermanischen Grundsprache* 4: 32–39.

———. 1956. *Kurzgefasstes etymologisches Wörterbuch des Altindischen.* Vol. 1. Heidelberg: Carl Winter Universitätsverlag.

McCarthy, Dennis J. 1969. "The Symbolism of Blood and Sacrifice." *Journal of Biblical Literature* 88 (2): 166–76.

———. 1973. "Further Notes on the Symbolism of Blood and Sacrifice." *Journal of Biblical Literature* 92 (2): 205–10.

McGhee, Robert. 1977. "Ivory for the Sea Woman." *Canadian Journal of Archaeology* 1: 141–49.

McGraw-Hill Editors. 1963. *Modern Chinese-English Technical and General Dictionary.* Vol. 3. New York: McGraw-Hill.

McLaughlin, Mary M. 1974. "Survivors and Surrogates." In *The History of Childhood*, 101–81. (L. deMause, ed.). New York: Psychohistory Press.

Mead, Margaret. 1947. *Male and Female.* New York: William Morrow.

———. 1977. "End Linkage: A Tool for Cross-Cultural Analysis." In *About Bateson* (M. C. Bateson et al., eds.), 170–231. New York: E. P. Dutton.

Megivern, J. J. 1963. *Concomitance and Communion.* Studia Friburgiensia, n.s., 33. Fribourg: Fribourg University Press.

Meillet, Antoine. 1920. "Les noms du 'feu' et de l'"eau' et la question du genre." *Mémoires de la Société de Linguistique de Paris* 21: 249–56.

———. 1964. *Introduction à l'étude comparative des langues indo-européennes.* Reprint. Alabama Linguistic and Philosophical Series, no. 3. Tuscaloosa: University of Alabama Press.

Meissner, Rudolf. 1921. *Die Kenningar der Skalden.* Germanische Beiträge und Hilfsbücher zur germanischen Philologie und Volkskunde. Vol. 1. Bonn: Kurt Schroeder.

Meletinskij, Eleazar. 1973. "Scandinavian Mythology as a System" (C. V. Ponomareff, trans.). *Journal of Symbolic Anthropology* 1: 43–57.

———. 1974. "Scandinavian Mythology as a System" (C. V. Ponomareff, trans.). *Journal of Symbolic Anthropology* 2: 57–78.

———. 1977. "Scandinavian Mythology as a System of Oppositions." In *Patterns of Oral Literature* (H. Jason and D. Segal, eds.), 252–60. The Hague: Mouton.

Melson, Robert. 1992. *Revolution and Genocide.* Chicago: University of Chicago Press.

Mieder, Wolfgang. 1982. "Proverbs in Nazi Germany." *Journal of American Folklore* 95 (378): 435–64.

———. 1983. "Sprichwörter unterm Hakenkreuz." In his *Deutsche Sprichwörter in Literatur, Politik, Presse und Werbung*, 181–210. Hamburg: Helmut Buske Verlag.

———. 1984. *Investigations of Proverbs, Proverbial Expressions, Quotations and Clichés.* Sprichwortforschung. Vol. 4. Bern: Peter Lang.

Miller, Daniel, and Christopher Tilley (eds.). 1984. *Ideology, Power, and Prehistory.* Cambridge: Cambridge University Press.

Miller, William Ian. 1990. *Bloodtaking and Peacemaking.* Chicago: University of Chicago Press.

Minkenberg, Michael. 1994. "Alte Politik, neue Politik, anti-Politik." *German Studies Association*, Dallas, Tex., 29 Sept.-2 Oct 1994.

Mintz, Sidney W. 1985. *Sweetness and Power*. New York: Penguin Books.

Misciattelli, Piero (ed.). 1913–22. *Le Lettere de S. Caterina da Siena*. 6 vols. Siena: Giuntini y Bentivoglio.

Moeller, Robert G. 1996. *Protecting Motherhood*. Berkeley: University of California Press.

Mommsen, Hans. 1991. *From Weimar to Auschwitz*. Princeton: Princeton University Press.

Monsen, Erling (ed.). 1932. *Heimskringla, or the Lives of the Norse Kings by Snorre Sturlason*. Cambridge: W. Heffer.

Montague, M. F. Ashley. 1937–38. "The Origin of Sub-Incision in Australia." *Oceania* 8: 193–207.

Montgomery, Rita E. 1974. "A Cross-Cultural Study of Menstruation, Menstrual Taboos, and Related Social Variables." *Ethos* 2: 137–70.

Moore, Henrietta. 1988. "Women and the State." In her *Feminism and Anthropology*, 128–85. Minneapolis: University of Minnesota Press.

Moore, Henrietta (ed.). 1990. *Space, Text, and Gender*. Cambridge: Cambridge University Press.

Mosse, George L. 1975. *The Nationalization of the Masses*. New York: Howard Fertig.

———. 1985. *Nationalism and Sexuality*. Madison: University of Wisconsin Press.

Motz, Karl. 1934. *Blut und Boden: die Grundlagen der deutschen Zukunft*. Berlin: Zeitgeschichte Verlag.

Muchembled, Robert. 1983. "Le corps, la culture populaire, et la culture des élites en France (XVe–XVIIIe siècles)." In *Leib und Leben in der Geschichte der Neuzeit* (A. E. Imhoff, ed.). Berliner historische Studien. Vol. 9. Berlin: Dunker and Humblot.

———. 1985. *Popular Culture and Elite Culture in France, 1400–1750* (L. Cochrane, trans.). Baton Rouge: Louisiana State University Press.

Müller, P. Iso. 1961. "Die Blut-Hostie von Münster. Die Entstehung eines vintschgauischen Wallfahrtsortes." *Der Schlern* 35 (7–8): 177–89.

Müller, Wilhelm (ed.). 1854. *Mittelhochdeutsches Wörterbuch*. Vol. 1. Leipzig: S. Hirzel Verlag.

Müller-Freienfels, R. 1936. *The German: His Psychology and Culture* (R. Hoffmann, trans.). Los Angeles: New Symposium Press.

Müller-Hill, Benno. 1988. *Murderous Science* (George R. Fraser, trans.). Oxford: Oxford University Press.

Münch, Ursula. 1992. *Asylpolitik in der Bundesrepublik Deutschland*. Opladen: Leske and Budrich.

Muralt, Johannes von. 1692. *Hippocrates Helveticus*. Basel: Im Verlag Emanuel and Johann Georg Konigen.

Neckel, Gustav. 1962. *Edda: die Lieder des Codex Regius nebst verwandten Denkmälern* (Hans Kuhn, ed.). Vol. 1, *Text*. 4th ed. Heidelberg: Carl Winter Universitätsverlag.

Needham, Joseph. 1959. *A History of Embryology*. 2d ed. Cambridge: Cambridge University Press.

Needham, Rodney. 1967. "Blood, Thunder, and the Mockery of Animals." In *Myth and Cosmos* (J. Middleton, ed.), 271–85. Garden City, N.Y.: Natural History Press.

Needham, Rodney (ed.). 1973. *Right and Left*. Chicago: University of Chicago Press.

Neugebauer, Hugo. 1953. "Der heilige Baum bei Nauders." *Tiroler Heimat* 17: 119–32.

Niedermeyer, H. 1974. "Über die Sakramentsprozession im Mittelalter." *Sacris Erudiri* 22: 401–36.

Noffke, Suzanne (trans.). 1980. *Catherine of Siena: The Dialogue.* New York: Paulist Press.

Nordal, Sigurdur (ed.). 1978. *Vǫluspá* (B. S. Benedikz and John McKinnell, trans.). Durham: Durham and St. Andrews Medieval Texts.

Nordstrom, Carolyn. 1991. "Women and War: Observations from the Field." *Minerva* 9 (1): 1–15.

———. 1996. "Rape: Politics and Theory in War and Peace." *Australian Feminist Studies* 11 (23): 147–62.

Nössler, Regina, and Petra Flocke (eds.). 1997. *Blut.* Tübingen: Konkursbuchverlag.

Offe, Claus. 1987. "Modernity and Modernization as Normative Political Principles." *Praxis International* 7 (1): 2–17.

O'Flaherty, Wendy Doninger. 1980. *Women, Androgynes, and Other Mythical Beasts.* Chicago: University of Chicago Press.

Oingt, Margaret of. 1965. *Les Oeuvres de Marguerite d'Oingt* (A. Duraffour, P. Gardette, and P. Durdilly, eds. and trans.). Publications de l'Institut de Linguistique Romane de Lyon 21. Paris: Belles Lettres.

Olujic, Maria. 1995. "Representation of Experience and Survival of Genocidal Rape in Croatia and Bosnia." International Conference on (En)Gendering Violence, Zagreb (Croatia). 27–28 October 1995.

O'Malley, John W. 1979. *Praise and Blame in Renaissance Rome.* Durham: University of North Carolina Press.

O'Neill, Mary R. 1984. "Sacerdote ovvero strione: Ecclesiastical and Superstitious Remedies in Sixteenth-Century Italy." In *Understanding Popular Culture: Europe from the Middle Ages to the Nineteenth Century* (Steven L. Kaplan, ed.), 53–83. New York: Mouton.

Onians, Richard Broxton. 1973 [1951]. *The Origins of European Thought About the Body, the Mind, the Soul, the World, Time, and Fate.* Reprint. Cambridge: Cambridge University Press.

Oosten, Jarich G. 1985. *The War of the Gods.* London: Routledge and Kegan Paul.

Ortner, Sherry B. 1974. "Is Female to Male as Nature Is to Culture?" In *Women, Culture, and Society* (M. Z. Rosaldo and L. Lamphere, eds.), 67–88. Stanford: Stanford University Press.

Ortner, Sherry B., and Harriet Whitehead (eds.). 1981. *Sexual Meanings.* Cambridge: Cambridge University Press.

Otto, Karl A. 1988. "Wenn über die Einreise der deutsche Stammbaum entscheidet." *Frankfurter Rundschau* 293 (16 Dec.): 14–15.

Ovid (Ovidius Naso, Publius). 1925–26 [1916]. *Metamorphoses* (F. J. Miller, trans.). 2 vols. Reprint. New York: Putnam.

Paechter, Heinz. 1944. *Nazi Deutsch: A Glossary of Contemporary German Usage.* New York: Frederick Ungar.

Page, Jake. 1981. *Blood: The River of Life.* Washington: U.S. News Books.

Die Päpstlichen Bullen über die Blutbeschuldigung. 1900. Munich: August Schupp.

Parker, Andrew, Mary Russo, Doris Sommer, and Patricia Yaeger. 1992. Introduction to their *Nationalisms and Sexualities* (ed.), 1–18. New York: Routledge.

Payer, Pierre J. 1984. *Sex and the Penitentials.* Toronto: University of Toronto Press.

Pelphrey, Brant. 1982. *Love Was His Meaning: The Theology and Mysticism of Julian of Norwich.* Salzburg: Institut für Anglistik und Amerikanistik.

Penney, Clara Louis. 1954. *The Book Called Celestina.* New York: Library of the Hispanic Society of America.

"Persistence of Ritual Blood Libel Charges." 1975. *Intellect* 103: 283–84.

Perusinus, Sebastian. 1866. "Life of Columba of Rieti." In J. Bollandus and G. Henschenius, *Acta sanctorum . . . editio novissima* (J. Carnandet et al., eds.). Vol. 5 (May), 153–217. Paris: Palmé.

Peter of Poitiers. 1841. "Sententiae." In *Patrologiae cursus completus: Series latina* (J.-P. Migne, ed.). Vol. 211, cols. 789–1280. Paris: Migne.

Peter, Rolf. 1937. "Erb- und Rassenpflege im neuen deutschen Strafrecht." *Volk und Rasse* 12 (9): 343–47.

Peters, Hermann. 1900. *Der Arzt und die Heilkunde in der deutschen Vergangenheit.* Leipzig: Eugen Diederichs.

Peuckert, Will-Erich. 1935. "Ritualmord." In *Handwörterbuch des deutschen Aberglaubens.* Vol. 7, 727–39. Berlin: Walter de Gruyter.

Pfaff, R. W. 1970. *New Liturgical Feasts in Later Medieval England.* Oxford: Oxford University Press.

Philipp, Wolfgang. 1980. "Asylmissbrauch—ein Problem der Wirtschaft?" *Frankfurter Allgemeine Zeitung* (1 Apr.).

Pisani, Vittore. 1951. "Vxor: Richerche di Morfologia Indoeuropa." In *Filologia Orientale Glottologia.* Vol. 3 of *Miscellanea G. Galbiati,* 1–38. Milan: Ultico Hoepl Editore.

Ploucquet, Wilhelm Gottfried. 1809. *Literatura medica digesta; sive repertorium medicinae practicae, chirurgicae atque rei obstetricae.* Tübingen: Johann Georg Cotta.

Pokorny, Julius. 1959. *Indogermanisches etymologisches Wörterbuch.* Vol. 1. Bern: Francke.

Polenz, Peter von. 1967. "Sprachpurismus und Nationalsozialismus." In *Germanistik—eine deutsche Wissenschaft* (E. Lämmert, W. Killy, K. O. Conrady, and P. von Polenz, eds.), 111–65. Frankfurt am Main: Suhrkamp Verlag.

Poliakov, Léon. 1974. *The History of Anti-Semitism.* New York: Schocken Books.

Polomé, Edgar C. 1969. "Some Comments on Voluspá, Stanzas 17–18." In *Old Norse Literature and Mythology* (E. Polomé, ed.), 265–90. Austin: University of Texas Press.

———. 1987. "Who Are the Germanic People? In *Proto-Indo-European* (S. N. Skomal and E. C. Polomé, eds.), 216–44. Washington, D.C.: Institute for the Study of Man.

Pontal, O. (ed.). 1983. *Les Statuts synodaux francais du XIII siecle. II: Les Statuts de 1230 a 1260.* Collection de documents inedits sur l'histoire de France, Section d'histoire médiévale et de philologie 15. Paris: Bibliotheque nationale.

Poovey, Mary. 1988. *Uneven Developments.* Chicago: University of Chicago Press.

Powicke, F. M., and C. R. Cheney (eds.). 1964. *Councils and Synods with Other Documents Relating to the English Church.* Vol. 2. Oxford: Clarendon Press.

Preus, Anthony. 1977. "Galen's Criticism of Aristotle's Conception Theory." *Journal of the History of Biology* 10: 65–85.

Proctor, Robert. 1988. *Racial Hygiene.* Cambridge: Harvard University Press.

Pseudo-Bonaventure. 1961. *Meditations on the Life of Christ* (I. Ragusa and R. B. Green, trans.). Princeton: Princeton University Press.

Puhvel, Joan. 1978. "Victimal Hierarchies in Indo-European Animal Sacrifice." *American Journal of Philology* 99: 354–62.

———. 1984. *Hittite Etymological Dictionary.* New York: Mouton.

Pulgram, E. 1958. *The Tongues of Italy.* Cambridge: Harvard University Press.

Rabinbach, Anson, and Jessica Benjamin. 1989. Foreword to *Male Fantasies,* by Klaus Theweleit. Vol. 2, ix–xxv. Minneapolis: University of Minnesota Press.

Rank, Otto. 1959. *The Myth of the Birth of the Hero.* New York: Vintage Books.

Ranke, K. 1978. "Blut." In *Reallexikon der Germanischen Altertumskunde.* Vol. 3, 77–78. Berlin: Walter de Gruyter.

Rappaport, Ernest A. 1943. "The Tree of Life." *Psychoanalytic Review* 30: 263–72.

———. 1975. *Anti-Judaism.* Chicago: Perspective Press.

———. 1991. "The Ritual Murder Accusation." In *The Blood Libel Legend* (A. Dundes, ed.), 304–35. Madison: University of Wisconsin Press.

Raum, Johannes. 1907. "Blut- und Speichelbünde bei den Wadchagga." *Archiv für Religionswissenschaft* 10: 269–94.

Rauschning, Hermann. 1939. *Hitler Speaks.* London: Thornton Butterworth.

Rechenbach, Horst. 1935. "Untitled." *Volk und Rasse* 10 (12): 376.

———. 1937. "Weckung der Blutskräfte im deutschen Bauerntum." *Volk und Rasse* 12 (6): 219–23.

Renfrew, Colin. 1979. *Problems in European Prehistory.* Cambridge: Cambridge University Press.

———. 1988. *Archaeology and Language.* New York: Cambridge University Press.

———. 1989. "They Ride Horses Don't They? Mallory on the Indo-Europeans." *Antiquity* 63: 843–47.

Reypens, L. (ed.). 1964. *Vita Beatricis.* Antwerp: Ruusbroec-Genootschap.

Rhein-Zeitung. 1980a. "Aufstieg zum Asyl-Land Nummer Eins." *Rhein-Zeitung* (1 Feb.).

———. 1980b. "Die Flut der Ausländer überfordert viele Städte." *Rhein-Zeitung* (2 Apr.).

———. 1980c. "Union fordert Änderungen im Asylrechts-Entwurf." *Rhein Zeitung* (25 June).

Riedl, Joachim. 1985. "Das Anderl vom Judenstein." *Die Zeit* 38 (13 Sept.): 74.

Zur Ritualmordbeschuldigung. 1934. Berlin: Philo Verlag.

Robbins, R. H. 1939. "The Anima Christi Rolls." *Modern Language Notes* 34: 415–21.

Roberts, Stephen H. 1938. *The House That Hitler Built.* New York: Harper.

Robinsohn, Jacob. 1896. "Das Blut." In his *Die Psychologie der Naturvölker,* 18–32. Leipzig: Wilhelm Friedrich Verlag.

Rochholz, Ernst L. 1856. *Schweizersagen aus dem Aargau.* Vol. 1. Aargau: H. R. Sauerländer.

———. 1862. Untitled. *Aargauer Nachrichten* (26 July): 40.

Róheim, Géza. 1945. *War, Crime, and the Covenant.* Monticello, N.Y.: Medical Journal Press.

———. 1949. "The Symbolism of Subincision." *American Imago* 6: 321–28.

Röhrich, Lutz. 1967. *Gebärde—Metapher—Parodie.* Wirkendes Wort. Vol. 4. Düsseldorf: Pädagogischer Verlag.

Rollins, Hyder E. 1921. "Notes on Some English Accounts of Miraculous Feasts." *Journal of American Folklore* 34 (134): 357–76.

Rommel, Manfred. 1989. "An Weltoffenheit gewinnen." *Die Zeit* 8 (17 Feb.), 4.

Rosenberg, Alfred. 1935. *Der Mythus des 20. Jahrhunderts.* Munich: Hoheneichen Verlag.

Rosenthal, Joel T. 1966. "Marriage and the Blood Feud in 'Heroic' Europe." *British Journal of Sociology* 17 (June): 133–44.

Ross, Anne. 1962. "Severed Heads in Wells." *Scottish Studies* 6 (1): 31–48.

Roth, Cecil. 1934. *The Ritual Murder Libel and the Jew.* London: Woburn Press.

Róth, Ernst. 1964. "Aus der Geschichte der Juden im Rheingebiet." In his *Festschrift zur Wiedereinweihung der alten Synagoge zu Worms* (ed.), 179–235. Frankfurt am Main: Ner Tamid Verlag.

Rothkrug, Lionel. 1979. "Popular Religion and Holy Shrines." In *Religion and the People, 800–1700* (J. Obelkevich, ed.). Chapel Hill: University of North Carolina Press.

Rothman, David J., Steven Marcus, and Stephanie A. Kiceluk (eds.). 1995. Introduction to their *Medicine and Western Civilization.* New Brunswick, N.J.: Rutgers University Press.

Rubin, Miri. 1991. *Corpus Christi: The Eucharist in Late Medieval Culture.* Cambridge: Cambridge University Press.

Rüsche, Franz. 1930. *Blut, Leben, und Seele.* Paderborn: Ferdinand Schöningh Verlag.

Sahlins, Marshall. 1983. "Raw Women, Cooked Men, and Other 'Great Things' of the Fiji Islands." In *The Ethnography of Cannibalism* (Paula Brown and Donald Tuzin, eds.), 72–93. Washington, D.C.: Society for Psychological Anthropology.

Salfeld, Siegmund. 1898. *Das Martyrologium des Nürnberger Memorbuches.* Berlin: L. Simion.

Salomon, Ernst von. 1930. *Die Geächteten.* Berlin: Rowohlt. Trans. under the title *The Outlaws.* New York: P. Smith, 1935.

Sanday, Peggy Reeves. 1986. *Divine Hunger.* Cambridge: Cambridge University Press.

Sanderson, Meredith. 1954. *A Dictionary of the Yao Language.* Zamba, Nyasaland: Government Press.

Sauers, Wolfgang Werner. 1978. *Der Sprachgebrauch von Nationalsozialisten vor 1933.* Hamburg: Buske.

Schell, O. 1893. "Woher kommen die Kinder? Eine Umfrage." *Am Ur-Quell* 4 (9–10): 224–26.

Schier, Kurt. 1963. "Die Erdschöpfung aus dem Urmeer und die Kosmogonie der Völuspá." In *Märchen, Mythos, Dichtung* (H. Kuhn and K. Schier, eds.), 303–34. Munich: C. H. Beck Verlag.

Schiller, Gertrud. 1971–72. *Iconography of Christian Art* (Janet Seligman, trans.). 2 vols. London: Humphries.

Schlette, Heinz R. 1959. *Die Lehre von der geistlichen Kommunion bei Bonaventura, Albert dem Grossen, und Thomas von Aquin.* Munich: M. Hueber.

Schmitz, H. J. 1958 [1898]. *Die Bussbücher.* 2 vols. Reprint. Graz: Akademische Druck und Verlagsanstalt.

Schneider, David W. 1968. *American Kinship.* Englewood Cliffs, N.J.: Prentice-Hall.

Schöner, E. 1964. *Das Viererschema in der antiken Humoralpathologie.* Wiesbaden: F. Steiner.

Schrader, O. 1904. "Über Bezeichnungen für die Heiratsverwandtschaft bei den indogermanischen Völkern." *Indogermanische Forschungen* 17 (1–2): 11–36.

Schrenk, Martin. 1971. "De sanguine: Blutmagie und Blutsymbolik." In *Et Multum et Multa* (S. Schwenk, G. Tilander, and C. A. Willemsen, eds.), 329–39. Berlin: Walter de Gruyter.

———. 1974. "Blutkulte und Blutsymbolik." In *Einführung in die Geschichte der Hämatologie* (K. G. v. Boroviczény, H. Schipperges, and E. Seidler, eds.), 1–17. Stuttgart: Georg Thieme Verlag.

Schrep, Bruno. 1983. "Totschlagen, alles totschlagen." *Der Spiegel* 37 (33): 72–73.
Schröder, Franz Rolf. 1931. "Germanische Schöpfungsmythen." *Germanisch-Romanische Monatsschrift* 19: 1–26.
———. 1953. "Balder und der zweite Merseburger Spruch." *Germanisch-Romanische Monatsschrift* 34, n.s., 3 (3): 161–82.
———. 1960. "Die Göttin des Urmeeres und ihr männlicher Partner." *Beiträge zur geschichte der deutschen Sprache und Literatur* (Tübingen) 82 (2–3): 221–64.
Schröder, Hein. 1934. "Farbiges Blut in Deutschland." *Volk und Rasse* 9 (5): 153–55.
Schröder, Karl (ed.). 1871. *Der Nonnen von Engelthal Büchlein von der Genaden Überlast.* Tübingen: Literarischer Verein in Stuttgart.
Schultz-Lorentzen, A. 1927. *Dictionary of the West Greenland Eskimo Language.* Copenhagen: C. A. Reitzels Forlag.
Schurig, Martin. 1744. *Haematologia historico-medica, hoc est sanguinis consideratio physico-medico-curiosa.* Dresden: Apud Fridericum Hekel.
Schuster, Daniel. 1970. "The Holy Communion." *Bulletin of the Philadelphia Association for Psychoanalysis* 20: 223–35.
Schütt, Peter. 1981. *Der Mohr hat seine Schuldigkeit getan.* Dortmund: Weltkreis Verlag.
Schwab, Julius. 1937. *Rassenpflege im Sprichwort.* Leipzig: Alwin Fröhlich.
Schwanitz, F. 1937. "Der Sippengedanke im germanischen Bauerntum." *Volk und Rasse* 12 (66): 249–52.
Schwartz, Martin. 1982. "Blood in Sogdian and Old Iranian." *Monumentum Georg Morgenstierne* II. Vol. 8, 189–96. Leiden: E. J. Brill.
Schwerdtfeger, Günther. 1980. *Welche rechtlichen Vorkehrungen empfehlen sich, um die Rechtstellung von Ausländern in der Bundesrepublik angemessen zu gestalten?* Munich: C. H. Becksche Verlagsbuchhandlung.
Sedgwick, Eve Kosofsky. 1992. "Nationalisms and Sexualities in the Age of Wilde." In *Nationalisms and Sexualities* (A. Parker et al., eds.), 235–45. New York: Routledge.
Seidel, Eugen, and Ingeborg Seidel-Slotty. 1961. *Sprachwandel im Dritten Reich.* Halle: Verlag Sprache und Literatur.
Senders, Stefan. 1996. "Laws of Belonging." *New German Critique* 67 (winter): 147–76.
Sennett, Richard. 1994. *Flesh and Stone.* New York: Norton.
Seremetakis, C. Nadia. 1996. "In Search of the Barbarians." *American Anthropologist* 98 (3): 489–511.
Shachar, Isaiah. 1974. *Die Judensau.* London: Warburg Institute.
Shapiro, Warren. 1988. "Ritual Kinship, Ritual Incorporation, and the Denial of Death." *Man,* n.s., 23: 275–97.
———. 1989. "The Theoretical Importance of Pseudo-Procreative Symbolism." *Psychoanalytic Study of Society* 14: 71–88.
Sherratt, Andrew, and Susan Sherratt. 1988. "The Archaeology of Indo-European." *Antiquity* 62: 584–95.
Showalter, Elaine, and English Showalter. 1970. "Victorian Women and Menstruation." *Victorian Studies* 14 (1): 83–89.
Siegel, Rudolph. 1968. *Galen's System of Physiology and Medicine.* New York: S. Karger.
Simpson, Jacqueline. 1962. "Mímir: Two Myths or One?" *Saga-Book of the Viking Society for Northern Research* 16 (1): 41–53.

————. 1963/64. "A Note on the Folktale Motif of the Heads in the Well." *Saga-Book of the Viking Society for Northern Research* 16 (2–3): 248–50.

Simrock, Karl J. 1865. *Die deutschen Volksbücher.* Vol. 12. Frankfurt am Main: H. L. Brönner.

————. 1878. *Handbuch der deutschen Mythologie mit Einschluss der Nordischen.* 5th rev. ed. Bonn: Adolf Marcus.

Skeat, Walter W. 1882. *An Etymological Dictionary of the English Language.* Oxford: Clarendon Press.

Skomal, Nacev, and Edgar C. Polome (eds.). 1987. *Proto-Indo-European.* Washington, D.C.: Institute for the Study of Man.

Smith, Carol A. 1995. "Race-Class-Gender Ideology in Guatemala: Modern and Anti-Modern Forms." *Comparative Studies in Society and History* 37 (4): 723–49.

Smith, W. Robertson. 1972. *The Religion of the Semites.* New York: Schocken Books.

Söhns, Franz. 1904. *Unsere Pflanzen.* 3d ed. Leipzig: B. G. Teubner.

Sonny, A. 1906. "Rote Farbe im Totenkult." *Archiv für Religionswissenschaft* (Leipzig) 9: 525–29.

Sorel, Georges. 1941. *Reflections on Violence* (T. E. Hulme, trans.). New York: P. Smith.

Spalding, Keith. 1957. *An Historical Dictionary of German Figurative Usage.* Vol. 2. Oxford: Basil Blackwell.

Der Spiegel. 1980a. "Deutschland: Da sammelt sich ein ungeheurer Sprengstoff." *Der Spiegel* 23 (2 June): 17–18.

————. 1980b. "Finished, aus, you go, hau ab. Ausländerwelle." *Der Spiegel* 25 (16 June): 32–35.

————. 1984. "Schleswig-Holstein: Früh bis Spät." *Der Spiegel* 3, 52, 65.

Sprenger, R. 1893. "Zum Bahrrecht: eine Umfrage." *Am Ur-Quell* 4 (12): 275–76.

Stachnik, Richard et al. (eds.). 1978. *Akten des Kanonisationsprozesses Dorotheas von Montau von 1394 bis 1521.* Cologne: Böhlau.

Stagel, Elsbet. 1906. *Das Leben der Schwestern zu Töss beschrieben von Elsbet Stagel* (F. Vetter, ed.). Deutsche Texte des Mittelalters 6. Berlin: Weidmannsche Buchhandlung.

Stahl, Georg Ernst. 1730. *De motus haemorrhoidalis, et fluxus haemorrhoidium, diversitate.* Paris: F. Horth Hemels.

Stählin, Otto (ed.). 1936. *Clemes Alexandrinus.* Vol. 1. Leipzig: Hinrichs.

Steinberg, Leo. 1983. *The Sexuality of Christ in Renaissance Art and Modern Oblivion.* New York: Pantheon Books.

Steinmueller, John E. 1959. "Sacrificial Blood in the Bible." *Biblica* 40 (2): 556–67.

Stemplinger, Eduard. 1927. "Blut." *Handwörterbuch des deutschen Aberglaubens.* Vol. 1, 1430–42. Berlin: Walter de Gruyter.

Stephens, John. 1972. "The Mead of Poetry." *Neophilologus* 56: 259–68.

Stern, Moritz (ed.). 1893. *Die Päpstlichen Bullen über die Blutbeschuldigung.* Berlin: S. Cronbach.

Stewart, Susan. 1993. *On Longing.* Durham, N.C.: Duke University Press.

Stiglmayer, Alexandra. 1994. *Mass Rape.* Lincoln: University of Nebraska Press.

Stobbe, Otto. 1866. *Die Juden in Deutschland während des Mittelalters.* Braunschweig: C. A. Schwetschke.

Storch, Johann. 1747a. *Unterricht vor Heb-Ammen.* Gotha: Mevius.

————. 1747b. *Von Kranckheiten der Weiber.* Vol. 2. Gotha: Mevius.

————. 1748. *Von Kranckheiten der Weiber.* Vol. 3. Gotha: Mevius.

————. 1749a. *Von Weiberkrankheiten.* Vol. 4, pt. 1. Gotha: Mevius.

————. 1749b. *Von Weiberkranckheiten.* Vol. 4, pt. 2. Gotha: Mevius.

————. 1750. *Von Weiberkranckheiten.* Vol. 5. Gotha: Mevius.

————. 1751a. *Von Weiberkranckheiten.* Vol. 6. Gotha: Mevius.

————. 1751b. *Von Weiberkranckheiten.* Vol. 7. Gotha: Mevius.

————. 1752. *Von Weiberkranckheiten.* Vol. 8. Gotha: Mevius.

Strack, Hermann L. 1900. *Das Blut im Glauben und Aberglauben der Menschheit.* 5th ed. Schriften des Institutum Judaicum in Berlin, no. 14. Munich: C. H. Becksche Verlagsbuchhandlung.

————. 1909. *The Jew and Human Sacrifice [Human Blood and Jewish Ritual].* New York: Bloch.

Strathern, Andrew. 1982. "Witchcraft, Greed, Cannibalism, and Death." In *Death and the Regeneration of Life* (M. Bloch and J. Parry, eds.), 111–32. Cambridge: Cambridge University Press.

Strathern, Marilyn. 1980. "No Nature, No Culture: The Hagen Case." In *Nature, Culture, Gender* (C. MacCormack and M. Strathern, eds.), 174–222. Cambridge: Cambridge University Press.

Ström, Folke. 1954. *Diser, Nornor, Valkyrjor.* Stockholm: Almqvist and Wiksell.

Stübe, R. 1924. "Kvasir und der magische Gebrauch des Speichels." *Festschrift Eugen Mogk,* 500–509. Halle: M. Niemeyer.

Sutton, Constance R. (ed.). 1995. *Feminism, Nationalism, and Militarism.* Washington, D.C.: Association for Feminist Anthropology/American Anthropological Association.

Szemerényi, Oswald. 1977. "Studies in the Kinship Terminology of the Indo-European Languages." *Acta Iranica* (Textes et Mémoires 7, Varia 1977) 16: 1–231.

Tacitus, Cornelius Publius. 1923. *The Germania* (D. R. Stuart, ed.). New York: Macmillan.

Tannahill, Ray. 1975. "The Red Elixir." In his *Flesh and Blood,* 56–74. New York: Stein and Day.

Taussig, Michael. 1992. *Mimesis and Alterity.* New York: Routledge.

Taylor, John Walter. 1979. "Tree Worship." *Mankind Quarterly* 20: 79–141.

Tegnaeus, Harry. 1952. *Blood-Brothers.* New Series Publication, no. 10. Stockholm: Ethnographic Museum of Sweden.

Temkin, Owsei. 1977. "The Scientific Approach to Disease." In his *The Double Face of Janus and Other Essays in the History of Medicine.* Baltimore: Johns Hopkins University Press.

Thass-Thienemann, Theodore. 1973. *The Interpretation of Language.* New York: Jason Aronson.

Theweleit, Klaus. 1987. *Male Fantasies.* Vol. 1, *Women, Floods, Bodies, History.* Minneapolis: University of Minnesota Press.

————. 1989. *Male Fantasies.* Vol. 2, *Male Bodies: Psychoanalyzing the White Terror.* Minneapolis: University of Minnesota Press.

Thomas à Kempis. 1956. *Le Manuscrit autographe de Thomas à Kempis et "l'Imitation de Jésus-Christ"* (L. M. J. Delaissé, ed.). 2 vols. Publication de Scriptorium 2. Paris.

Thompson, E. A. 1965. *The Early Germans.* Oxford: Clarendon Press.

Thompson, Stith. 1955/58. *Motif-Index of Folk Literature.* 6 vols. 2d rev. and enl. ed. Copenhagen: Rosenkilde and Bagger.

Thurston, Herbert. 1952. *The Physical Phenomena of Mysticism.* Chicago: Regnery.

Tilly, Charles. 1970. "The Changing Place of Collective Violence." In *Essays in Theory and History* (M. Richter, ed.). Cambridge: Harvard University Press.

Timm, Klaus. 1964. "Blut und die rote Farbe im Totenkult." *Ethnographisch-Archäologische Zeitschrift* 5: 39–55.

Todd, Malcolm. 1975. *The Northern Barbarians: 100* B.C.–A.D. *300*. London: Hutchinson Library.

———. 1992. *The Early Germans*. Oxford: Blackwell.

Todorov, Tzvetan. 1990. "Measuring Evil." *New Republic* (19 Mar.), 31.

Toporov, V. N. 1973. "L'albero universale." In *Richerche Semiotiche* (J. M. Lofman et al., eds.). Vol. 43, 148–201. Turin: Nuova Biblioteca Scientifica.

Trachtenberg, Joshua. 1943. *The Devil and the Jews*. New Haven: Yale University Press.

Trexler, R. C. 1974. "Ritual in Florence." In *The Pursuit of Holiness in Late Medieval and Renaissance Religion* (H. A. Oberman and C. Trinkhaus, eds.), 200–264. Leiden: Brill.

Trier, Jost. 1973. *Aufsätze und Vorträge zur Wortfeldtheorie* (A. van der Lee and O. Reichmann, eds.). The Hague: Mouton.

Trumbull, H. Clay. 1885. *The Blood Covenant*. New York: Scribner.

———. 1896. *The Threshold Covenant, or the Beginning of Religious Rites*. New York: Scribner.

Tubach, Frederic C. 1969. *Index exemplorum: A Handbook of Medieval Religious Tales*. Folklore Fellows Communications 204. Helsinki: Suomalainen Tiedeakatemia.

Turner, Brian S. 1984. *The Body and Society*. Oxford: Basil Blackwell.

Turner, Victor W. 1965. "Colour Classification in Ndembu Ritual." In *Anthropological Approaches to the Study of Religion* (M. Banton, ed.), 47–84. London: Tavistock.

———. 1967. *The Forest of Symbols*. Ithaca: Cornell University Press.

———. 1974. *Dramas, Fields, and Metaphors*. Ithaca: Cornell University Press.

Turville-Petre, Gabriel. 1964. *Myth and Religion of the North*. London: Weidenfeld and Nicolson.

Ur-Quell. 1893. "Untitled." *Am Ur-Quell*, no. 4.

Ury, Heinrich von. 1700. *Bauern-Practica oder Wetter-Büchlein*. N.p.: n.p.

Ussher, Harland. 1983. "The Slipper on the Stair." In *Cinderella* (A. Dundes, ed.), 193–99. New York: Wildman Press.

Vasmer, Max. 1953. *Russisches Etymologisches Wörterbuch*. Heidelberg: Carl Winter Universitätsverlag.

Vauchez, André. 1981. *La Sainteté en Occident aux derniers siècles du moyen âge d'après les procès de canonisation et les documents hagiographiques*. Rome: Ecole Française de Rome.

Vaux, Peter of. 1865. "Life of Colette." In J. Bollandus and G. Henschenius, *Acta sanctorum . . . editio novissima* (J. Carnandet et al., eds.). Vol. 1 (March), 538–88. Paris: Palmé.

Virgil (Vergilius Maro, Publius). 1960. *Virgil. Aeneid*. 2 vols. (H. R. Fairclough, trans.). Cambridge: Harvard University Press.

Vitry, James of. 1867. "Life of Mary of Oignies." In J. Bollandus and G. Henschenius, *Acta sanctorum . . . editio novissima* (J. Carnandet et al., eds.). Vol. 5. Paris: Palmé.

———. 1890. *The Exempla; or, Illustrative Stories from the "Sermones Vulgares" of Jacques de Vitry* (T. F. Crane, ed.). London: D. Nutt.

———. 1972. "De sacramentis." In *The "Historia occidentalis" of Jacques de Vitry* (J. F. Hinnebusch, ed.), 192–246. Spicilegium Friburgense 17 (Freiburg).

Voigt, Gerhard. 1967. "Zur Sprache des Faschismus." *Das Argument* 9 (43): 154–65.

————. 1974. "Bericht vom Ende der 'Sprache des Nationalsozialismus.'" *Diskussion Deutsch* 9: 445–64.

Vondung, Klaus. 1979. "Spiritual Revolution and Magic." *Modern Age* 23 (4): 394–402.

Voragine, Jacopo da. 1900 [1483]. *The Golden Legend; or, Lives of the Saints as Englished by William Caxton*. London: J. M. Dent.

Walpole, A. S. 1922. *Early Latin Hymns*. Cambridge: Cambridge University Press.

Wander, Karl-Friedrich W. 1964. *Deutsches Sprichwörter Lexicon*. Vol. 4. Darmstadt: Wissenschaftliche Buchgesellschaft.

Warner, Richard. 1791. *Antiquitates Culinariae*. London: Blamire.

Wassermann, Rudolf. 1992. "Plädoyer für eine neue Asyl- und Ausländerpolitik." In *Aus Politik und Zeitgeschichte* [Beilage zur Wochenzeitung Das Parlament], no. 9 (21 Feb.): 13–20.

Wasserschleben, F. W. H. 1851. *Catholic Church: Die Bussordnungen der abendländischen Kirche*. Halle: Ch. Graeger Verlag.

Weber, Max. 1947. *The Theory of Social and Economic Organization* (A. M. Henderson and T. Parson, trans.). New York: Oxford University Press.

Weiss, Konrad. 1993. "Untitled." *Das Parlament* (11 June): 4.

Weniger, Ludwig. 1919. *Altgriechischer Baumkultus*. Leipzig: Dieterich.

Wenzel, S. 1978. *Verses in Sermons*. Medieval Academy of America Publication 87. Cambridge: Cambridge University Press.

Westfeling, V. (ed.). 1982. *Die Messe Gregors des Grossen*. Cologne: Schnütgen Museum der Stadt Köln.

Wiedemann, Karl Alfred. 1892a. "Das Blut im Glauben der alten Aegypter." *Am Ur-Quell* 3 (4): 113–16.

————. 1892b. "Das Blut in den frühmittelalterlichen Bussbüchern." *Am Ur-Quell* 3 (6): 182–83.

————. 1923/24. "Der Blutglaube im alten Agypten." *Archiv für Religionswissenschaft* 22: 58–86.

Wiegand, Eberhard. 1937. "Rasse, Volk, Wirtschaft." *Volk und Rasse* 12 (1): 39–40.

Wildenthal, Lora. 1994a. "Citizenship in the German Empire." International Conference of Europeanists, Chicago (1 Apr).

————. 1994b. "Colonizers and Citizens." Ph.D. diss. Department of History, University of Michigan, Ann Arbor.

Wilkins, D. (ed.). 1737. *Concilia Magnae Britanniae et Hiberniae*, A.D. *446–1718*. London: R. Gosling.

Williams, Brackette F. 1995. "Classification Systems Revisited." In *Naturalizing Power* (S. Yanagisako and C. Delaney, eds.), 201–36. New York: Routledge.

Wirsung, Christoph. 1520. *Ain hipsche tragedia*. Augsburg: Sigismund Grym and Max Wersung.

Wood, Charles T. 1981. "The Doctor's Dilemma: Sin, Salvation, and the Menstrual Cycle in Medieval Thought." *Speculum* 56 (4): 710–27.

Wülker, Heinz. 1937. "Erbgutauslese im Bauerntum." *Volk und Rasse* 12 (6): 234–41.

Wunderlich, Eva. 1925. *Die Bedeutung der roten Farbe im Kultus der Griechen und Römer*. Giessen: Alfred Töpelmann Verlag.

Wünsche, August. 1905. *Die Sagen vom Lebensbaum und Lebenswasser*. Ex Oriente Lux. Vol 1, nos. 2/3. Leipzig: Winckler.

Wyss, Gottlieb. 1915. "Die Stimme des Blutes." *Schweizer Volkskunde* (Basel) 5 (1–2): 9–10.

————. 1917. "Stimme des Blutes." *Schweizer Volkskunde* (Basel) 7 (1–2): 12.

Young, Jean I. (trans.). 1964. *The Prose Edda of Snorri Sturluson.* Berkeley: University of California Press.

Yuval-Davis, Nira, and Floya Anthias. 1989. *Women-Nation-State.* New York: St. Martin's Press.

Zedler, Johann H. 1735. *Grosses vollständiges Universal-Lexicon aller Künste und Wissenschaften.* Vol. 11. Halle: J. H. Zedler.

———. 1737. *Grosses vollständiges Universal-Lexicon aller Künste und Wissenschaften.* Vol. 15. Halle: J. H. Zedler.

———. 1745. *Grosses vollständiges Universal-Lexicon aller Künste und Wissenschaften.* Vol. 31. Halle: J. H. Zedler.

Zika, C. 1988. "Hosts, Processions, and Pilgrimages in Fifteenth-Century Germany." *Past and Present* 118: 25–64.

Zimmels, Hirsch J. 1956. *Magicians, Theologians, and Doctors.* London: Oxford University Press.

Zingerle, Ignaz D. 1891. *Sagen aus Tirol.* 2d rev. ed. Innsbruck: Wagnersche Universitäts-Buchhandlung.

Zvelebil, Marek, and Kamil V. Zvelebil. 1988. "Agricultural Transition and Indo-European Dispersals." *Antiquity* 62: 574–633.

Index